African Health Leaders
Making change and claiming
the future

Peln and Meny
mh lo l mh e
Ny
Nan hn 2014

African Health Leaders

Making change and claiming the future

Edited by

Francis Omaswa and Nigel Crisp

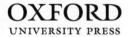

OXFORD

UNIVERSITY PRESS

Great Clarendon Street, Oxford, OX2 6DP,
United Kingdom

Oxford University Press is a department of the University of Oxford.
It furthers the University's objective of excellence in research, scholarship,
and education by publishing worldwide. Oxford is a registered trade mark of
Oxford University Press in the UK and in certain other countries

© Oxford University Press 2014

The moral rights of the authors have been asserted

First Edition published in 2014

Published in the United States of America by Oxford University Press
198 Madison Avenue, New York, NY 10016, United States of America

British Library Cataloguing in Publication Data

Data available

Library of Congress Control Number: 2014938493

ISBN 978–0–19–870332–7

Printed and bound by
CPI Group (UK) Ltd, Croydon, CR0 4YY

Dedication

For our wives
Catherine Omaswa and Siân Crisp

Foreword: Her Excellency Dr Nkosazana Dlamini-Zuma

As Africans we must celebrate improvements in health and the people who have made them happen, but we must also claim our own future for ourselves.

There are many wonderful stories here of how people throughout Africa have worked to improve health—drawing on the strengths of communities, creating innovative ways of delivering services, designing new roles for health workers, and calling on help from partners internationally. This rich experience enables us to see how, country by country, we can move towards our goal of offering health care to all our people.

Written by Africans, this book is essential reading for African health leaders who want to build on our own traditions and experience. It is also a vital orientation for partners who want to know how they can best support our efforts in a spirit of global solidarity.

Her Excellency Dr Nkosazana Dlamini-Zuma
Chairperson of the African Union Commission

Foreword: Dr Judith Rodin, Dr Mark Britnell, and Dr Paul Fife

This book, *African Health Leaders: Making Change and Claiming the Future,* is a timely celebration of African leadership in health at a time when many African countries are growing rapidly and playing an increasingly prominent role in world affairs.

But despite these advances, Africa is still facing some of the worst health challenges in the world—from HIV/AIDS and malaria to staggering levels of maternal and child mortality. To address these problems head on, African health leaders are taking new approaches to problem solving, forming new and productive collaborations within their own nations, and joining with partners across the globe to transform entire health systems.

Yet, despite all we can learn from these visionaries, they remain all but unknown outside of the African continent. Little has been written by or about them, and their insights and experiences have been largely hidden from the rest of the world.

Until now. This book, written primarily in the words of African health leaders themselves, tells the story of how these leaders are tackling issues in their own countries—and, in doing so, are often sparking exciting new innovations in health and health care for the rest of the world. It is an invaluable source of information for individuals and organizations currently working in, or planning to work in, Africa—and also has a great deal to teach the global community about how we can improve health in our own countries.

We are delighted to have played a part in supporting the production of this book. By celebrating the achievements of Africa's recent past, we are better positioned to unlock the opportunities of its future.

Dr Judith Rodin, President, Rockefeller Foundation
Dr Mark Britnell, Global Chairman for Health, KPMG
Dr Paul Richard Fife, Director, Department for Global Health,
Education and Research

Contents

Part 4 **Making the best use of all the talents**

Part 5 **Health for the whole population—leaving no-one behind**

Part 6 **The future**

Abbreviations

3TC	Lamivudine
ACHEST	African Centre for Global Health, and Social Transformation
ACRiA	AIDS Care and Treatment Research in Africa
ADAC	African Dialogue on AIDS
ADF	African Development Forum
AIDS	Acquired Immune Deficiency Syndrome
AMSA	Association of Medicals Schools in Africa
APOC	African Programme for Onchocerciasis Control
ART	Anti-Retroviral Therapy
AU	African Union
AUC	African Union Commission
AZT	Zidovudine
BEmONC	Basic Emergency Obstetric and Neonatal Care
CARMMA	Campaign for the Accelerated Reduction of Maternal Mortality in Africa
CBDAs	Community Based Distributor Agents
CBHI	Community Based Health Insurance
CDDs	Community Directed Distributors
CDTI	Community Directed Treatment with Ivermectin
CHAM	Christian Health Association of Malawi
CHC	Community Health Committee
CHEWs	Community Health Extension Workers
CHMWs	Community Health Midwives

CHN	Community Health Nurses
CHU	Community Health Unit
CHV	Community Health Volunteers
CHW	Community Health Worker'
CON	Community Ophthalmic Nurse
CSDH	Commission on Social Determinants for Health
DAC	Development Assistance Committee
DALYs	Disability Affected Life Years
DFID	The UK's Department for International Development
DMHIS	District-wide Mutual Health Insurance Schemes
DSA	Department of Social Affairs
ECOWAS	Economic Community of West African states
EmOC	Emergency Obstetric Care
EPI	Expanded Programme of Immunization
FDI	Foreign Direct Investment
GAF	Global AIDS' Fund
GAVI	Global Alliance for Vaccines and Immunization
GFATM	Global Fund to Fight Aids, TB, and Malaria
GHIs	Global Health Initiatives
GHWA	Global Health Workforce Alliance

GNP	Gross National Product
GPRS	Ghana Poverty Reduction Strategy
GVAP	Global Vaccine Action Plan
HAART	Highly Active Anti-retroviral Therapy
HHA	Harmonization for Health in Africa
HRH	Human Resources for Health
IAPB	International Agency for the Prevention of Blindness
ICEH	International Centre for Eye Health
ICT	Information and Communications Technology
IKS	Indigenous Knowledge Systems
IMR	Infant Mortality Rate
JCRC	Joint Clinical Research Centre
LEb	Life Expectancy at Birth
MDGs	Millennium Development Goals
MDR-TB	Multi-Drug Resistant TB
MHO	Mutual Health Organization
MRC	Medical Research Council
NCDs	Non-Communicable Diseases
NDC	National Democratic Congress
NHIF	National Health Insurance Fund
NHIL	National Health Insurance Levy
NHIS	National Health Insurance System
NIPRD	Nigerian Institute for Pharmaceutical Research and Development
NGDOs	Non-Governmental Development Organizations
NGOs	Non-Governmental Organizations
NPP	New Patriotic Party
NRCATM	National Reference Centre for African Traditional Medicine
NTDs	Neglected Tropical Diseases
NVP	Niverapine

OAFLA	Organization of African First Ladies Against AIDS
OAU	Organization for African Unity
OCP	Onchocerciasis Control Programme
ODA	Official Development Assistance
OLS	Operation Life Line Sudan
OOPS	Out-of-Pocket Payments
OOR	Onchocerciasis Operational Research
ORID	Other Related Infectious Diseases
PAT	Progress Assessment Tool
PEPFAR	President's Emergency Plan for AIDS Relief
PMPA	Pharmaceutical Manufacturing Plan for Africa
PMTCT	Prevention of Mother to Child Transmission
RCE	Regional Centres of Excellence
RCSB	Royal Commonwealth Society for the Blind
RECs	Regional Economic Communities
REMO	Rapid Epidemiological Mapping of Onchocerciasis
ROTP	Regional Ophthalmic Training Programme
SAMSS	sub-Saharan African Medical School Study
SANAC	South African National Aids Council
SEN	State Enrolled Nurses
SHI	Social Health Insurance
SOMA	Senior Ophthalmic Medical Assistants
SRH	Sexual and Reproductive Health
SSA	sub-Saharan Africa
STAC	Scientific and Technical Advisory Committee
SWAp	Sector Wide Approach

TAC	Treatment Action Campaign
THE	total health expenditure
TRIPS	Trade Related Aspects of International Property Rights
TREAT	The Regional Expansion of Anti-retroviral Therapy
UCI	Universal Childhood Immunization
UNFPA	United Nations Population Fund
UNAIDS	Joint United Nations Programme on HIV/AIDS
UNISA	University of South Africa
USAID	United States Agency for International Development

UTH	University Teaching Hospital
V/CHW	Village or Community Health Worker
WFME	World Federation for Medical Education
WHO	World Health Organization
WIPO	World Intellectual Property Organization
XDR-TB	extensively drug resistant TB

Contributors

The editors

Dr Francis Omaswa is the Executive Director of the African Centre for Global Health and Social Transformation (ACHEST), Chancellor of Busitema University, and Chair of the African Platform on Human Resources for Health. He was Special Adviser to the WHO Director-General and founding Executive Director of the Global Health Workforce Alliance (GHWA). He was the Director-General for Health Services in the Ministry of Health in Uganda, when he coordinated and implemented major reforms in the health sector in Uganda, including the introduction of Swaps, quality assurance, and decentralization. He has a keen interest in low-cost rural health service delivery and spent five years testing models for this at the Ngora hospital in Uganda. He was founding chair, and later Vice-Chairman, of the Global Stop TB Partnership; was one of the architects of the Global Fund to Fight AIDS, TB, and Malaria and served as Chair of the Portfolio and Procurement Committee of the Board; he was founding President of the College of Surgeons of East, Central and Southern Africa, a member of the steering committee of the High Level Forum on health-related MDGs; and

was Chair of the GAVI Independent Review Committee, among other commitments. Dr Omaswa is a graduate of Makerere Medical School, Kampala, Uganda.

Lord Nigel Crisp is an independent crossbench member of the House of Lords where he co-chairs the All Party Parliamentary Group on Global Health. He was Chief Executive of the NHS in England—the largest health organization in the world with 1.4 million employees—and Permanent Secretary of the UK Department of Health between 2000 and 2006. Previously he was Chief Executive of the Oxford Radcliffe Hospital NHS Trust. Lord Crisp chairs Sightsavers, the King's Health Partners' Global Advisory Board, The Zambia UK Health Workforce Alliance, and the Uganda UK Health Alliance. He is an Ambassador for the eHealth Foundation, a Senior Fellow at the Institute for Healthcare Improvement, a Distinguished Visiting Fellow at the Harvard School of Public Health, and an Honorary Professor at the London School of Hygiene and Tropical Medicine. His book *Turning the World Upside Down—the search for global health in the 21st century* describes what high-income countries can learn from low- and middle-income ones and takes further the ideas about partnership and mutual learning he developed in *Global Health Partnerships*, his 2007 report for the Prime Minister. He described his experience in running the NHS in *24 Hours to Save the NHS* – the Chief Executive's account of reform 2000–06.

The authors

Dr Uche Amazigo is a public health specialist and leader in tropical parasitic disease control and community directed health interventions—and one of the few female Africans to head a UN agency. She holds a PhD from Vienna University (Austria), DTM&P from Bernhard-Nocht Institute of Tropical Medicine (Germany), and was a Takemi Fellow at the Harvard School of Public Health (USA). For over 25 years, she has made numerous valuable contributions to health research and disease control. Her pioneering work on onchocerciasis (river blindness) in rural Nigeria revealed startling results about the social isolation and disability caused by onchocercal skin disease. This discovery fundamentally changed international perceptions of onchocerciasis, forming the scientific basis for the African Programme for Onchocerciasis Control (WHO/APOC), established in 1995. After joining WHO/APOC in 1996, her relentless championing of a

community directed treatment approach for drug delivery proved highly successful, community involvement being the foundation for APOC's success. APOC Director from 2005–11, she coordinated the control of river blindness in sub-Saharan Africa. She is a Trustee of Sightsavers, TY Danjuma Foundation, and other organizations responsible for setting global health policies and research agenda. In 2013, she received an honorary DSc degree from the University of KwaZulu-Natal, Durban, South Africa, and won the Prince Mahidol Award 2012 in Public Health.

John Paul Bagala is President of the Federation of African Medical Students' Associations (FAMSA) and a student at Gulu University Faculty of Medicine in Uganda. He is also an Ambassador of the Global Health Learning Opportunities, Association of American Medical Colleges, and a member of the coalition to prevent maternal mortality due to unsafe abortion in Uganda. He was the founding President of the United Nations' Association of Uganda Gulu University chapter 2011–12; the Medical Students' Chair of the Child Health Now Campaign, World Vision 2012–13; and has participated in conferences in Africa and abroad.

Dr Agnes Binagwaho was appointed Minister of Health of the Republic of Rwanda in 2011 after serving as Permanent Secretary since 2008. She practiced medicine in public hospitals before joining Rwanda's National AIDS Control Commission as Executive Secretary in 2002. She has a Master's in Paediatrics and specialized in emergency, neonatology, and the treatment of HIV/AIDS. Dr Binagwaho chaired the Rwandan Paediatric Society and is a member of the Editorial Board of Public Library of Science, and the Harvard University *Health and Human Rights Journal.* She sits on the international advisory board for The Lancet Global Health journal. She co-chaired the Millennium Development Goal Project Task Force on HIV/AIDS and Access to Essential Medicines for the Secretary-General of the United Nations under the leadership of Professor Jeffrey Sachs. She was the global co-chair of the Joint Learning Initiative on Children and HIV/AIDS. She is a member of the Global Task Force on Expanded Access to Cancer Care and Control in Developing Countries. Dr Binagwaho has published on a wide range of topics, including human rights' policies and implementation of health programmes. She serves also as a senior lecturer in the Department of Global Health and Social Medicine of Harvard Medical School and as a Clinical Professor of Paediatrics at the Geisel School of Medicine at Dartmouth College. She received an Honorary Doctor of Sciences from Dartmouth College.

Clarisse Bombi Lamnyan is a senior nurse with a Bachelor of Nursing Science Degree from the University of Buea, Cameroon. She is presently employed as a nurse tutor and a nurse clinician by the Cameroon's Ministry of Public Health. In 2012, Clarisse was awarded a Commonwealth Professional Fellowship to spend 3 months at the Commonwealth Nurses' Federation in the United Kingdom, further developing her skills in leadership; communication and networking; and organizational governance and management in order to enhance her contribution to nursing and health in her own country. In 2009, Clarisse received the Young Nurse Award, which enabled her to attend and address the delegates at the 2009 Commonwealth Nurses' Federation Biennial Conference, which held in Botswana. Back home, Clarisse is a member of the Cameroon Nurses Association where she serves as the assistant secretary of the association.

Susana Edjang works at the Executive Office of the Secretary-General of the United Nations where she is Project Manager of the Secretary-General's signature movement Every Woman Every Child to advance the health MDGs. Previously she worked at the UK Parliament as an advisor on global health and climate change. Susana is the co-founder of the Zambia UK Health Workforce Alliance and HIFA-Zambia, networks to advance understanding and support for Zambia's national health plans; and was a senior manager at the Tropical Health and Education Trust, where she led a four-fold growth of partnerships between UK health intuitions and their counterparts in developing countries. She is on the Council of the Royal African Society, and is a trustee of Progressio, a development charity. Susana is the co-author of *Working in International Health* (Oxford University Press, 2011).

Dr Peter Eriki is Director of Health Systems for ACHEST. He previously served as a WHO country representative for over 15 years in several priority African countries, including Angola, Kenya, and Nigeria. He played a significant role in the revitalization of immunization programmes in Nigeria, which had threatened to derail the global polio eradication effort. For this achievement he was rewarded the Paul Harris Fellowship by Rotary International. Dr Eriki has also worked with the Ministry of Health in Uganda in various positions including Medical Officer, Medical Superintendent, TB Consultant, and Director of the TB Control Programme; he did research in TB &HIV interaction and taught medical students. Dr Eriki is a graduate of Makerere University, where he also obtained a Master's Degree in Internal Medicine and has an MPH from Harvard.

Dr Hannah B. Faal was born in Calabar, Nigeria, and obtained the MBBS of the University of Ibadan in 1970 and the Fellowship in Ophthalmology of the Royal College of Surgeons of Edinburgh in 1975. She also holds Fellowships of the West African College of Surgeons and the Royal College of Ophthalmologists. She moved to The Gambia in 1980 with her late husband and established the national eye care programme. This contributed in 1998 to the founding of VISION 2020 The Right to Sight, a global initiative of WHO and the International Agency for The Prevention of Blindness, of which she became the President. Dr Faal has been an advisor to WHO, served on ophthalmology professional bodies, eye health boards, and expert advisory panels and holds several visiting lectureships. She has published widely on major causes of blindness, community eye health and eye care programming, human resource development, and health systems. She is a recipient of several awards, including the Order of The Republic of The Gambia. Working for Sightsavers from 1988, she provided support to Sightsavers' field programmes and retired in 2010 as programme development adviser but continues to provide consultancy services. She is Chairperson of the African Vision Research Institute and a member of the Calabar Institute of Tropical Disease Research and Prevention.

Advocate Bience Gawanas is the Special Advisor on Social Issues to the Namibian Minister of Health and Social Services. She was elected Commissioner for Social Affairs at the African Union in 2003 and again in 2008. Her portfolio of issues included health, HIV/AIDS, population, migration, welfare of vulnerable groups, culture, sport, and labour. She previously worked as a lawyer at the Legal Assistance Centre, a human rights NGO, and was lecturer on gender law at the University of Namibia. She was also Chair of the Law Reform and Development Commission, Member of the Board of the Namibian Central Bank and Ombudswoman of Namibia until 2003. As the Commissioner of Social Affairs, she developed policy instruments and programmes, including the Social Policy Framework, the Maputo Plan of Action on Sexual and Reproductive Health and Rights, the Migration Policy Framework for Africa, Plan of Action on Drug Control and Crime Prevention, the Charter for the African Cultural Renaissance. She launched the African Union's Campaign on Accelerated Reduction of Maternal Mortality in Africa (CARMMA), mobilizing global, regional, and country-level support and refocusing attention on women's health. Bience Gawanas has served on the UNAIDS Global Task Team; the Task Force for Scaling-Up of Education and Training of Health Workers; the Global Commission on HIV and the Law; the Commission on Accountability and Information on Women's and Children's Health; the Global Steering Committee on Universal Access; and the Lancet–Oslo University Commission on Global Governance for Health. She has an LL.B Honours from the University of Warwick, a Barrister Degree from Lincolns Inn, and an Executive MBA from the University of Cape Town.

Professor Catherine Odora-Hoppers holds a South African Research Chair in Development Education at the University of South Africa having previously been a technical adviser on Indigenous Knowledge Systems to the Parliamentary Portfolio Committee on Arts, Culture, Science and Technology. Professor Hoppers is a scholar and policy specialist on International Development, education, North–South questions, disarmament, peace, and human security. She has been a Distinguished Professional at the Human Sciences Research Council; an Associate Professor at the University of Pretoria; a visiting Professor at Stockholm University (Sweden); and a recipient of an Honorary Doctorate in Philosophy from Orebro University (Sweden) and an Honorary Doctorate in Education from Nelson Mandela Metropolitan University in South

Africa. She is a Fellow of the African Academy of Sciences (AAS) and a member of the African Academy of Science Advisory Council on the Social Sciences. She was given the Presidential Medal of Honour by the President of Uganda in 2013 for her academic research and leadership.

Dr Patrick Kadama is the Director for Health Policy and Strategy at ACHEST, where he leads in health policy and strategy analysis, strengthening African engagement in global health, tracking and sharing lessons in health development, and supporting institutional capacity building for better health outcomes. Prior to joining ACHEST, he was with the World Health Organization as Health Systems' Adviser in Geneva, where he supported countries with policy advice and in working with global health initiatives and has gained deep insights in country health systems. Before joining WHO he was Commissioner for Health Planning and Development in the Ministry of Health in Uganda and was involved in the development of new Health Policy and Health Sector Strategic plans, including the introduction of Sector Wide Approaches (SWAp) and long-term National Health Financing Strategy and rolling it out to district health authorities and agencies. Dr Kadama is a graduate of Makerere Medical School and holds an MPhil from the London School of Hygiene and Tropical Medicine in Health Planning and Financing.

The Honourable Miatta Barlay Kargbo became Minister of Health and Sanitation in Sierra Leone in February 2013. Ms Kargbo is a Board member of the UNAIDS Programme Coordinators Board and Rollback Malaria Board. Previously, Ms Kargbo had served as Adviser to the President of the Republic of Sierra Leone, advising on policy issues, driving change, and providing strategy and implementation oversight of the government's development agenda across: Health and Sanitation, Labour and Social Security, Social Welfare, Gender and Children's Affairs, the National AIDS Commission and Information and Communication. Born in Sierra Leone, Ms Kargbo holds a degree in Information Technology (Howard University, DC), and a Master's in Business Administration (Butler University, IN). Her background covers both the public and private sectors, and she is a Six Sigma Black-Belt, specialized in helping companies and governments enhance performance through strategic process improvements, accelerated innovation, and streamlined operations.

Dr Chisale Mhango is Senior Lecturer in Obstetrics and Gynaecology at the College of Medicine in Malawi. Before taking this position he was Director for Reproductive Health Services in Malawi's Ministry of Health. During his post-graduate training in London, he spent the elective year at the Centers for Disease Control in Atlanta, Georgia, training in public health. He has since worked for the United Nations' Population Fund and the World Health Organization, promoting women's health in the Africa Region, and later at the African Union secretariat, developing continental policy frameworks for women's health in Africa region before his government recalled him to lead the national Sexual and Reproductive Health programme. This meant implementing the policies that he developed with Commissioner Bience Gawanas through the Maputo Plan of Action, which was endorsed by the Conference of African Ministers of Health in 2005. Having realized the great influence politicians and traditional leaders have on their constituents, Dr Mhango enlisted Vice-President Joyce Banda as National Safe Motherhood Ambassador, and worked with traditional leaders to mobilize their people for safe motherhood. To this day Dr Mhango continues to work with traditional leaders in Malawi in support of President Joyce Banda's Safe Motherhood Initiative.

The Honourable Dr Pascoal Mocumbi was Prime Minister of the Republic of Mozambique from 1994 to 2004. Prior to that, he headed the Ministry of Foreign Affairs for eight years and the Ministry of Health for 6 years. He received his medical degree from the University of Lausanne, did his internship in Switzerland, and practiced medicine as an obstetrician and gynaecologist in hospitals throughout Mozambique. As Prime Minister he led the establishment in Mozambique of the National AIDS Council to coordinate the implementation of the national HIV response. Dr Mocumbi is committed to the importance of public health as an essential arm of sustainable development; he has expertise in health systems and women's' health issues. As Health Minister he established the MCH nurse career and initiated the training of non-physician health professionals in delivering life-saving emergency obstetrics. As Prime Minister he contributed to the substantial progress in fighting poverty and improving human development, and to the transformation of a war-torn Mozambique into one of the most well-governed and fastest growing economies of Africa. Dr Mocumbi served on the WHO Task force on Health and Development from 1989 to 1998, and he is the WHO Good Will Ambassador for Maternal, Newborn, and Child Health of the African Region and Chair of the African Medical Research Foundation (AMREF). He has been active in global health initiatives, serving, amongst other things, on the Coordinating Committee of the Global HIV Vaccine Enterprise, as a Commissioner on the WHO

Commission on the Social Determinants of Health, and as a Board member of the Alliance of Health policy and Systems Research (AHPSR) and the Women's Health Coalition. He is a Foreign Associate of the Institute of Medicine.

The Honourable Professor Gottlieb Lobe Monekosso is a former Minister of Public Health of Cameroon, Director Emeritus of the WHO African Region, and Professor Emeritus of Medicine. Professor Monekosso has spent a lifetime devoted to teaching, practice, and research in clinical medicine and public health in Africa. He attended school in Lagos, Nigeria, studied medicine at Guy's Hospital (1948–53) and the School of Tropical Medicine in London. After house appointments at Guy's, he was Resident in medicine at the University College Hospital, Ibadan (1954–58); then lecturer in Makerere College, Uganda (1958–60); Research Fellow, University College West Indies; Associate Professor and Vice Dean, Ibadan (1960–63); Professor and head of the department of medicine, University of Lagos (1963–68). He was foundation Dean of the Faculty of Medicine, University College Dar es Salaam, Tanzania (1968–70) and of the University Centre for Health Sciences, Yaounde, Cameroon (1969–78). He subsequently became a resident consultant for WHO in Geneva with missions in Asia, Africa,

and Latin America (1979–80), WHO Representative, Commonwealth Caribbean (1980–85) from where he was elected WHO Regional Director for Africa (1985–1995). He retired to Cameroon in 1995 and was Minister of Public Health from 1997 to 2000. Professor Monekosso has published many papers and a number of books, and travelled widely internationally. Currently he runs a small foundation 'Global Health Dialogue' in Buea, Cameroon. In 2012 he was awarded the Queen Elizabeth II Gold Medal.

The Honourable Dr Aaron Motsoaledi was one of the South African Health leaders interviewed by Lord Nigel Crisp for Chapter 18. He has been Minister of Health in South Africa since 2009. He was formerly the Member of the Executive Council of Limpopo for, in turn, transport, agriculture, environment and education. Dr Motsoaledi trained as doctor in Natal and practiced in the small rural town of Jane Furse before entering government as a member of the Limpopo Provincial Legislature from 1994 to 2009. He has served in many health roles, as well as within the Legislature and the ANC.

Dr Peter Mugyenyi (MB ChB, DCH, FRCPI, FRCP Edin) was born in South-Western Uganda and studied Medicine at Makerere University in Kampala and specialized in paediatrics in Britain. He worked in Lesotho, UK, and the Middle East before returning to Uganda in 1989. Currently, he is the Director of the Joint Clinical Research Centre (JCRC), Uganda's centre of excellence in AIDS research, care, treatment, and prevention, and the Chancellor of Mbarara University of Science and Technology in Uganda. He has authored many scientific papers in peer-reviewed medical journals, contributed chapters to a number of medical textbooks, and made numerous presentations in international scientific conferences. He is author of *Genocide by Denial: How Profiteering Killed Millions* (Fountain Publishers, 2008) and *A Cure Too Far; The Struggle to end HIV* (Fountain Publishers, 2012). Dr Mugyenyi is a Fellow of the Royal Colleges of Physicians of Ireland and Edinburgh and also a Fellow of the Academy of Sciences of Uganda, Africa, and the Academy of the developing World. Internationally, he has served as a board member of several national and international organizations in Africa and USA. He has won a number of awards in recognition of his role in the fight against AIDS.

Dr Ndwapi R. Ndwapi is currently the Manager of the Ministerial Strategy Office of the Ministry of Health in Botswana. The Ministerial Strategy Office has overall responsibility for ministry strategy in the key areas of Project Management; Coordination of Donor Funding; Performance Improvement; Outsourcing; and Public Private Partnerships. Until recently Dr Ndwapi was The Director of Clinical Services, a position that gave him the responsibility of overseeing all of Botswana's 26 public hospitals and more than 500 free standing public outpatient clinics. Dr Ndwapi's core training is in internal medicine, with an interest in infectious disease. He therefore has extensive experience in the treatment of HIV disease in the public sector, having been one of the co-founders of the first wholly government-funded anti-retroviral therapy clinic in Africa. He has previously held the position of Operations Manager for the Botswana National Anti-retroviral Therapy Programme. He is a current member of the HIV/AIDS National Clinical Advisory Committee of the Botswana Ministry of Health. He has also previously served in a clinical advisory role in antiretroviral therapy for the Nelson Mandela Foundation. Dr Ndwapi is cited as an author in numerous clinical publications on HIV and AIDS.

Dr Frank Nyonator (MB ChB; MPH; FGCPS) is Dean of the School of Public Health, University of Health and Allied Sciences Ghana. He was previously the Ministerial Advisor on Health Systems' Strengthening and Director, Human Resource for Health Development for the Ministry of Health in Ghana. He was Acting

Director-General of the Ghana Health Service from June 2011 to November 2012. He has held many public service posts including being the Volta Regional Director for the Ghana Health Service and Health Systems' Advisor for the WHO Country Office in Abuja, Nigeria. He has served on many expert advisory groups internationally including the Technical Steering Committee of the Child and Adolescent Health Department, WHO; the GAVI Alliance Independent Review Committee; and served as Vice-Chair of the UNICEF/UNDP/World Bank/WHO Special Programme for Research and Training in Tropical Diseases. He is a Founding Member of Health Systems' Action Network and a member of the Global Health Council, American Public Health Association, Population Association of America, Ghana College of Physicians and Surgeons, and Ghana Medical Association. Dr Nyonator's research interests and experience are in health systems and health service provision, especially using new technologies, and he has authored and co-authored many publications on these issues.

Dr Kelechi Ohiri is the Senior Adviser to the Minister of Health in Nigeria and the Lead for the Saving One Million Lives' Initiative. In this position, he has followed his passion for improving health outcomes, especially for the poor, through improving access to primary care;

strengthening clinical governance for better quality of care; and unlocking the potential of Nigeria's Private Health Sector. In addition, he works on social policy issues including social safety nets. He was previously with McKinseys and the World Bank, which he joined as part of the Young Professionals' Programme. Dr Ohiri has written policy papers, academic publications, and has co-authored two books on health systems. He is on the Board of the WHO's Alliance for Health Policy and Systems' Research and the Nigeria Hub for the Centre for Health Markets' Innovation. He is also a 2013 Archbishop Tutu Leadership Fellow of the African Leadership Institute and a recipient of the Emerging Public Health Professional award from Harvard University. Dr Ohiri has a Medical Degree from the University of Lagos, a Master of Public Health degree from Harvard University, as well as a Master of Science Degree in Health Policy and Management, from Harvard University.

Dr Luis Gomes Sambo has been the WHO Regional Director for Africa since 2005, having previously been Director of Programme Management, Director of the Division of Health Services' Development, Coordinator of the Health-For-All strategy, and WHO Representative for Guinea Bissau. Prior to joining WHO, he was the Vice-Minister of Health of Angola, having earlier held various health leadership positions in the country. He has published over 50 articles in peer-reviewed journals. He is member of: the Angolan Medical Association, the Public Health College of the Portuguese Medical Association, Scientific Board of the Centre of Advanced Studies on Medical Education—University Agostinho Neto, Royal Society of Medicine, Editorial Board of the Global Library of Women's Medicine, UK Systems' Society, and the International Society of Systems' Science. Some of his awards include: *Doutor Honoris Causa* by the Universidade Nova de Lisboa and by the University of Kinshasa; '*Officier de l'Ordre National de la Valeur de la République du Cameroun*'; '*Commandeur de l'Ordre National du Mérite du Benin*'; '*Officier de l'Ordre National du Burkina-Faso*'; '*Chevalier de l'Ordre Croissant Vert de l'Union des Comores*; *Commandeur de l'Ordre de Madagascar*; Public Health golden medal *by the Republic of* Níger; '*Paul Harris Fellow*' of Rotary International; the Silver Plate award by the Angolan Medical Association; and an official *Commendation by the Government of Angola.* Dr Sambo has a PhD in Management from the University of Hull, a Degree in Medicine from the University of Angola, and a Diploma in Public Health from the Portuguese Medical Association.

Dr Nana A.Y. Twum-Danso is a public health and preventive medicine physician with fourteen years of experience in global health policy, strategy development, programme design, project management, implementation, monitoring, and evaluation. She is currently a Senior Programme Officer in the Maternal, Neonatal, and Child Health Division of the Bill and Melinda Gates Foundation, where she develops and manages grants to improve health outcomes at scale in several African countries. Prior to that, she led a nationwide quality improvement initiative to reduce maternal and child mortality in Ghana while working for the Institute for Healthcare Improvement. She has a Bachelor's Degree in Biochemical Sciences and a medical degree, both from Harvard University, and a master of public health degree in Health Policy and Management from Emory University.

Dr Miriam Khamadi Were is a medical doctor and Public Health specialist. While her main focus is health, she is also Chancellor of Moi University and Chairperson of the Governing Council of Great Lakes University of Kisumu, GLUK. Currently, Were is a member of the Independent Expert Review Group on Women's and Children's Health, which monitors performance of the UN Secretary General's Global Strategy for Women's and Children's health; a member of the Champions for an HIV-Free Generation; a member of the Global Health Workforce Alliance (GHWA), and a Trustee of the Kenya Medical Women Association. She formerly chaired Kenya's National AIDS Control Council, and the African Medical and Research Foundation Board. She worked at UNICEF, WHO, and UNFPA following a period of teaching Community Health in the University of Nairobi Medical School. Her work has been honoured internationally through The Queen Elizabeth II Gold Medal for Public Health, the Hideyo Noguchi Africa Prize, and Knight of the French Legion of Honour. Kenyan honours include recognition as SHUJAA (Hero) in Public Health Scholarship and by naming her Goodwill Ambassador for Community Health Strategy. She has honorary doctorates from Moi University, Kenya; Ochanomizu University, Japan, and De Paul University, Chicago.

Part 1

Overview of African health leaders

Chapter 1

Introduction to Part 1: Overview

Francis Omaswa and Nigel Crisp

This chapter provides an overview of the structure and contents of the book. It begins by explaining why the book was written and goes on to describe the context and particular challenges facing African health leaders. It shows how the book is organized into six parts, which bring out the key themes and describes the leaders from three different generations who have contributed to it.

A celebration of the past and a vision for the future

We decided to produce this book for three very simple reasons. It is first, and above all else, about recognizing and celebrating African leadership in health.* Second, it describes in practical terms how African Leaders have successfully improvised and innovated, building on the strengths of their communities, to improve the health of their people. Third, it sets out a vision for the future, which shows how a new relationship can be created with international partners and demonstrates how insights and experiences from Africa can help improve health globally. We hope, too, that it will be an inspiration to Africans to claim the future for themselves.

Most accounts of health and healthcare in sub-Saharan Africa are written by foreigners. This book redresses the balance. It is written by Africans who have themselves led improvements in their own countries and describes many of the features of leadership, policy, and implementation that have been involved. It is about Africans re-claiming their place as leaders in health.

Health leaders in sub-Saharan African countries face some of the most demanding challenges anywhere in the world. Disease, poverty, the legacy of colonialism including the post-colonial power imbalance and, all too often, conflict and political instability, combine to make improving health and healthcare

---

* This book is primarily about sub-Saharan Africa. We mean sub-Saharan Africa when refer-ring to Africa unless we state otherwise. We are also very conscious that sub-Saharan Africa is made up of 49 different countries with different cultures, circumstances, and histories and will make the distinctions between countries apparent wherever necessary.

extraordinarily difficult. Nevertheless, in chapter after chapter, health leaders describe how they have made progress. There are many lessons here for the rest of the world.

The authors demonstrate how social and cultural issues can inhibit or accelerate improvement and, using their understanding of these issues, describe how they have mobilized communities and individuals with stunning results. As Professor Miriam Were of Kenya says in Chapter 8 'Through this approach, health-promoting and disease-preventing norms develop in the community' and 'If it doesn't happen in the community, it won't happen in the nation'.

In leading change, the authors invariably have had to identify and make the best use of the assets they have to hand, developing new practices and bringing new people and resources into play. In Chapter 12, for example, Dr Pascoal Mocumbi describes how as Mozambique's Minister of Health after the revolution of 1974—when there was an exodus of Portuguese doctors—he faced such a shortage that he decided to train non-medical *Tecnicos de Cirurgia* to do emergency obstetric surgery. They continue to operate successfully today not only in Mozambique, but in other African countries as well. This is an example of an African innovation that has now been formalized by the World Health Organization (WHO) under the name of Task Shifting and is beginning to be applied in developed countries.[1]

Author after author has also shown how health relates to everything else in their society—from education and the environment to the economy and future prosperity of the country. Health has to be part of all policies, integrated into the national poverty reduction and development plans. Others have had to argue, as Dr Aaron Motsoaledi, the South African Minister of Health, describes in Chapter 18 that 'You soon won't have enough people to build the roads or other investments unless you tackle HIV/AIDS'. Health can't be treated just as a separate department or enterprise. It affects and is affected by everything else.

Taken together, these and other approaches create what amounts to a distinctive vision for health in sub-Saharan Africa where 'Health is made at home' from the complex intermingling of behaviour, customs, science, education, and economic factors. Good health starts with, and is created by, individuals, their families, and communities and is supported, where necessary, by the skills, knowledge, and technology of the professionals; not the other way round. Health is the domain of the people more than of the professionals. Government has a role in setting the framework and in making sure all sectors contribute to the health and well being of the population. It is an approach that is reflected in, and reinforced by, the different ways in which major policies, such as universal health coverage, are being developed in different countries.

International organizations, development partners, foreign NGOs, and private businesses play major roles in health and healthcare in most sub-Saharan African countries with differing degrees of success. As these writers demonstrate, African leadership can enable foreign agencies and individuals working in Africa to avoid all those misunderstandings and misinterpretations of culture and context, which lead to wasted efforts and frustrated hopes.

More importantly, it is time to change the relationship between sub-Saharan Africa and development partners and the wider world. As Francis Omaswa writes in Chapter 2, 'Africans went to . . . institutions and countries begging for advice and for money and we got both but in exchange for certain core values'. Africans were the junior partner in all these partnerships and a sense of dependency was created. Now, however, the world has moved on.[2] The future is about interdependence and co-development. Richer and poorer countries both need each other and can learn from each other.[3]

Africa may be undergoing a renaissance but all is not rosy.[4] There are overpowerful elites, corruption, appalling inequalities between rich and poor and, all too often, between men and women, and some harmful traditional practices remain a challenge. Poverty persists and health problems are more complex and diverse than anywhere else on earth. Globalization and growth are bringing many benefits in education, health, and wealth; but these are accompanied by plagues of fast foods and obesity, new forms of foreign exploitation and economic exclusion.

The leaders writing in this book are very aware of these issues: Professor Monekosso writes in Chapter 14 of the importance of ensuring that 'health policies are not those of the intellectual elite but that they represent the needs and wants of local populations'; Dr Agnes Binagwaho, Minister of Health for Rwanda, argues in Chapter 17 that 'when you focus on the poorest first, you take the rest with you. When you focus on where the greatest gaps are, you make the biggest gains'; whilst Clarisse Bombi describes in Chapter 23 the need to control corruption in the health sector.

The structure of the book

The book has six parts, which each address a different theme. Each part, after this first one, begins with a short introduction to the theme written by the editors, which is followed by two or three accounts from leaders of specific projects or programmes they led in their countries. The final chapters of each part are written by authors with a broader oversight of Africa—such as the Regional Director of the African Region of the WHO and the former Commissioner for Social Affairs for the African Union—and offer a wider and deeper analysis of the themes under discussion.

- **Part 1: Overview** sets the scene, describing some of the history of the last few decades and the challenges facing African health leaders (Chapters 1 and 2).

- **Part 2: The greatest challenges** describes the highest profile challenges facing Africa in the Millennium Development Goals; shows how these have been confronted in two countries and sets this against the background of the wider epidemiological and policy environment (Chapters 3 to 6).

- **Part 3: All the resources of the community** shows how, in very different circumstances, health leaders in different countries have mobilized the community to tackle endemic problems ranging from hygiene and basic health awareness to river blindness and other neglected tropical diseases; it concludes with a discussion of the wider social and political context (Chapters 7 to 10).

- **Part 4: Making the best use of all the talents** deals with human resources. It describes how inspirational leaders have trained and developed health workers and volunteers to their maximum potential to enable them to deliver high-quality services to their communities and concludes with an account of how professional education has developed alongside service development and a chapter about the role of indigenous knowledge systems (Chapters 11 to 15).

- **Part 5: Health for the whole population—leaving no-one behind** focuses on Universal Health Coverage and describes the progress being made, using rather different approaches, in three different countries; it concludes with an overview of how health policy and health systems have developed within the wider economic context (Chapters 16 to 20).

- **Part 6: The future** begins with contributions from younger and future leaders about their experiences and their hopes and fears for the future; draws out common themes from the book as a whole; describes a vision for what health and healthcare could be like in Africa in the future; and concludes with three actions that will help make it happen (Chapters 21 to 24).

A book of this length cannot cover every part of Africa or every topic, we have, therefore, used the introduction to each part as a way of drawing attention to important topics that aren't covered in detail and to provide the context for the following chapters.

The authors

There are many impressive and inspiring health leaders in the countries of sub-Saharan Africa and we could not include them all. Our selection is broadly representative at best. There are contributors here from 14 African countries; 13 are men and 10 women. Most trained as doctors but there are also nurses, physiotherapists, policy makers, administrators, sociologists, lawyers, and scientists. Five are, or have been, ministers, including a Prime Minister, there are two WHO Regional Directors and five have held very senior positions in regional and global organizations. In addition there are quotations from a number of other leading Africans.

All are Africans and all but two live in Africa today. Most, however, have trained or worked abroad, reflecting the lack of opportunities in their own countries. Others have been in exile abroad at times of struggle, either against foreign colonialists or as a result of national politics, and at least one has been a political prisoner. Their life experiences are very different from those of their peers in most of the rest of the world.

Each of the chapters are written by the leaders themselves except for Chapter 18, which is based on conversations with South African health leaders, including Dr Aaron Motsoaledi, the South African Minister of Health. In addition, the penultimate chapter is a composite of views from younger and future leaders about their experiences and their hopes and fears for the future.

There are also many references to other African leaders in these pages, some of whom are sadly no longer alive. Appendix 1 offers a brief overview of the contributions made by African health leaders to global institutions and organizations.

The past, present, and future are all represented in these chapters: with accounts from the 1970s and 1980s; chapters by serving ministers and leaders; and contributions from younger people about how they see the world, and their hopes and fears as current and future leaders. Authors range in age from their 20s to their 80s. They offer interestingly different perspectives, which mirror the way Africa has changed over the generations from the people leading the reconstruction of their countries after colonialism to the experienced and increasingly confident leaders of today, and on to the world citizens of tomorrow with their different expectations of Africa and of its place in the world. We are very grateful to them all but sorry we could not include more.

The people represented here are all leaders, people who get their hands dirty and make things happen rather than being pure policy makers, academics, or commentators. Some, but not all, have published in research journals; few have published more widely. More generally, it is noticeable how few African leaders publish. We hope that this book will encourage more to do so.

The editors

Dr Francis Omaswa is a Ugandan doctor who, in common with many of the authors, has lived and worked abroad, as well as in his own country, and held high office abroad. In Chapter 2 he sets the scene for this book, offering an overview of the last 40 years and more and, in the last chapter, paints a vision for the future.

Lord Nigel Crisp is British and a former NHS Chief Executive and Permanent Secretary of the UK Department of Health. He has wide experience in health globally, has worked in a number of African countries, and has written extensively on partnership and co-development. His role as editor has been facilitative, drawing out connections and placing the contributions within the wider context of global health.

We are both extremely grateful to all the contributors; to the many people who have offered advice and help, and to our colleagues at Oxford University Press. We would particularly like to acknowledge and thank Siân Crisp for her help with editing and proof reading, Elisabeth Oywer who provided us with information on nursing in Africa, James Hakim for his insights on research, and Dr Yogan Pillay, Johannes Kgatla, Dr Oliver Johnson, and Lucy Irvine for their help with specific chapters. Above all, we are very grateful to our families for their understanding, love and support.

Acknowledgments

We are very grateful to the Rockefeller Foundation for hosting Francis Omaswa at their Bellagio Conference Centre whilst he wrote some of his chapters, NORAD for supporting ACHEST, and KPMG for its help with publishing and launching this book in Cape Town, London and New York.

References

1 World Health Organization. *Task Shifting; Global Recommendations and Guidelines.* World Health Organization, 2007.

2 Report of the Commission for Africa. *Our Common Interest.* March 2005.

3 **Crisp N.** *Turning the World Upside Down—the Search for Global Health in the 21st Century.* CRC Press, 2010.

4 **Dowden R.** *Africa: Altered States, Ordinary Miracles.* Portobello Books, 2008.

Chapter 2

Health leadership in Africa

Francis Omaswa

In this chapter Dr Omaswa describes the challenge facing African health leaders in stark terms: 'Until and unless we Africans, individually and collectively, feel the pain and the shame of our condition, we will not have the commitment to take the actions needed to right the situation.' This is a fitting introduction to a chapter in which Dr Omaswa describes developments in Africa from his own experience over the last 40 years and, in particular, the way in which relationships between donors and African countries has simultaneously helped improve health and slowed down the development of national capacity and systems. This account sets the scene for the following chapters in which individual leaders describe the way they have struggled with this complex relationship as they have worked to improve health in their own countries.

Health leadership in Africa in context

My experience growing up in Africa was very hopeful. The rural village where I grew up was secure and peaceful. Law and order was assured by the clan heads and the local chiefs. The schools were well run by missionaries and funded by the colonial administration and the local governments. I graduated from the prestigious Makerere Medical School where the students lived a very good life.

My first job was at a small up-country hospital where my salary was good enough to live on, to buy a car on hire purchase, and to build a house back in my village home. The hospital was well-equipped, with medical supplies, running water and electricity, and I enjoyed my work. The public service was managed by Ugandans funded by the Uganda economy and there were no donors. There were expatriate doctors in some of the hospitals, including my hospital and at the university teaching hospital in Kampala. Indeed at this time, Africans had great expectations for their post-independence future.

Idi Amin captured power in 1971 in Uganda during my very first year of public service and things started to fall apart in that country. In Uganda we have tended to blame almost everything that has gone wrong on Idi Amin. However, other countries in the region without Amin-like leaders also declined at the same time. The whole of sub-Saharan Africa experienced a decline accelerated by military dictatorships, fuelled and condoned by the Cold War between the West and the Soviet Union, and compounded by the collapse of commodity prices and the sharp rise in the price of oil. The net result was a mismanaged Africa with bankrupt and collapsed economies, on her knees as a beggar for aid in order to provide basic services to her populations and to make a new beginning economically, socially, and politically.

The new beginning that Africa aspires to, with a view to exit from the legacy of the period of economic decline and bad governance, is being played out against a background of five crippling factors:

1 High levels of poverty among her people: with poverty figures according to the World Bank ranging from 30% to 70%.

2 High population growth that is applying extreme pressure on social services: school classrooms are overcrowded with implications for the quality of education, and health facilities are overflowing with patients with implications for access to basic healthcare. Both are key issues in poverty alleviation.

3 The population structure with 50% being below the age of 15 years represents a high dependency ratio. All educated Africans with jobs feel this very much, as we do not only take care of our immediate families but are also expected to support lots of members of the extended family with paying school fees, marriages, and funerals. If one African is generous enough to support many relatives, there are many who will leave everything to be taken care of and will do little or nothing for themselves.

4 A culture of tolerance of the unacceptable has become normal; the demand side for quality services is weak, which in itself perpetuates the status quo. When things go wrong, the population and their leaders just shrug their shoulders and say 'What to do? What do you expect? This is Africa' We will come back to this point later.

5 The fifth crippling factor is the dependency of African countries on outsiders for development assistance and, worse still, for solutions, to provide essential social services, including healthcare to their populations.

Herein lies the origins and some of the root causes of many problems that bedevil Africa today. Africans went to the Bretton Woods' institutions[1] and to other institutions and countries begging for advice and for money and we got both, but in exchange for certain core values. Africans lost self-respect, self-confidence, and self-determination. In order to get the much needed money, African technocrats and politicians accepted being humiliated by their donor counterparts and were forced to accept and implement solutions that they knew would not work. The new order dictated that Africans were told what to do and how by foreign technocrats and politicians who did not have the same depth of understanding of the African situation as the locals. Studies were frequently commissioned as part of analytical work to define the problems and identify solutions. Often, however, these were designed and carried out by external experts whose contextualization of the issues was misplaced, resulting in the generation of findings and recommendations that were out of context and solutions that did not solve the problems.

I know of many such examples. A recent World Bank report '*The Labor Market for Health Workers in Africa: new look at the crisis*' makes damning assertions on its section on the Performance of African health workers that lack contextualized insights into the reasons for the behaviour patterns of African health workers. For example, the report states: 'The inefficiency of health workers is associated with absenteeism and shirking. "On any given day, 37 percent of health workers in Uganda are absent from work for no apparent reason". '[2]

The fact is that Ugandan health workers are, in general, very responsible individuals and are not fools. When they stay away from their jobs it must be for a good cause, such as supplementing the low pay and coping with other deserving and relevant responsibilities. A trusted insightful researcher would have been able to establish the root causes of this alleged 'absenteeism'. Further, the report is disparaging and derogatory; failing to acknowledge the outstanding and heroic performance of many African health workers who save lives daily under difficult conditions and for which a Ugandan nurse has been nominated for the Nobel Prize and two other Ugandan health workers have won awards for outstanding performance during the 2nd and 3rd Global Forum on HRH.

In other examples, inexperienced and young donor technocrats prescribed solutions that were blatantly wrong. An example was a one-man mission by a 29-year-old employee of the Global Fund to Fight Aids, TB, and Malaria (GFATM) to Uganda in 2003 to appraise the level of readiness of the country to receive the first disbursement of a grant from the GFATM. He arrived with many 'non-negotiable positions' and was speaking in a style that made it clear that he was in charge, and left no room for discussion and clarifications. We took him from the Ministry of Health to the Minister of Finance who told him: 'Young man at my level everything is negotiable', without much effect. We took him to meet the President of the country who quizzed him about his qualifications and age, and asked why he was not listening to the local position, without much effect.

In the end the young man directed that Uganda could apply for only $6 million out of a possible grant of over $240 million. A few months later at the World

Health Assembly, the Executive Director of GFATM, while addressing Health Ministers, used Uganda as an example of a country that had access to a large grant but applied for only a small amount. We, of course, objected to this at the meeting and later in writing, and got an apology from the Executive Director of the GFATM. As a result of this type of treatment, wrong solutions have been imposed on Africa and, further, the implementation of the correct solutions was often interfered with by project and programme supervisors who did not have sufficient understanding of the intricacies and context of the local situation.

Loss of self-confidence, self-respect, and self-determination, and the humiliation of being forced to implement solutions that Africans knew to be wrong, have resulted in an insidious and malignant psychological demoralization of many African leaders and populations. A mindset has emerged that combines disempowerment, loss of self-confidence, and loss of the 'can do' attitude.

The opposite attributes were prevalent just before and after independence in many African countries. At that time a significant number of African economies were strong and donor dependence was negligible in these countries. Public servants, including health professionals, were well paid and health systems were efficient and well led by empowered, confident, and motivated Africans. I had the privilege to work in such a system in Uganda. Miriam Were (who contributes Chapter 8 to this book) argues that the legacy of the humiliations previously accumulated during centuries of slavery and colonialism accelerated the entrenchment of this new disempowerment and demoralization.

The disempowered syndrome suffered by African leaders and populations has had another devastating consequence: the erosion of a sense of ownership and accountability. As in the case of the dependent members of the extended family, if donors are paying for African health, the emergency that led to begging is perceived as being addressed and taken care of by someone else, so we can all relax a bit or divert our attention and concentration to another emergency. This represents eroded ownership and accountability.

The net result of decades of mismanagement—and despite the benefits of development assistance—is that Africa now finds herself at the bottom of the world league in human development indices. Africa has 11% of the world's population but carries a disproportionate 25% of the global disease burden, 49% of maternal deaths, 50% of under-five mortality, 67% of the HIV burden, and 85% of the malaria burden. It has 1.3% of the global health workforce and spends only 3% of the world's total expenditure on health.[3] Why should this situation be allowed to persist? Does anyone care? Until and unless we Africans, individually and collectively, feel the pain and the shame of our condition, we will not have the commitment to take the actions needed to right the situation.

The foundation that makes ownership and accountability by Africans an imperative is the thesis that sustainable change is inherently endogenous and must come from within the country, the community, the people, or individuals who are the beneficiaries of the change. As Thoraya Obaid, former Executive Director of the United Nations Population Fund has said, 'Only that change that comes from the communities themselves is sustainable'.[4] Or, as Miriam Were writes in Chapter 8, 'In Africa if it doesn't happen in the communities, it doesn't happen'.

Due to the variety of factors described here, including natural disasters, wars, and famine, Africa has become a continent for global pity. It is deemed not to be able to take care of itself and to be in need of outside help for both resources and, worse still, for ideas and solutions as well. This is what needs to change: we all need to create conditions that enable Africans to regain confidence in themselves and to own and be committed to provide the leadership needed to cause the change that we desire. Friends and partners from outside only come to help, they cannot do it for us.

For years I have participated in conversations among African leaders talking to ourselves about our disempowered status. We have talked loudly, when we are alone, but in whispers when non-Africans are in earshot. It is now time for this conversation to come out into the open, moving from whispers to genuine dialogue for all concerned: Africans, our friends, and our enemies.

I set up ACHEST (the African Centre for Health and Social Transformation) in 2009 to help create and contribute to this dialogue. In pursuit of this, ACHEST convened African institutions in 2009 and established the African Health Systems Governance Network (Ashgovnet) that now conducts a bimonthly online health systems' Governance Forum in which Africans and partners participate. This forum has provided an opportunity for genuine dialogue on various topics, such as ownership and accountability, closing the implementation gap, creating synergies, and working with donors.

Here are some messages from the Ashgovnet[5] governance forum: Godfrey Sikipa of Zimbabwe, observed that:

> The fact that we were having this honest discussion is indeed testimony that Africans are taking up their rightful role as the prime actors and movers in the efforts to improve the health of Africans. I would like though, to caution ourselves that as we debate and share ideas, thoughts and suggestions; we should avoid the temptation of blaming everyone else for our (Africans) problems and situation. The only way we can move forward and remedy things is for US as African individuals, institutions and governments) to do some serious 'introspection' in order to identify our weaknesses (and strengths) that we need to address in order to move forward faster and be the respected, efficient and authoritative leaders and coordinators that we want rest of the world to view us as.

I could not agree more with this position. As a surgeon, it has always been my principle to take the blame personally for any mistakes and complications that happen to my patients. In the event that it was my assistant or another member of the team that primarily caused the problem, I have to ask myself the question, 'What do I have to do now or in the future to make sure that the same error does not happen again to another of my patients?'. Similarly, the primary responsibility for fixing Africa's condition rests with we Africans and not with the rest of the world.

The African situation is looking better and I see light at the end of the tunnel. Leadership and coordinated action is critical now more than ever for a sprint finish that will propel Africa to a state of irreversible progress and to becoming an equal and respected member of the international community and no longer a subject for pity. The African Union (AU) has transformed itself from an institution that focused on decolonizing and ridding Africa of apartheid into a development and people-centred institution. Unlike the predecessor, Organization of African Unity, the AU is constituted not only by governments, but also by civil society and is positioned to be the interface between Africa and the rest of the world. Military governments are no longer tolerated and the score card of the AU in championing Africa's health is commendable, as will be illustrated later.

Africa is hopeful again, as was the case during the immediate post-independence period. The *Economist* magazine in May 2000, wrote a commentary under the title '*Hopeless Africa*'; ten years later in December 2011, this magazine had to eat its words and wrote another commentary titled '*Rising Africa*'. According to the World Bank, African economies are growing at an average of 5–6% annually and eight of the ten fastest growing global economies are in sub-Saharan Africa. There are discoveries of viable deposits of oil, gas, and minerals in 34 African countries. I have travelled widely in Africa over the years. There was a time when African cities were dead quiet and dirty with a lethargic population. Today, I see different African cities: cleaner, more and taller buildings, people walking in them with a purpose.

A key determinant of Africa's future is what happens to the youth bulge: 50% of country populations are below the age of 15 and 70% below 30 years of age. The potential of reaping a demographic dividend of the youth bulge adds to the hopefulness, while at the same time also posing the threat of a disaster if not well managed. Evidence shows that for a demographic dividend to be harvested there needs to be a drop in the birth rate, which in turn reduces the dependency rate. For this to happen, effective primary healthcare services should be made widely accessible. It is also important for the youth to receive good-quality secondary and tertiary education.

African leaders and leadership in health have an enormous role to play in a new Africa, a hopeful Africa, where Africans recognize that the responsibility for making Africa an equal player in the global community rests primarily with Africans. In the next few pages I will illustrate how African leadership for health can be brought into play at individual, family, community, sub-national, national, regional, and global levels.

Leadership, governance, and management for health in Africa

Africa has well-established coordination structures in the health sector. We have the African Union one of whose objectives is 'to work with relevant international partners in the eradication of preventable diseases and the promotion of good health on the continent'.[6] The African Union Commission (AUC) has a department and a team led by a Commissioner for Social Affairs with Health Specialists. There are five Regional Economic Communities (RECs), which have active health secretariats for East, Central, West, and Southern Africa. There are also two WHO Regional offices in Brazzaville and Cairo. The UN family and other partners in Africa also have a coordination structure known as Harmonization for Health in Africa (HHA) with a secretariat based alongside the WHO African Region. On top of these, there are specialized African health institutions that act as centres of excellence in various fields and are in official relations with the AUC, RECs, and the WHO Regional Offices and routinely play the role of expert resources to these bodies. There are also active African Professional Associations in various health specialties. There are universities, research centers and academies of science with potential to act as additional African resources.

These agencies have access to African governments, including ministers and heads of state and governments. I have seen many of these institutions work well over many years. Others, of course, have not. However, both the good and the bad are all too often undermined and bypassed by international organizations. I know that many Westerners will say that they have evidence of corruption in governments and amongst officials in Africa. This is undeniable and very important. However, this should not mean that everyone should be treated the same. As this book demonstrates, there are very many effective and honest leaders in Africa. Why are they and the authentic African structures they work within not be the entry point for international partners?

I discuss the main parts of this structure in the next few sections: looking in turn at the AU and at national governments and their relationships with local organizations and professionals. I go on to discuss international partnerships and the wider global picture.

The African Union

African leaders through the Organization for African Unity (OAU) took an interest in health from the 1980s onwards and have adopted several declarations and commitments. These include: the 1987 Declaration on Health as the Foundation for Socio-Economic Development; the 1992 and 1994 Dakar and Tunis Declarations on HIV; the 1996 Addis Ababa Declaration and the African Plan of Action Concerning the Situation of Women in Africa in the Context of Family Health.

The AU, which took over from the OAU, has built upon this tradition and several African Heads of State and Government summits have been convened exclusively to deliberate on the health of African people. The health agenda has featured frequently and prominently in the summits in recent years. These include the Abuja Declaration on Roll Back Malaria in Africa (2000) and the Abuja Declaration on HIV/AIDS, Tuberculosis, and Other Related Infectious Diseases (ORID) (2001). Maternal and child health has been discussed several times, culminating in the Kampala Declaration of 2010, among others.

The key role of leadership in African health was underscored at the African Development Forum (ADF) held in Addis Ababa in December, 2000 titled 'AIDS: The Greatest Leadership Challenge'. As it said at the time 'For the first time, there was a focus on leadership at all levels from youth to traditional chiefs, women to people infected with the disease, and academia to Heads of State.'[7] This noteworthy event paved the way for the Abuja summit in April and the UNGAS in New York in June, 2001 on HIV.

The Forum defined leadership for health as 'a position of power and authority, with corresponding responsibility, over an organized institution, collectivity or community. For leadership to be more than simply presiding over an inert group or organization, it must also have the component of agency, the ability to affect change or to resist change'.[8] This Forum highlighted the need for exceptional, personal, moral, political, and social commitment to the leadership needed to combat the HIV pandemic. This was illustrated by concrete examples of how individual leaders such as President Kenneth Kaunda had changed the face of the HIV fight in Zambia by announcing publicly that his own son had died of HIV, and the personal interest and leadership demonstrated by President Yoweri Museveni in leading a national awareness campaign that led to the dramatic reduction of prevalence in Uganda from a high of 18% to 6% in few years.

This forum also pointed out the important leadership role of 'high government officials' (whom I describe below as 'techno-professionals') and stated that they 'carry the primary responsibility for policy development and implementation. They have the capacity and authority for legislation, execution of policy, and allocation of resources to muster appropriate actions.'[9]

The recommendations of the ADF are now mainstreamed into the Economic Commission for Africa programmes for regional integration, sustainable development, and empowerment of women.

There have also been examples of leadership taking countries completely in the wrong direction, and of lack of leadership that have wreaked havoc in some African countries and which the AU appeared helpless to do anything about. Notable and tragic examples include the prolonged denial of the existence of HIV by the leadership of South Africa and the struggle to vaccinate children against polio in Nigeria.

National governments

National governments in all countries have the ultimate responsibility and accountability for population health and this cannot be delegated. Most international agreements, conventions, and treaties assume that it is governments that are responsible for assuring the health of their populations and that compliance with international health regulations are the responsibility of national governments. This is seen in the composition, for example, of the United Nations, the World Health Organization, and the African Union, all of which have national governments as constituent member states.

In terms of providing health services, most national constitutions contain some language concerning the right of citizens to basic health services. It is the constitutional responsibility of the government to fulfill that obligation. This stewardship role of government means that it has the responsibility to ensure that arrangements to provide basic health services are in place and that other conditions that enable people to be as healthy as possible prevail in the country. In other words, it has to create an effective health system that will ensure that the following five components are addressed: (1) personal and family health-care services, (2) public or population health services, (3) health research, (4) that health is streamlined into all the policies of other sectors, and (5) ensure that there is a skilled health workforce in the country to deliver these services.

The WHO has identified leadership and governance as one of the six building blocks for health systems. Indeed, it is the most important given its impact on all the others. Unfortunately, it is also the most neglected. This is a complex area that involves championing the health agenda among the general population, negotiating with various interest groups and with other government sectors for funds, personnel, space, and visibility. It is country and context specific, being rooted in local history, culture, power balances, and the resource base. It calls for vision as well as courage and perseverance and demands skill sets in communication, advocacy, and the generation, interpretation of data and evidence and its dissemination to the right audience at the right time.

This leadership and governance role generally rests with the Minister and Ministry of Health but it also calls for leadership from the top echelons of government: the head of state and government, the Prime Minister, and the political party all providing support to the Minster of Health. It requires strong technical leadership from techno-professional leaders, inside the Ministry and across government, and the support of the local health partners outside the government. Strong ministries of health are critical to the achievement of national health goals. There is evidence to show that it is the countries with strong, confident, and clear local leadership that are able to stay the course in implementing home-grown policies, and are also making the most progress towards achieving the MDGs.[10] Their stories are part of this work and this book. This evidence is reflected in international research, which shows that it is precisely this issue of governance that is the most important for sustained improvement.[11]

Despite the central role of ministers and ministries, they are still generally overlooked when investments are being made and initiatives are being designed to strengthen health systems. On top of this, the turnover rate of ministers of health is high with short tenure periods, averaging 3.9 years on the job, and many come without any preparation for the onerous leadership roles expected from them. In a study that I led with Dr Jo Ivey Boufford, there was strong support amongst ministers and stakeholders for an executive leadership development programme for new ministers, leadership support for sitting ministers, and the establishment of a virtual information resource centre on health systems' stewardship and governance.[12]

I have been involved in the Aspen Institute's Ministerial Leadership Initiative and, with my co-editor Nigel Crisp, in Harvard's Ministerial Leadership Forum, both of which have been very effective in providing support for ministers from low- and middle-income countries around the world. However, there is still a long way to go to build awareness among politicians, policy makers, and the public, of the importance of stewardship and governance in strengthening health systems, and the critical role of ministers and ministries of health. Selection of such individuals and their motivation are often the source of failure of African health leadership. Tools for their induction and for them to perform their functions should be made available through far more extensive and wide-reaching executive leadership development programmes, which need to be well contextualized for Africa and individual countries by Africans and other international experts with experience of working with the international community.

Governments cannot delegate the responsibility for stewardship of health systems but government action alone is insufficient. Governments need to work closely with an ever increasing array of other actors in health. These include NGOs and civil society, advocacy groups, private sector and business, academia and think tanks, professional associations, media, parliaments, and development partners. Ministers of health and other African and international health leaders who were interviewed for the study mentioned above, strongly emphasized the importance of organizations both in and outside of government that can provide needed expertise and resource to ministries of health. The study noted that every country needs to cultivate and grow a critical mass of individuals, groups, and institutions that interact regularly among themselves and with their governments, parliaments, and civil society as agents of change, holding each other and their governments to account, as well as providing support and collectively ensuring that the visibility of the national health agenda remains prominent in the national psyche and culture.

These organizations, we called them Health Partner Resource Organizations, are well positioned to support government in policy formulation and implementation, health service provision, and enhancing governance and stewardship. They can also work with ministries to create a culture of evidence-based policy and practice, and hold each other accountable for results. A mapping study of five countries (Kenya, Malawi, Mali, Tanzania, and Uganda), by ACHEST found that there were organizations active in all the countries that were ready to partner with their governments and that the governments were ready to work with them. However, the evidence also showed that this did not always happen effectively.

It is clearly vital that countries develop a critical mass of these partnerships as recommended in our study and, in so doing, build effective local institutions and governance arrangements.[13]

The leaders of the HRPIs and government officials are the techno-professionals who are knowledgeable but, in my experience, often do not demonstrate the bold leadership that should make them stand out as change agents in their societies and communities. There are obvious and impressive examples, such as the authors of chapters in this book. However, all too often, the techno-professionals watch and tolerate wrong things in their midst and fear or fail to speak out on the side of the people and the common good. Leadership is largely left to politicians, some of whom have the legitimacy of holding elective positions, while others are aspiring to be elected, and both groups have vested personal interest.

I would argue that the technocrats and professionals as a group have let Africa down. Why? These policies and resolutions adopted by political leaders are crafted by techno-professionals and implementation strategies are designed by them. It is the techno-professionals who understand how the technologies work and monitor implementation success or failures round the world. They attend many meetings all over the world on health issues but most go back home to business as usual. They have the statistics on mortality and morbidity rates and can interpret the significance of these in terms of suffering, deprivation, and premature death, including the economic and social ramifications. Yet the sense of urgency and the outrage the situation calls for is nowhere to be seen or heard. The absence of leadership and the complacency of the techno-professionals is disturbing. Many have left Africa for greener pastures.

Partnerships for health development

The relationship between Africa and its development partners has gone through many phases ranging from encounters with adventurous explorer Europeans, to religious missionaries, and to traders and the colonialists. Following independence, there was a cautious relationship at the background of which was the Cold War. Then Africa suffered the economic collapse already described and became a beggar. During the beggar period, African countries accumulated debts, which became unbearable and earned these countries the derogatory title of Highly Indebted Poor Countries (HPICs).

During this phase, there was chronic tension between the donors and the aid recipients. Donors inserted themselves into government offices of African countries to make sure that the aid was used to the satisfaction of the donors. Priority setting was generally controlled by the donors and resulted in the disempowerment syndrome, misunderstandings, and frustrations that have been described already. It was Africans who pushed for a new way of managing aid, which led to a series of conferences in Monterey and Rome and culminated in the crafting of the Paris Declaration on Aid Effectiveness in which Africans made an effective contribution. Credit also goes to the leadership of the OECD countries who were active supporters of the development of the new partnership principles enshrined in the Paris Declaration on Aid Effectiveness.

A major turning point was the transformation by Africans of the OAU into the African Union, the establishment of the NEPAD initiative with a vision to spearhead new thinking, ownership, and sharing in all fields and balanced partnership with the international community. The African Peer Review Mechanism was adopted by heads of governments and states as an accountability mechanism. On top of this, was the revival of the theme of the African Renaissance first described by Cheikh Anta Diop in a series of essays *'Towards the African Renaissance: Essays in Culture and Development, 1946–1960'* (Trans. Egbuna P. Modum. London: The Estate of Cheikh Anta Diop and Karnak House, 1996) and advocated by presidents Thabo Mbeki, Olusegun Obasanjo, Abdoulaye Wade and Bouteflika. It called for African renewal in self-pride and a commitment to self-determination.

President John Kufour of Ghana, at the launch of the Thabo Mbeki Foundation, provides a useful perspective when he states 'We should bear in mind however that the renaissance is not an event or project whose success must be measured at a predetermined time. It must be seen as a whole movement, a whole crusade that will result in unearthing all that is beautiful, adorable and unique of Africa'.[14] The renaissance movement is real and alive. There are annual renaissance conferences in South Africa, there is an *International Journal of African Renaissance Studies*, and an African Renaissance Institute of Science and technology, among several other initiatives.

Indeed the level and quality of policy debate among Africans has improved. There is a call for intellectual work on African problems to shift from international institutions to Africa. At least on paper, there is no doubt that Africans have demonstrated leadership and ownership of the process towards transformation of Africa. There have been equally promising commitments from the international community to increase development assistance and to adhere to agreed partnership principles. Africa has featured regularly at the meetings of the G8 countries and we have seen the Commission for Africa. There have been promises of increased development assistance and at the same time calls for Africans to strengthen governance and accountability capacities.

The discussion on partnerships for health development in Africa has been dominated by the relations between African governments and donors through bilateral government to government arrangements and multilateral institutions, such as the World Bank, IMF, African Development Bank, European Union Commission, and the UN Family. Global Health Initiatives (GHIs), such as the Global Fund to Fight Aids, TB, and Malaria (GFATM) and the Global Alliance on Vaccines and Immunization have also emerged as major routes for donors to channel funds to Africa for health development. There are also GHIs that specialize in providing technical support and coordination, not money, such as the UNAIDS, Global Stop TB Partnership, Roll Back Malaria, the Global Health Workforce Alliance (GHWA), and others.

Over the years I have had an exceptional opportunity to work intensively in this space in different capacities. For nearly two decades I was a senior civil servant in Uganda; during six of these years I served as Director General of Health Services and was directly responsible for donor coordination in the health sector in the country. At this same time, I was also active on the global scene and was one of the architects who created the Global Stop TB Partnership; I was elected as first Board Chair and later served as Vice Chair. Uganda was at the forefront in the establishment of the GFATM. The Ugandan Minister of Health, Hon. Dr Crispus Kiyonga, was elected as first Board Chair and I was an active technical contributor during the negotiations and later served as the Chair of the Board Portfolio and Procurement Committee. I have also served for one year as the chair of the GAVI Independent Review Committee that reviewed applicants for grants and makes recommendations to the Board for awards. I also served in several global and regional committees and participated at the crafting of the famous Paris Declaration on Aid Effectiveness in February, 2005. A few months later, I was appointed to a position at the WHO Headquarters as the founding Executive Director of the GHWA. I have also served as an adviser to a number of developed country governments.

From this vantage point I have seen my own country of Uganda's relationship with partners go full circle from being very bad to being a 'donor darling' and back to bad again over a decade or so. I have also observed the good intentions of those populations in donor countries who support development assistance budgets and the hopes of the populations in Africa to whom development assistance is targeted. I have observed the aspirations of the Paris Declaration sometimes take a back seat.

The subject of good donorship is difficult and vexed. At the implementation level, donor and aid recipient representatives often have tensions and regularly trade accusations against each other. Aid recipients are concerned about the possible loss of ownership and leadership for priority setting, while donors are concerned that they want to see more results for their money and want a role in priority setting. The rules of engagement, however, are well articulated in the Paris Declaration on Aid Effectiveness and the Accra Accord, where 'country leadership' is the core guiding principle of good donorship. However, the question that is at the heart of the debate is: 'If countries lead, will donors follow?'. Will this happen in practice?

There is evidence that where countries are clear and strong about what they want to achieve, donors actually follow and these are the countries making the most progress in achieving health goals. These achievements are incentives to donors to provide more support. Where countries do not have explicit health policies and strategies, or are not strong and have no individuals able to articulate these clearly, then donors want to argue for what they believe to work better, which gets interpreted as taking over ownership and country leadership. Donors have to account to their taxpayers and need evidence of success and positive results from the aid recipients for accountability and to justify additional allocations. Countries are sometimes desperate for the money and fear to lose it by appearing strong or challenging donor positions during negotiations. I have also seen donor representatives who are too strong, appear to know everything, are patronizing and push their own positions on timid 'beggar' countries— sometimes at variance with official donor country guidelines. I have heard donors say that they want to be led. Regrettably, I have also seen countries where local partners are either too weak or are lacking commitment.

Clearly, the situation is complex. Building trust between donors and aid recipients is the key to a productive relationship. Yet nurturing this trust can be tough, has to be learnt, needs touch, takes time to earn, and is easy to lose. Individuals of high calibre who are committed to genuine development are required from both sides and need to be prepared for their roles. Mutual respect and clear separation of roles and responsibilities are other pillars upon which this trust is built and sustained. Structures and instruments for managing the relationship are essential and should be institutionalized; examples include committees and other forums for regular joint reviews and for resolving conflicts which inevitably occur.

Africa will need donors for some time to come and I am convinced from my own experience that 'if countries lead, donors will follow'. This is only possible, however, where you have Africans who are committed, willing, and able to lead and, of course, willing to be held accountable. As Amartya Sen has written: 'Ultimately development or progress of a community or country is associated with independence or freedom from being controlled by others or by external factors'.[15]

My co-editor, Nigel Crisp, has argued that rich and poor countries need to learn from each other in health and that we should talk about co-development not international development in the future.[16] This would be a formula for a very different relationship and is nowhere more relevant than when we turn to technical assistance and capacity building.

The purpose of technical assistance and capacity building is to provide interim support that enables the recipient country or institution to achieve an objective and/or to develop the capacity to become capable of undertaking the same tasks independently and on their own. Ideally, it should aim at developing the capacity of the partner so that the further technical assistance becomes unnecessary. It is helpful to think of capacity existing in a country or an institution when there are capabilities to achieve desired social, economic, political or cultural objectives without being controlled by others or by external factors. It presupposes that there are tools, skills, staff, infrastructure, structures and systems that are blended to deliver the expected outputs.

While it is easier to acquire tools, skills staff, and infrastructure, the structures and systems for management and governance (coordination, communication, negotiation, monitoring, and evaluation) are harder, require socio-cultural interventions, and take longer to achieve. For capacity building to be owned and sustained, these structures and systems cannot be dropped in from outside but need to be grown from within the institutions and countries, taking into account the history, culture, resource base, and politics. This is where many current well-meaning capacity building initiatives fail. Enthusiastic partners import wholesale practices that work in other contexts and transplant them on weak, unknowing recipient structures and systems, and they work for short periods and fail.

Two contextual issues are of particular importance: (1) the recipient resource base and (2) the social and cultural environment. In a study of 20 years of USA government investments in leadership and capacity building in the health sector in Uganda, carried out by ACHEST in 2010, we found that the leadership capacity building initiatives failed to take into account the fact that the local resource base for sustainability of the initiatives was not given due attention and, therefore, the capacities that were developed withered soon after the ending of the capacity building grants. Similarly, the ability of the district staff to manoeuvre around the political and social environment, such as nepotism and corruption, was not factored into the training of the local health leaders whose capacity was being developed. As a result, a lecturer from one of the top management schools stated 'We train leaders and managers in new public management concepts based on market principles. But when they get back to their posts in civil service, the environment does not allow them to apply what they have learnt'.[17] This simply means that the correct training was not provided.

In a similar study of technical assistance and capacity development in Cambodia, Martin Godfrey et al.[18] found that the 'Cambodia's experience since 1993 suggests that most projects in such a situation are donor-driven in their identification, design and implementation, to the detriment of capacity development. Connected with this is the chronic underfunding of government in such an economy, which hinders implementation of projects and threatens post-project financial sustainability.'

Sridhar Devi identifies seven challenges in donor aid, all related to capacity building and two of them are relevant to this discussion:

1 Over-emphasis on new players (UN organization, bilateral agencies, international NGOs, private foundations) rather than reforming and strengthening existing institutions and capacities. HRPIs are in all countries and have stronger promise of building sustainable capacity from within the country and the institutions and understanding the local culture and politics better.

2 Channelling funds through northern organizations, thereby denying capacity development of indigenous institutions.[19]

There seems almost to be a concerted effort to eliminate or reduce the role of government and local organizations in aid management.

In this debate, the US government through the Global Health Initiative and USA Forward has expressed commitment to transfer more ownership and support to African institutions. There is, however, fierce lobbying against this from the current beneficiaries. Other OECD countries started to move in this direction earlier, although some of them still contract northern organizations to carry out work that can be better done by African institutions.

The quality of such assistance is yet another issue. During my tenure as donor coordinator at the Ministry of Health (MOH) in Uganda, we had some excellent assistance from partner countries but we also had some very poor quality assistance. This has led to some technical assistance or TA being characterized as being about technical apprentices who do not have more skills than the local experts and have come to learn or technical associates who are on a long vacation, happy to be around but not contributing much to the institution, or technical agents who mostly watch and report what is going on.

Africa has witnessed a massive invasion of international NGOs. In many African cities, there are NGO boulevards and enclaves, usually in the most posh and up-market areas, and they drive the most elegant and expensive vehicles. What are they all doing in Africa with those assets? Whilst many may be doing an excellent job, we must question the roles and motivations of some. Some of these NGOs have missions that are serving interests that are not necessarily aligned with local or national or African interests. I have watched leaders of such NGOs use young and sometimes older Africans who have been coached to speak for the NGO at international meetings pushing agendas that they do not fully understand. I have also argued with international NGOs that believe that they have an equal mandate and legitimacy as local NGOs to represent Africa and to speak for African populations because they are registered locally and have a local governance structure.

Most African experts agree that partnerships, North to South, in Africa are essential for accelerating development and learning from each other. Many country health systems are not optimally benefiting from the many centres of excellence that exist worldwide. Young, upcoming professionals have to go north, while they could more cheaply and with greater relevance benefit from sister institutions and mentors in Africa or, increasingly, in other low- and middle-income countries. There is an obvious need to develop these partnerships further as part of the wider development of health in Africa.

Africans on the world stage

Action on health takes place in countries, yet it is heavily influenced by the global environment. As we have seen with SARS or avian and swine flu, a single health event in one place in one country can have far-reaching consequences for health in other parts of the world within a short time, and impact not only health but also the global economy. Practices and behaviour from one part of the world get transmitted to other parts of the world for better or for worse. For example, dietary practices of developed countries have been copied by Africans, resulting in a sharp rise in diabetes among African populations. There are also health challenges that need multi-sector and multi-national responses, such as the health consequences of climate change. There is now a great need for improved health governance globally to ensure that all these sorts of issues are handled both effectively and equitably.[20] The World Health Organization was created to play the central role in this as the UN specialized agency for health. WHO has two regional offices in Africa and is in every country. There are other members of the UN family with health mandates including UNICEF, UNFPA, UNAIDS; other multilateral players like the World Bank, ILO and the World Trade Organization; and many new Global Health Initiatives.

Africans have increasingly played roles as leaders in these organizations over the years beginning from an inauspicious start. An African has been head of the African Region of the WHO since 1965 (before that the post was occupied by a Portuguese) but no other African was able to take on one of the top jobs in these organizations for several years thereafter. One of the first, Dr Ade Lucas, recalls how in 1977 the President of the World Bank, Robert McNamara, was not prepared to have him as Director of the joint Special Programme for Research and Training in Tropical Diseases and only relented a year later.[21]

Worse still is the story of how Dr Ransome Kute from Nigeria was a candidate for the post of Director General of the WHO in 1988 and seen by many outsiders as an excellent choice. He had been told publically that he would receive the votes of a number of delegates, including from the African Region. However, in the event nobody voted for him. Because he received no votes at all, it was very obvious that everyone had broken their promises. The African delegate who did not vote for him didn't return to his home country after the elections and got employed by WHO in another region.

Appendix 1 provides short biographies of Africans who have held some of these top appointments and shows how over the years the numbers have increased, with both men and women taking on these appointments. Today the heads of UNAIDS and UNFPA are both Africans, with others taking on leadership roles such as Deputy Director General of WHO and the Executive Director of the Roll Back Malaria Partnership.

Several of the accounts in this book reflect on the way Africa and Africans have been seen in a very negative light globally. Dr Peter Mugyenyi's description in Chapter 4 of how, as recently as 2001, it was considered unfeasible for Africans to be given anti-retroviral drugs for AIDS because they wouldn't take them consistently because 'they tell the time by the sun' is a case in point.

It is not just about individuals. Things may have improved but we need to do far more to improve the way Africans represent themselves globally. I am delighted to have seen African Health Ministers go to the World Health Assembly during three consecutive years and push through resolutions on health workers that were not on the original agenda during each of those years. Africans were angry over the practice of recruitment agencies from developed countries going to hotels in African cities to recruit and take away health workers who were trained using public funds from poor African tax payers. The issue was emotive: ministers provided leadership, and technical support was provided to the ministers by techno-professional members of their delegations to draft and circulate the resolutions.

However, I have also attended meetings at the United Nations, the World Health Assembly, and the Global Fund where Africa was getting a raw deal. We were not prepared for the debates as well as we should have been and decisions were made that we did not support, because we did not come with evidence to defend our position and did not speak with one voice. On top of this, African delegations to the global meetings are stretched. Africans go to the World Health Assembly or to the Global Fund meeting with two or three delegates, while the US government will come with a delegation of 30–40 people, and the Americans come to these meetings with very clear positions negotiated and agreed at home before delegations leave for the global meetings.

African leaders often have to think on their feet at these meetings and have to be all over the place all day. They get exhausted and their performance is affected. On top of this, African officials, while at home, have got so many things calling for their attention; they sometimes get on the plane to go to a very important international meeting and might be reading their conference papers on the plane.

One of the reasons why ACHEST was created was to respond to this challenge. During the online Governance Forum discussions of the African Health Systems Governance Network advice was given by Professor Lucas on how to improve African performance and benefits from international events. There are four steps:

1 **Preparation**: to what extent are the representatives attending the conference prepared to engage meaningfully in the discussion at the meeting? To what extent have they reviewed relevant documents and consulted other experts within and outside the Ministry? To what extent are they prepared to define and express the national position at the meeting?

2 **Participation**: to what extent is the national delegation able to make meaningful contributions to the discussions keeping in mind the responsibility to implement agreed decisions?

3 **Dissemination**: to what extent are the reports from the conference and the national plan disseminated to all those who need to know within and outside the Ministry?

4 **Implementation**: has a feasible plan been developed to implement the decisions of the conference?[22]

In the worst cases, the delegate admits that he was assigned the task at 5 a.m. to proceed to the conference and read the paper on behalf of the minister! The official report is filed away. Nothing happens until another conference is organized.

It is also very disappointing to see the way that some ministries ignore national experts in the process of managing information and planning implementation. The 'international airport syndrome' often occurs: the national expert is flying out to another country to provide technical assistance to another country, whilst a foreign expert is arriving at the same airport to advise the government on the same subject.

Individuals, families, and communities

Several of the chapters in this book make use of the skills of communities and rely on strong family and local bonds. These ties and traditions must undoubtedly remain at the heart of the way we as Africans improve health in our countries. However, African countries and communities are changing and we need to discover and develop new ways of harnessing these traditional strengths and applying them to the new world. In the meantime, however, it is important to consider what is happening here and now in our communities, and how the changing environment is affecting even on the most traditional communities.

Individuals live their lives in private and in public. They make choices in lifestyles that have consequences for their personal, household, and community health; independently or in consort with others. It is these same individuals who, depending on their place in society, make choices for others too. This may be as heads of households and extended families, political or civic leaders in the community or in government. This is why it becomes critical for children in families and during school days to grow up recognizing how important the life choices are that they make in everyday life and how these impact on themselves, their families and communities. Individuals should grow up with positive attitudes to health-seeking behaviour and personal responsibility for their own, their family and their community health. This is where the roles of parents; both mother and father, assume the highest importance.

If the father smokes at home, the children will smoke too; if he takes too much alcohol, children often follow; if he is violent, the children will likely be violent too. The opposite is equally true. Well-run homes generally produce well-behaved children and responsible citizens who can be relied upon to have healthy families in their own homes and community as adults. The food that children grow up eating at home often ends up as preferred food as adults. Therefore, correct dietary habits, a very important determinant of health outcomes, are created at home with important implications for the future health of individuals, communities, and populations. The role of mothers here becomes paramount, including in the area of personal and domestic hygiene.

Yet today, Africans as individuals, families, and communities face serious challenges to the concept that the home is the place to ensure that ill health is avoided and good health is promoted. I grew up in a rural agro-pastoralist community in Okunguro village, Mukura sub-county in a rural part of Eastern Uganda. We ate food that we grew ourselves, mostly millet, greens, sweet potatoes, peas, and ground nuts, cooked with traditional seasoning and no cooking oil. There was plenty of milk from a large herd of our own cows, and very occasionally there was meat and chicken when important visitors came, and during feasts such as Christmas. There was also occasional smoked fish that my grandmother caught with other women from a nearby lake. On this type of diet, there is absolutely no worry about cardiovascular diseases, such as heart attacks or diabetes. As a doctor, I have done post-mortem examinations on adults from these populations and the blood vessels in their bodies, including hearts, are like those of children: smooth and clean with no atheroma.

The children from this part of Uganda never suffered from *kwashiorkor* or other forms of malnutrition. Unfortunately, my childhood diet is now generally viewed as low prestige. The population now admires fried food, meat with fat, roast pork with salt, soft drinks, sugar. Cassava and sorghum have replaced millet because they grow more easily, and the local green vegetable 'eboo' is no longer popular. The peas are sold for money and the largest cow population in the country was rustled during the civil war and there is no milk. Children suffer from malnutrition and there are regular food shortages related to erratic rains, poor agricultural practices, and population pressure on land.

The population was physically trim from farm work, but now a sedentary life and desk work, associated with being large with abdominal fat, is considered to be cool. These are the challenges that health leaders in Africa face today. How do they navigate their way against strong currents that are washing away sound African societal values? The roots of these currents are old, dating from colonial days, and religious and cultural imperialism that came together and that saw African practices broadly as inferior or even worse: evil and sinful.

African communities are also less cohesive today than two to four decades ago. There has been a massive creaming-off of the most able members of these rural communities to the cities and to distant lands round the world as professionals and as part of the irresistible pull of urbanization experienced the world over. Those who have stayed behind have less power and influence and are considered by the youth as out of touch and, indeed, their self-confidence has been eroded to the extent that they are looking out to follow what is coming from those kith and kin from the cities.

The youth in particular are disillusioned and uncooperative. The level of education in rural areas has increased in quantity but declined in quality. Most children go to primary school but less than half complete full primary school. The dropout rates for girls are much higher than for boys but both groups leave school unprepared for life. The education system will not have provided them with new skills to exit from peasantry but at the same time it will not have provided them with skills to remain as peasants. They have scorn for agriculture but cannot find other jobs. They look to a sedentary and relaxed life yet they have no resources to afford that. They are reluctant to conform to cultural practices and will avoid participating in funerals and clan meetings. They will be found in groups along highways, playing cards, taking alcohol and other drugs. They may be married but leave the care of their wives and children to their parents. Above all they are averse to guidance and criticism.

Several decades ago, the situation was different; communities were more cohesive. The clan heads were respected and they governed the extended family effectively. When I completed primary school, I was well prepared to remain a peasant as I had been taught how to grow crops, manage the cattle, and the household chores for men. The same applied to my sisters who were familiar with female roles. The community and village was administered by an appointed civil servant as administrator, the local chief, who knew the village thoroughly and ensured that all households in the communities complied with the public health act: domestic hygiene with clean homesteads, pit latrines, nutrition and granaries for food security, checked that girls were old enough to marry, settled disputes for law and order, and so on. Today, governance at local level has, in many African countries, been politicized. The administrators, and also often the governors responsible for policy, are elected. These elected leaders find it difficult to enforce laws as their political status calls also for popularity among the population in view of future elections for which votes from the community will be needed. As a result the health and other laws are not enforced, with negative implications for community and population health and general social order.

The study on Ministerial Health Leadership and its 'Strong Ministries for Strong Health Systems Report', pointed out that the countries that are making steady progress in achieving MDGs are those with strong governments and strong social order, which require all citizens to conduct their personal and community life within agreed community parameters in a similar way to the management of villages and community led by the colonial village chief. The societal indiscipline condoned by elected community leaders is a major threat to achieving population health goals and presents a leadership challenge in many African countries. Accountability metrics should be institutionalized at this and all other levels of government.

At its best, the routine governance of society should be the foundation of the health system by ensuring that laws, regulations, and good practice are complied with by all: that homesteads are hygienic, mothers attend antenatal clinics, children are immunized, the nearest health facility has required personnel and supplies, the referral system is in place, the correct food crops are grown and stored properly, all children are going to school, the rural road network is maintained, law and order is enforced, and so on. This should be the job description of the village or community administrator as the very first frontline health worker. The roles of the general administrative cadres must include and prioritize health and such officials need management skills and authority and not health training.

Embedding health goals and aspirations in routine governance of society will facilitate the achievement of health in all policies objective, address social determinants of health, and deliver sustainable health outcomes. This is how countries such as Eritrea, Rwanda, Cuba, Iran, and China have been able to improve health indices in a relatively short time. Compliance with public health regulations and other rules in the communities are in fact enforced more rigorously in developed countries than in many African countries that I know.

The future

In this chapter I have attempted to describe the context within which African health leaders work and to illustrate how the can-do attitude, so evident in many countries at the time of independence, was replaced across much of Africa by a despondency and a dependency. Today, we have something of a renaissance but to take advantage of it we need change. We need Africans to see themselves and the world differently and to deal positively with all the issues I have raised in this chapter. We need the international community and our friends and partners throughout the world also to see Africa and the world differently and to behave accordingly. We also need to create together new approaches to health and new health systems which are fit for the twenty-first century.

The following chapters describe the work of so many brilliant leaders who have overcome these difficulties in their particular environment and role. The final part of the book looks to the future and to a time when we can all, as Africans, realize our right to health as part of our wider freedom to live our lives as citizens of this great continent and the world.

Acknowledgments

Text extracts from African Development Forum: '*Aids: The Greatest Leadership Challenge*', copyright © 2000 Economic Commission for Africa (ECA), reproduced with permission of the United Nations, available from <http://213.55.79.31/adf/adf2000/index.htm>.

References

1 **Articles of Agreement of the International Monetary Fund (1945).** International Monetary Fund, Washington, D.C.

2 **Soucat A, et al.** quoting Chaudhury et al. *The Labor Market for Health Workers in Africa*, 2013, p.41. <elibrary.worldbank.org/doi/pdf/10.1596/978-0-8213-9555-4>.

3 **Kinney MV et al.** (2010) Sub-Saharan Africa's mothers, newborns, and children: where and why do they die? *PLoS Med* **7**(6): e1000294. doi:10.1371/journal.pmed.1000294. Published June **21**, 2010.

4 **Obeid T.** Statement at African Union Heads of State and Governments Summit meeting, Kampala, July 2010.

5 **African Health Systems Governance Network (Ashgovnet).** Governance Forum, 2013. <www.achest.org>.

6 **Constitutive Act of the African Union.** <www.uneca.org/Portals>.

7 **African Development Forum.** *Aids: The Greatest Leadership Challenge*, 2000 <http://213.55.79.31/adf/adf2000/index.htm>.

8 **African Development Forum.** *Aids: The Greatest Leadership Challenge*, 2000 <http://213.55.79.31/adf/adf2000/index.htm>.

9 **African Development Forum.** *Aids: The Greatest Leadership Challenge*, 2000 <http://213.55.79.31/adf/adf2000/index.htm>.

10 **Omaswa F, Boufford J.** *Strong Ministries for Strong Health Systems.* ACHEST, New York Academy of Medicine, January 2010.

11 **Balabanova D, McKee M, Mills M.** '*Good Health at Low Cost' 25 Years On.* Rockefeller Foundation and London School of Hygiene and Tropical Medline, 2011.

12 **ACHEST and the New York Academy of Medicine.** *Strong Ministries for Strong Health Systems*, January 2010, p. 9.

13 **ACHEST and the New York Academy of Medicine.** *Strong Ministries for Strong Health Systems*, January 2010, p.22.

14 *Africa's Renaissance—Dream or Reality?* Former president John Kufuor at the launch of the Thabo Mbeki Foundation. NEPAD Transforming Africa, 2010. <www.nepad.org>.

15 **Sen A.** *Development as Freedom.* OUP, 1999.

16 **Crisp N.** *Turning the World Upside Down—the Search for Global Health in the 21st Century. CRC Press,* 2010.

17 **Omaswa F and Okuonzi S.** *Leadership Capacity Enhancement in the Health Sector in Uganda.* Study Report, 2010. <www.achest.org>.

18 **Godfrey M, et al.** *World Development,* 30 **(3):** 355–73, 2002. <www.elsevier.com/locate/worldde>.

19 **Sridhar D.** Seven challenges in international development assistance for health and ways forward. *The Journal of Law, Medicine and Ethics,* 38(3): 459–69, 2010.

20 **Frenk J, Moon S.** Governance challenges in global health. *New England Journal of Medicine* 368(10): 936–42, 2013.

21 **Lucas AO.** *It was the Best of Times.* BookBuilders, 2010, p. 16.

22 **Omaswa F.** *Discussions in Stewardship and Leadership of Health Systems in Africa,* 2013. <www.achest.org>.

Part 2

The greatest challenges

Chapter 3

Introduction to Part 2: The greatest challenges

Francis Omaswa and Nigel Crisp

This chapter describes the greatest challenges facing countries in sub-Saharan Africa. It highlights the Millennium Development Goals against the background of the whole range of issues that need to be confronted by health leaders. It sets the scene for two compelling chapters written by leaders in Uganda and Malawi about their country's achievements. These are complemented by an authoritative account by Dr Luis Sambo, the WHO Regional Director, of the state of health and healthcare in Africa.

The greatest challenges

The Millennium Development Goals (MDGs) have very largely set the current health priorities for Africa with their targets for reductions in HIV/AIDS, TB, malaria, and child and maternal mortality, among others. They have been the focus of extraordinary amounts of African and international activity, and have led to great improvements for millions of people. However, as the United Nations MDG report for 2013 says, accelerated progress and bolder actions are needed. It concludes that Africa has halted the spread of HIV/AIDS, TB, and malaria but that, despite good progress, Africa still has the greatest burden of child and maternal ill health and mortality.[1]

Part 2: The greatest challenges opens with two accounts, one from Uganda and one from Malawi, of how African leaders have tackled the epidemics of HIV/AIDS and maternal mortality, respectively, in their countries. They are followed by Chapter 6 written by Dr Luis Sambo, who describes the wider epidemiological and policy context.

As Dr Sambo shows, Africa has to deal with a very wide range of health problems that go far beyond the MDGs. The WHO's African Region now has about 12% of the world's population but carries more than 25% of the burden of disease. The 2010 Global Burden of Disease Report demonstrates the scale and spread of the problems and, crucially, how they are changing very dramatically and rapidly.[2] South Africa, to take one typical example, faces epidemics of non-communicable diseases such as diabetes and heart and respiratory disease and trauma, as well as epidemics of the MDG targets of maternal mortality and communicable diseases.[3] There are also 13 so-called Neglected Tropical Diseases (NTDs) such as guinea worm, elephantitis, and river blindness that affect large populations.

Ill-health, trauma, pregnancy related problems, and disease in Africa are all made far worse by poverty and wider social issues such as conflict, poor education, and social division, some of which are the direct legacy of colonialism. Health leaders, as a few examples from this book show, have to work to improve health under very adverse conditions. In Chapter 12 Dr Pascoal Mocumbi describes decisions he took as Health Minister in Mozambique during the civil war. His neighbour, Dr Aaron Motsoaledi, is working to address the historical inequalities in South Africa where 17% of the population consume 85% of the health spend. Meanwhile in The Gambia, Dr Hannah Faal had to work out how to deliver eye care in a region where colonial boundaries have split the same peoples into different jurisdictions with different laws and languages.

Underlying all of this is the impact of population growth. World population has grown by more than a billion since the MDGs were agreed in 2000; Africa meanwhile has grown at about double the pace of the rest of the world and added about a third to its population or 250 million extra people.[4] This, of course, represents the opportunity for a 'demographic dividend' of young workers able to contribute to economic and social growth. It equally represents a potential disaster of over-crowding and under-employment and all that they may bring. Health leaders have their part to play in making sure the opportunity is taken and disaster is avoided.

There is also the fundamental issue of resources. There has been an enormous growth in aid expenditure on health in recent years but this has done little to address global inequalities. Despite this greater share of aid, the mobilization of Western support, the Commission for Africa and much more, Africa still has very small proportions of the world's health resources and of the world's health workers to take on its vast burden of disease. Moreover, by 2011 all but one African country had failed to meet their own target, which they set themselves in Abuja in 2001, that they would each spend 15% of annual government expenditure on health.[5] Resourcing remains a vital issue.

The MDGs have focused efforts on particular diseases and problems, and have led to big improvements. There is, however, much more to do to achieve some of them, with the reduction in maternal mortality in particular still far behind target. They also served to displace other important issues. Declaring anything a priority necessarily creates non-priorities, bends resources in their direction, and can disadvantage others. There has been a great deal written in recent years about how these 'vertical programmes' of the MDGs have attracted resources at the expense of others and, unintentionally, damaged other vital health programmes.

As Dr Sambo shows, the debate is moving on. The emerging priorities are about health systems strengthening and universal health coverage. They bring with them new emphasis on areas such as non-communicable diseases, disability, and mental health. As we write, there appears to be a gathering consensus that what should replace the MDGs after 2015 will be something that 'leaves nobody behind' and gives everyone the opportunity to 'live their lives with dignity'.[6] The question now is how to achieve these new goals. Three leaders—from South Africa, Rwanda, and Ghana—describe how their countries are working towards these aims in Part 5 of this book and show how they are designing their systems to match the specific needs and circumstances of their countries.

There has been an explosion of interest in health in Africa in the last 20 years with many foreign governments and informal and formal groups seeking to play their part in improvement. The benefits are obvious and visible in the improving health status of individuals and populations. This outpouring of good will has, however, also led to problems of coordination as well as to the welcome focus on the priorities, has created misunderstandings as well as harmony amongst partners and, sadly, led in some situations to competition and zealotry about aims and methods.

Foreign and international contributions to health in Africa are, and have been, enormous and quite unprecedented. They should be celebrated. Our focus here, however, is on African leadership and the recognition that ultimately it is Africans who are carrying the continuing burden of healthcare in every clinic and hospital, and governments and ministries of health who have the legal responsibility for healthcare. It is also Africans who, through their out-of-pocket expenditure and government funds, pay by far the largest share of health costs.

The WHO, the other UN agencies such as UNICEF, UNDP and UNFPA, and the African Union (AU) play major roles. In 2006, under the leadership of Commissioner Bience Gawanas, Commissioner for Social Affairs, the AU began the Campaign for Accelerated Action on Maternal Mortality in Africa (CARMMA), which brought African leadership to the problem. It encouraged countries to support each other, to learn and share experience, and to commit to faster improvement. Dr Chisale Mhango refers to the campaign in Chapter 5, whilst Commissioner Gawanas has contributed Chapter 10 to the book.

As Francis Omaswa said in Chapter 2, 'Africans went. . . . begging for advice and for money and we got both but in exchange for certain core values. Africans lost self-respect, self-confidence and self-determination'. These things need to be re-captured and the balance between partners needs to be re-set.

Our stance as editors is very simple. Our starting place is the needs of the poorest and most vulnerable in society and the understanding that these are most effectively articulated by those nearest to them—if, of course, they cannot speak or be heard by themselves. We recognize that local institutions and national governments can get things wrong and, tragically, may be corrupt. However, in all the countries where we have worked we have always been able to identify local leaders of passion and integrity. These are the people we try to place at the centre of dialogue about what needs to be done in a country. They are the focus of this book.

This introduction is followed by accounts by two such national health leaders who needed to persuade others to help them improve health in their countries. In the first, Dr Peter Mugyenyi (Chapter 4) had to confront attitudes that 'the use of anti-retroviral drugs in Africa was unfeasible'. In the second, Dr Chisale Mhango (Chapter 5) worked hard to convince traditional leaders to support improvements in maternal health. Both cases are about how to achieve delivery of improvements in a particular social context, rather than about clinical or scientific evidence and treatment. In the one case the barrier was American and other Western attitudes to Africans, in the other it was about traditional Malawian attitudes to women.

References

1 United Nations. *The Millennium Development Goals Report*, 2013.

2 **Murray CJL, et al.** *Global Burden of Diseases, Injuries and Risk Factors Study 2010 (GBD 2010)*; initial findings reported in *The Lancet*, December 2012.

3 **Lawn J, Kinney M.** *The Lancet South Africa Series Executive Summary Core Group: Executive Summary for the Series*; the Lancet, August 2009.

4 UN. *World Population Prospects: the 2012 revision*. UN, June 2013.

5 WHO. *The Abuja Declaration: Ten Years On*, March 2011.

6 High Level Panel on the Post-2015 Development Agenda. *A New Global Partnership to Eradicate Poverty and Transform Economies through Sustainable Development* July 2013.

Chapter 4

Pioneering work on HIV/AIDS in Uganda

Peter Mugyenyi

Director of the Joint Clinical Research Centre in Kampala, Uganda

When Dr Peter Mugyenyi returned to Uganda from exile in 1989 he found a country struggling with the biggest AIDS epidemic in the world. This chapter describes how he and colleagues set about trying to tackle the disease in their own country through health education and prevention campaigns, collaborative research, and, ultimately, treatment. Through the work of the Joint Clinical Research Centre and active support from the country's President, Uganda took the lead in many aspects of research and development. Over time, it became clear that the biggest challenge was to secure access for Ugandans and Africans more generally, to the treatments that were becoming available at the turn of the century. They had to confront attitudes that the use of antiretroviral therapy (ART) in Africa was simply unfeasible—and demonstrate that it was indeed both possible and essential to do so. Ultimately, Dr Mugyenyi was successful in his advocacy; ART became available and successful services were established throughout the country—and Uganda served as a model for many other countries in Africa. Now, however, there is a continuing need for investment and development to maintain and build on these successes.

Slim disease: a new disease in Uganda

Scatterings of cases of a new and mysterious disease first occurred in Uganda's rural district of Rakai in late 1970s. Alarmed residents noticed that sufferers almost always wasted away, failed to respond to any medical treatment, and inevitably died. On account of the severe emaciation of the victims, 'slim' was the name coined for the new plague.

At about the same time, the male homosexual communities in the US cities of New York and Los Angeles, were also startled by an outbreak of a rare form of fatal pneumonia and Kaposi's sarcoma—a cancer not previously endemic in the

United States. No immediate connection was made between these events in the most dissimilar communities and settings imaginable, especially as the affected Rakai populations were exclusively heterosexual, while in the USA heterosexuals seemed to be spared.

It was not until 5 June 1981 that the United States' Center for Disease Control (CDC) issued its first warning about the outbreak, which in the following year was better defined as Acquired Immune Deficiency Syndrome (AIDS). A few years later slim was confirmed to be AIDS. As HIV spread across the world, especially in sub-Saharan Africa (SSA) it soon became apparent that AIDS was one of the most complex infectious diseases of recent history, which involved a myriad of issues that extended beyond medicine, into human rights, patents, and access to medicines.[1]

Tackling the epidemic: the first stages

By 1989, when I started work at Mulago, Uganda's national referral hospital, after 13 years in exile, the infection had spread to all parts of the Uganda, and the country was the most AIDS affected in the world. My first day at work was distressing. I found the children's ward overflowing with very sick children, many of them sharing beds and others lying on the floor, and yet many others were outside awaiting admission! Most of the children were shrivelled and grossly emaciated, with redundant skin hanging on spidery limbs. Intermittent wailings of mothers from different parts of the ward was a constant reminder of the appallingly high death rate. Many mothers and some staff looking after the children did not look healthy. When the children on the ward were tested, we were horrified to discover that almost all of them were HIV positive, yet we had neither treatment nor resources to make any difference.

From the mid-1980s and throughout the 1990s, the situation deteriorated as HIV spread throughout the country, shadowed by high death rates. Poorly equipped and grossly understaffed hospitals with no treatment to offer struggled in vain to cope with overwhelming AIDS patients, many of them lying in corridors and dying in droves. Meanwhile, the people plunged into despair, as desperate patients resorted to taking ineffective herbal medicines, even including soil that an old woman claimed was an AIDS cure.[2]

The Joint Clinical Research Centre (JCRC) was started at the height of the AIDS crisis in 1991, to try and find a scientific solution to the scourge. To maximize scarce resources, JCRC was formed by bringing together Makerere University, which contributed researchers; the Ministry of Health, which provided policy guidance; and the Ministry of Defence, which vacated their operational offices to serve as the centre's base.

As I took the leadership of the new centre, the newly constituted board made it clear that what they expected out of JCRC was an AIDS cure, but apologized that they were unable to provide the necessary resources because the country faced dire economic constraints. Therefore, the JCRC had to raise its own funds to do the job. But with only four laboratory technologists, one doctor, and a couple of administrative aides to help me take on one of the toughest medical assignments, we faced an uphill task. Whenever I worried that the exercise may be futile, I would think of the sheer carnage due to AIDS, and realize that throwing in the towel was never going to be an option. Even if we failed to find a cure, we could hope to, at least, find some scientific means of alleviating the agony and find out whether the numerous remedies claimed to treat AIDS, which had suddenly flooded the country, were effective or not.

The Uganda success in prevention

From the late 1980s, the only good news out of the AIDS quagmire started emerging. Uganda was making unprecedented progress in the prevention of HIV. This achievement was the initiative of President Museveni who led a countrywide campaign of mass information, education, and communication (IEC). At almost all rallies Museveni addressed, he always included a message about AIDS aimed at inducing behavioural change. The official media, especially the radio, which reached the vast majority of the people, was brought on board. All news broadcasts on radio Uganda started and ended with the beating of the traditional alarm drums warning of impending danger, immediately followed by a sombre booming voice: 'Beware of a looming danger of the killer disease—AIDS![3]

While many countries vehemently denied the existence of AIDS, Uganda promoted a policy of openness, which, besides reducing stigma, also created a conducive atmosphere that encouraged many international NGOs, and the formation of local ones like The AIDS Support Organization (TASO) that joined in the fight against HIV. With donor and government support, numerous billboards and posters sprang up in all parts of the city and major highways, warning about AIDS and communicating prevention messages, including the use of condoms, focused on reducing sexual transmission—the main route of infection. The key messages were later abbreviated in a catchy adage—ABC (A for Abstinence, B for Be faithful and C for Condoms). In 1989 the first AIDS counselling and testing centre was opened in Kampala, and later services were extended upcountry as people were encouraged to come forward for voluntary HIV tests.

Realizing that the enormous task of preventing HIV was beyond the capacity of the ministry of health alone, a multi-sectoral strategy involving all stake

holders, including all government ministries, NGOs, religious and civil organizations, was adopted and a new multi-disciplinary Uganda AIDS Commission
(UAC) was set up to coordinate the activities.

The net result of the sustained campaign was amazing. From early 1990s
Uganda became the first country to reverse the vastly escalating HIV rates at the
time when the trend in the rest of SSA was for a relentless rise. HIV prevalence
mainly based on data from sentinel sites, in 1990 to 1992 ranged from 14% to
30% but by the end of 1990s the rate had come down to an average of 6.2%.

Although the decline in HIV rates was undoubtedly a prevention success, it
was still not enough to reduce the AIDS carnage, because over a million
Ugandans were already infected and many of them in urgent need of life saving treatment. The rate of 6.2% remained unacceptably high and was begging
for additional preventive measures together with effective treatment, which
throughout the 1990s remained inaccessible in Africa.

The treatment breakthrough—but not for Africa

By 1994 hope of finding an effective AIDS treatment was fading as a handful of
ARV drugs that had been discovered had all individually failed to control the
HIV virus effectively. A breakthrough came in 1995 when it was found that in
triple combination, ARVs were so effective that the new treatment was excitedly
dubbed Highly Active Anti-Retroviral Therapy (HAART).

In July 1996 the Vancouver International AIDS Conference celebrated the
discovery of HAART, which transformed AIDS in rich countries from a death
sentence to a manageable chronic infection. Despite shouldering close to 90%
of the world's disease burden, resource-constrained countries (especially Africa,
home to over 70% of the cases) remained without access to the new drugs
because of the unaffordable price tag of US$14 000 annually per patient.

Within a mere four years of HAART being available in rich countries, AIDS
death rates in developed countries had dropped by an incredible 84%. As
demands for access increased and a growing multitude of activists launched
worldwide protests, some donors insisted that the use of ARV drugs in Africa
was unfeasible because of lack of infrastructure and technical expertise, which
made their safe and effective use impossible. The high level of adherence and
precision timing then considered vital for successful ART use and minimiza-
tion of HIV resistance was said to be unachievable in Africa. Such claims were
lent credence by some highly qualified people in influential positions like
Dr Andrew Natsios, the former chief of the United States Agency for International Development (USAID), who in 2001 justified to the US Congress why
the agency opposed giving ARVs to Africans with HIV:

If we had [HIV medicines for Africa] today, we could not distribute them. We could not administer the program because we do not have the doctors, we do not have the roads, and we do not have the cold chain . . . . In many parts of Africa, people do not know what watches or clocks are. They do not use Western means to tell time. They use the sun . . . . You say, take it at 10 o'clock, they say, what do you mean 10 o'clock?[4]

Building capacity

Despite the humble beginning, and meagre funds, the role of the JCRC—which was, as it were, scrambled expressly to urgently fight the AIDS scourge—was to grow, extend beyond the borders of Uganda, inspire, and help increase access to care and treatment throughout the resource-constrained countries. JCRC pioneering work in the use of ARVs in Africa goes back to 1991 when the centre carried out the first study using Zidovudine (AZT)—the world's first ARV drug. Using self-generated funds from services to private patients and allowable overheads from research grants, JCRC established basic infrastructure, including laboratories, and set up necessary logistics that made it possible to test and introduce new drugs as they became available. In 1996 JCRC started using HAART for the small number of patients who could afford it on their own. Soon after, JCRC introduced PCR (polymerase chain reaction) technology to measure viral loads so as to better monitor the response of our patients to HAART. As donors and governments still declined to support AIDS treatment in Africa, inevitably, out of hundreds of thousands in need of immediate therapy, it was only a tiny number of rich Ugandans who had access. However, this was a unique opportunity to build capacity by training staff in HIV science and use of ART.

Contrary to widespread belief that ART use in Africa was unfeasible, we demonstrated that they could be safely used, and we daily carried out laboratory monitoring tests that were also said to be impossible in African conditions and with the same outcome for our patients as their counterparts in the West.[5] We further showed that ARV drugs could be scaled up, by successfully establishing a network of ART clinics and laboratories in the provinces—a model that later proved vital for nationwide rapid scale up of ART.

By the year 2000 it was common knowledge that effective treatment for AIDS existed and an increasing number of poor desperate patients besieged JCRC begging for ARVs to save their lives. Despite opposition by branded drugs manufacturers, and threats of punitive reaction, we took a decision to import and use low-cost generic ARVS from Cipla of India to save the lives of our patients, thus making JCRC the first institution to introduce generic ARVs in Africa. The numbers accessing ARVs in Uganda increased from a few hundreds to almost 1000, as for the first time some middle-class Ugandans could afford the price.

However, even though generic drugs were cheaper, their cost was still unaffordable to the vast majority of the patients in the country, and appeals for international help continued.[6]

On the research side, JCRC carried out the first HIV vaccine trial in Africa and further widened the HIV research agenda by establishing partnerships with local and international institutions, including those in the USA, Europe, and Japan.[7] We obtained a grant from Rockefeller and Doris Duke Foundations to start African Dialogue on AIDS (ADAC) and AIDS Care and Treatment Research in Africa (ACRiA) programmes that aimed at building capacity in SSA, by sharing experience in scaling up best HIV and TB care and treatment practices and providing first research opportunities for young African researchers. Under these projects I led teams of African doctors and scientists to many SSA countries and the Caribbean, holding workshops sharing experiences and discussing the way forward in management of the epidemic in developing countries. Many young African scientists got their first opportunity to carry out research on HIV/AIDS and we were gratified when the majority of them later succeeded in competing for independent research grants—a capacity which they previously lacked. Others became leaders in their countries AIDS treatment and prevention programmes.

We got an opportunity to define the serious nature of the epidemic better when my colleagues Ahmed Latif, Sulaymane Mboup, and I, carried out an in-depth study on the state of HIV/AIDS in SSA starting in 2000. We found that the entire region, with the exception of a few states in West Africa, was devastated by a rapidly escalating HIV epidemic with very high mortality rates, and yet remained without access to life-saving HAART well over five years after its discovery. The epidemic had adversely affected developmental and social programmes, undermined health services, retarded economic production and capacity of governments in Africa. We found that Africa was losing many of her youths, including some of her most educated, skilled manpower, with a net effect of curtailing human capital development.

As parents died, a rapidly increasing number of orphans shadowed the escalating death rates and continuing spread of the epidemic. Out of 25 million Africans then estimated to be living with HIV, over 4.5 million were newly infected within the previous year alone. Africa with only 10% of the world's population had 70% of the disease burden and over 11 million AIDS orphans; 2 million of them infected with HIV.

These grim data demonstrated that the AIDS catastrophe in Africa constituted a state of emergency and a moral imperative, and we called upon donors and the international community to come urgently to Africa's aid by providing ARVs to save the lives of millions dying of preventable deaths and increasing support for a robust preventive programme. Citing the JCRC example, we dismissed the myth that ART use in Africa was impossible. We presented our findings to an international meeting held in Kampala in April 2001, which included WHO, UNAIDS (Joint United Nations Programme on HIV/AIDS), US National Institute of Health, NGOs, donors, and some governments.

International response

Initial international response to the epidemic in Africa was dismal, a situation that led to worldwide protests. Activists decried the failure of global action, and demonstrated against TRIPS (Trade Related Aspects of International Property Rights) and patents' laws under which the pharmaceutical companies maintained exorbitant prices of ARVS. Protest parades mushroomed in many capitals of the world as activists besieged pharmaceutical companies and venues of G8 meetings. That bleak period became a very busy time for me as I travelled to many parts of the world, to present data illustrating the rapidly deteriorating AIDS crisis in Africa, and to appeal for ARV treatment. I used the JCRC treatment model to demonstrate that the often cited constraints of infrastructure and human resources were not insurmountable.

From 1996, UNAIDS held a series of meetings in Geneva involving pharmaceutical companies, in which I was a regular participant. They aimed at finding ways of increasing ART access to resource-constrained countries. The result was the establishment of the UNAIDS ARV Drugs Access Initiative in November 1997. When this failed to either reduce cost or increase access, a follow-on initiative, named Accelerated Access Initiative was announced in May 2000, but this too flopped.[8]

For too long, rich countries turned a blind eye to the disaster, while increasingly devastated poor countries suffered. Yet if the rich countries had reacted immediately, the epidemic could have been nipped in the bud especially in areas where it had not taken a firm hold in 1990s.[9]

Global AIDS fund (GAF)

Hope that action was finally being taken to alleviate the AIDS catastrophe originated from the G8 meeting held in Okinawa, in July 2000. A follow-on meeting involving African heads of states and Kofi Annan the UN Secretary General was held in Abuja, in April 2001. The meeting proposed the establishment of Global AIDS Fund (GAF) to channel funds to fight the disease. Subsequently, a United Nations General Assembly special session on AIDS, held in June 2001, endorsed the proposal. This undertaking was a worldwide effort and all nations, rich or poor, were invited to make pledges in line with their capacities. However, the commitment of rich countries was lukewarm. For instance, it was estimated that to be effective the fund needed at least $7 billion immediately; but the USA initially offered only $200 million, while France committed only $150 million. Hardly any country acted with the kind of urgency that the catastrophic situation demanded.

On 1 December, World AIDS Day 2003, UNAIDS announced plans to reach three million people living with AIDS in developing countries by the end of 2005, which became known as the '3 by 5 initiative', a low target considering the much larger numbers who would be excluded.

President's emergency plan for AIDS relief (PEPFAR)

While the rich countries quickly adopted HAART as the AIDS standard of care, by the year 2002, seven years after its discovery, millions of Africans were still dying from what in developed countries had become an easily treatable chronic disease. Then suddenly in November, I was invited to the White House to participate in a discussion with a panel of US experts and technocrats gathered to consider the feasibility of ART in resource-constrained countries and help form the basis of what would later become PEPFAR. I realized that I would be up against a tide of disapproval by many infectious disease experts and some highly influential members who still insisted that AIDS treatment in Africa was virtually impossible.

The predominant opinion at the time advocated the same old, easy to implement options, including limited preventive programmes and the cheap Cotrimaxazole prophylaxis that were the favourite of most donors and yet had little impact on the epidemic. The key to changing these deeply held views was to refocus attention on the real priorities that would make a difference.

We had already demonstrated ART scale-up feasibility with the extension of AIDS treatment to several rural districts. We and other sister African countries could use this model to rapidly scale up treatment and save millions if funds were made available. There were also some religious groups to contend with, as some of them advocated for sexual abstinence as the only acceptable intervention. In addition, the strong pharmaceutical lobby was also fighting to protect their ARV drugs' monopoly and guarantee their profits, and they objected to cheaper alternatives. Yet, without lower cost generic ARV drugs it was difficult to envision how millions of people in immediate need of ARVs could be successfully treated. I explained that no AIDS intervention in Africa with over a million people in immediate need of therapy would make any meaningful impact unless it addressed the critical issue of treatment.

JCRC had also trained a number of laboratory technologists and healthcare providers to work in rural clinics, which we had established, thus providing additional evidence that constraints could be overcome. The continuing carnage of millions in Africa due to AIDS, when they could be saved constituted a moral imperative—a catastrophe that the US was in a position to end.

Eventually, President Bush and his team of advisors concurred and the bleak AIDS situation in Africa was changed.[10] A few months later, at the annual US State of the Union address on 28 January 2003, he made the following historical pronouncement:

> Today, on the continent of Africa, nearly 30 million people have the AIDS virus—including 3 million children under the age 15. There are whole countries in Africa where more than one-third of the adult population carries the infection. More than 4 million require immediate drug treatment. Yet across that continent, only 50 000 AIDS victims—only 50 000—are receiving the medicine they need . . . . Many hospitals tell people, you've got AIDS, we can't help you. Go home and die. In an age of miraculous medicines, no person should have to hear those words . . . . Tonight I propose the Emergency Plan for AIDS Relief—a work of mercy beyond all current international efforts to help the people of Africa.

I was right there as a specially invited guest, when the US President made this now famous PEPFAR announcement.

My passionate assertion that use of ART would succeed in Africa was soon after put to the test when in November 2003 JCRC was selected to become the first PEPFAR-funded organization in Africa to scale up ART.[11] We hit the ground running with our project named The Regional Expansion of Antiretroviral Therapy (TREAT). We aimed at building capacity and establishing a framework for a quality and equitable countrywide ART access programme. TREAT brought other partners on board, including Ministry of Health and NGOs, including faith-based hospitals. Over the next few years we established seven regional centres of excellence (RCEs), which housed advanced laboratories serving each of Uganda's main regions. Within five years we had also renovated 50 main satellite clinics, to accommodate the surging numbers of AIDS patients. In addition, we established an additional twenty outreach clinics to serve hard to reach areas where the need for AIDS services was most acute.

We built new clinic extensions with laboratory spaces in Kalangala (the biggest island on Lake Victoria) to serve the big fishing community, known to have very high HIV prevalence, and built others in the war-torn northern region, where HIV was on a steep rise as well as western and far eastern parts of the country where we provided new space for doctors to treat surging numbers of AIDS patients.

An ARV drugs and laboratory reagents logistics system was put in place, as was a training programme. In 2004–2005 alone, TREAT trained 1143 healthcare providers. By the end of 2005, 35 satellite clinics had been established, and by 2008 the number had risen to over 50 with 15 outreaches. By 2009, when TREAT ended, over 80 000 patients had been initiated on therapy and more than twice the number were in care in all regions of the country. Our plan envisaged improving all the clinics that we established, ensuring best practices and then gradually transitioning them back to Ministry of Health and other healthcare providers closer to their homes or workplaces. Currently over 600 000 out of 1.4 million people living with HIV in Uganda and just over 1.7 million out of an estimated 5.7 million South African PLWHIV are receiving ARVs.[12]

We are gratified that our pioneering work in some way inspired widespread use of ART in Africa, which saved millions of lives, and personally I am humbled by the fact that President Bush found the role I played at the initiation of PEPFAR worth acknowledging in his book *Decision Points*.

To date PEPFAR remains one of the most successful humanitarian projects in terms of lives saved and health services strengthened that it has built in Africa.

The future

Although ARVs are highly effective, they are not a cure. All available ARV drugs have so far failed to completely clear the virus from the body, and no breakthrough is in the pipeline. Scientists in continuing the search for a cure are pursuing various approaches, including trying to flush the virus out of its sanctuaries (such as resting cells) or trying to activate the reproductive circle—a stage when HIV is most vulnerable to ARV drugs. But so far the elusive virus has to date lived up to its reputation. Also still elusive is an HIV vaccine, as all those candidate vaccines so far tested have failed. Therefore, there is still much more work ahead before a definitive solution is found for HIV/AIDS.[13]

As Africa has become the biggest user of ARV in the world, so it will inevitably harbour the biggest numbers of resistant viruses in the near future. This requires new drugs to which the continent currently has no access. This once again brings back the issue of patents and TRIPS in as far as they will adversely affect future drugs' access. There is need for international agreements on TRIPS that will ensure access to essential and emergency medicines to the poor.

Recent scientific evidence has shown that ARVs are also effective for prevention of HIV transmission.[14] The discordant couples study (where one partner is infected with HIV), coded HPTN 052 trial found that early initiation of ART in HIV-positive individuals reduced the transmission risk to the HIV-uninfected partner by a staggering 96%! This and other emerging evidence advocate for urgent need for universal ART access. Currently only just over 50% of those in need in Uganda are getting ART. Besides millions of lives that would be saved, the benefits also include the millions of new HIV infections that would be prevented.

In conclusion, the AIDS epidemic is not over and remains a leading killer in many countries in SSA. Recent epidemiological data from Uganda, which demonstrated early success in prevention, has shown a disconcerting upward HIV incidence trend. This is a strong warning against complacency and a call for strengthened preventive initiatives. Meanwhile, millions of people in need of ARVs are still not accessing them. And the commitment of donors to increase funding for AIDS treatment to achieve universal access is questionable. To succeed in controlling the epidemic requires the world's governments and donors to make an irrevocable long-term commitment to raise the necessary funds to address the still blazing killer plague by embracing and implementing all the scientifically proven preventive and treatment strategies.

References

1 **Serwadda D, et al.** *Slim disease: a new disease in Uganda and its association with HTLV-III infection. Lancet,* 1985 Oct. 19; **2**(8460): 849–52.

2 **Blumenkrantz D.** *Thirty tons of soil:* Nanyonga's *Divine Panacea,* Nov 1989.

3 **Green E, et al.** What happened in Uganda? Declining HIV prevalence, behaviour change, and the national response; in Hogle JE: *Lessons Learned—Case Study,* 2002. <www.unicef.org/lifeskills/files/WhatHappenedInUganda>.

4 Committee on International Relations, 2001. The United States war on AIDS. Hearing before the Committee on International Relations, House of Representatives, 107th Congress, 1st session, 7 June 2001. <http://commdocs.house.gov/committees/intlrel/hfa72978.000/hfa72978_0.HTM>. Accessed 21 August 2013.

5 **Attaran A.** Adherence to HAART: Africans take medicines more faithfully than North Americans. *PLoS Med,* 2007; **4**(2): e83. <doi:10.1371/journal.pmed.0040083>.

6 **Ferriman A.** Doctors demand immediate access to antiretroviral drugs in Africa. *BMJ* 2001; **332**:1018, 28 April 2001.

7 **Mugyenyi PN.** *HIV Vaccines: The Uganda Experience.* Elsevier Science, 2002.

8 The UNAIDS Pharmaceutical Industry Initiative. Health Gap Coalition Position Paper: 'Questioning the UNAIDS/Pharmaceutical Industry Initiative: Seven months and counting . . .'. Presented at the UNAIDS PCB in Rio, 13 December 2005. <http/www.globaltreatment.access.org/content/press_release/2000>.

9 **Mugyenyi PN.** *Genocide by Denial.* Fountain, 2008.

10 **Donnely J.** The Presidents emergency plan for AIDS relief: how George W. Bush and aides came to 'think big' on battling HIV. *Health Affairs,* 2012; **31**(7): 1389–96.

11 **Mugyenyi PN, et al.** Scaling up antiretroviral therapy: experience of the Joint Clinical Research Centre (JCRC) access programme. *ACTA Academica Supplementum,* 2006: 216–41. Perspectives on public sector antiretroviral access.

12 UNAIDS World AIDS Day Report, 2012 <www.unaids.org/en/unaids/jc2434>.

13 **Mugyenyi PN.** *A Cure Too Far.* Fountain, 2013.

14 WHO/UNAIDS joint press release. *Groundbreaking trial results confirm HIV treatment prevents transmission of HIV.* <www.who.int/entity/hiv/mediacentre/trial_results/en/index.html>. Accessed 15 May 2011.

Chapter 5

Mobilizing the community against maternal death— the Malawi community champion model

Chisale Mhango

Senior Lecturer in Obstetrics and Gynaecology at the College of Medicine in Malawi; previously Director for Reproductive Services in Malawi's Ministry of Health

Dr Mhango is a former head of Reproductive Health Services for Malawi and Medical Officer of Health for the African Region of the World Health Organization (WHO) and United Nations Population Fund (UNFPA). He remains heavily involved in improving maternal health as an academic at the University of Malawi and a supporter of the President's initiative on Safe Motherhood. In this chapter he describes how he took on the challenge of reducing maternal mortality in one of the least resourced countries in Africa through a mixture of clinical measures, service organization, and mobilizing the community. He describes how African Union (AU) and WHO policies were important in shaping plans and how international partners helped support and resource Malawi's plans. The community and community leaders have been central to the success in Malawi. Traditional leaders, chiefs, have played a very big role in giving maternal health greater priority and in changing behaviours amongst men as well as women. As Dr Mhango says, like other scientifically trained people he was constantly surprised at how well traditional leaders understood the issues and how forcefully they were willing to confront resistance to change, whether it came from the churches or from individuals. As a leader Dr Mhango was not afraid to take unpopular decisions where the evidence was clear: over the use of non-medical personnel, for example, in providing injectable contraceptives to women or in banning traditional birth attendants from delivering babies. There have been big improvements in maternal health in Malawi and a foundation laid for much more to come.

Maternal mortality in Malawi

Malawi is a low-resource country in sub-Saharan Africa with an economy that is predominantly agricultural. Of 16 million people, 80% live in rural areas. Adult literacy rate for women is 59% as compared to 69% for men. Females comprise 51% of the total population. Childbearing starts early with a mean age at first childbirth at 19 years.[1]

Healthcare infrastructure

Malawi is geographically divided into 28 districts. Administratively, the districts are subdivided into Traditional Authorities (T/As). Traditional Authorities, headed by hereditary chiefs, are composed of villages, which are the smallest administrative units. The Ministry of Health (MOH) has divided the country into five healthcare zones that supervise healthcare in the 28 districts. Healthcare management nonetheless is decentralized to the district.[2,3]

The health services are provided by three main agencies, notably the government, the Christian Health Association of Malawi (CHAM), and statutory bodies and private sector. All healthcare is free of charge in public health facilities operated by the government. To cater for the indigent population residing in the catchment areas of CHAM health facilities, service agreements have been signed between government and CHAM to provide free maternity services in their facilities; government reimburses CHAM for services provided.

The country has a democratically elected government with an independent judiciary. For the rural people, however, the hereditary traditional leaders guide their social lives, settle disputes, and give out land. The traditional leaders, therefore, have great influence on the behaviour of their constituents, including on how they relate to central government.

Malawi has one of the highest maternal mortality ratios in the world at 460 maternal deaths per 100 000 live births. The 2005 Emergency Obstetric Care (EmOC) needs assessment study reported that ruptured uterus and obstructed labour were the most common causes of maternal deaths, accounting together for 36% of all maternal deaths recorded. This was followed by postpartum sepsis (19%), obstetric haemorrhage (14%), hypertensive disease of pregnancy (8%), and complications of unsafe abortion (5%).[4]

Clinical strategies for tackling maternal mortality

Heading the department of reproductive health, I proposed a strategy to address each one of these as follows: to reduce incidence of prolonged labour and ruptured uterus we revised the partograph so as to simplify its use and increase compliance for routine monitoring of labour. I enlisted the support of zonal safe motherhood coordinators, with whom I had quarterly meetings in the national Maternal Death Confidential Enquiry meetings to enforce the routine use of the partogram.

To address haemorrhage I resisted the adoption of distribution of misoprostol to women attending antenatal care, which would have enabled them to take it when they delivered outside the health facility, for two reasons: first, studies[5,6,7] reported that oxytocin was superior to misoprostol and, second, I wanted to meet the MDG5 target of providing skilled attendants to at least 80% of the women at childbirth by 2015.[8] I thought that providing the option of a home delivery with misoprostol would prevent the reaching of this target. Instead, I had the misoprostol registered not only for management of postpartum haemorrhage, but also for post-abortion care as well as for medical abortion, despite the fact that safe abortion was not yet liberalized. In addition I introduced the policy of keeping all women delivering in health facilities for at least two days after delivery to eliminate the chances of primary haemorrhage occurring after an earlier discharge. Further, all women delivering at home were to report to the nearest health facility for assessment to exclude retained products of conception and manage any injuries sustained during childbirth.

For puerperal sepsis my department introduced the policy of early postnatal care. This meant that all women, whether they delivered at the health facility or at home, were to report with their newborns at the nearest health facility for assessment within the first week childbirth. I reckoned that by this time signs and symptoms of early infection in the mother and the baby could be detected and thereby facilitate early treatment.

I was also getting reports that the driver of the puerperal sepsis deaths was HIV. In 2000 it was estimated that a sixth of maternal deaths were related to HIV/AIDS.[9] My department had collaborated with the HIV department to introduce a policy of routine offer of HIV screening for all pregnant women when they presented for antenatal care with the option to opt out of the test if they did not want to know their HIV status. Many politicians spoke against this policy in parliament and I decided that I would reverse the policy only if data revealed that women were shunning antenatal care for fear of being tested for HIV. I was delighted that the coverage for antenatal care continued to rise and that hardly any women opted out of the test. Using this approach, the country rapidly expanded access to anti-retroviral therapy (ART) for pregnant women in hard-to-reach areas throughout the country. There followed a more than fivefold increase in the numbers of pregnant women being enrolled on ART in the first quarter of full nationwide implementation.[10,11]

During a UNICEF/WHO regional meeting in Nairobi in 2010, I led the Malawi delegation to adopt a new policy on Prevention of Mother to Child

Transmission (PMTCT). Under WHO's 2010 PMTCT ARV guidelines, countries could only choose between two prophylaxis regimens for pregnant women living with HIV, notably those with CD4[12] greater than 350 cells/mm^3: Option A and Option B.[13] Under Option A, women received anti-retroviral prophylaxis AZT during pregnancy starting from 14 weeks gestation. At onset of labour, single-dose niverapine (NVP) was taken orally and thereafter AZT/3TC daily and through the first 7 days postpartum. Option B, on the other hand, had a simpler clinical flow in which all pregnant and lactating women with HIV were offered triple anti-retroviral drugs (ARVs) from 14 weeks gestation and continued until 1 week after cessation of breastfeeding. At the end of breastfeeding, those women would discontinue the prophylaxis until the CD4 fell below 350 cells/mm^3 when ART would be commenced. Malawi was the only country at this meeting that opted for the new option referred to as Option B+, in which all pregnant women with HIV infection were offered life-long ART, regardless of their CD4 count starting from the day they tested positive. This was a challenge considering that Malawi is a low resource country. This, however, resulted in much lower viral loads by the time of delivery thereby eliminating HIV as a driver of puerperal sepsis.

To address hypertensive disease of pregnancy, use of magnesium sulphate was introduced to replace diazepam and other agents. All patients were to be managed at district and higher levels of care. Patients presenting with the condition at lower level of care were to be given the loading dose of magnesium sulphate and then immediately transferred to a higher level of care for continued management.

Expansion of the Basic Emergency Obstetric and Neonatal Care (BEmONC) sites increased the service outlets for comprehensive post-abortion care. The main strategy for reducing complications of unsafe abortion, however, was the taking of family planning services to the community, as indicated below. At that time unmet need for family planning was 28%[14, 15] and safe abortion was not liberalised.[16]

Healthcare workforce shortages

The shortage of the healthcare workforce is one of the major constraints for effective delivery of healthcare services in Malawi. At national level, there are only 40% of required nurse/midwife technicians, 47% of registered nurses, 28% of clinical officers, and 43% of medical doctors.[17] Nonetheless, significant progress has been made lately to reduce maternal mortality as can be seen from Fig. 5.1.

Among the factors that have helped Malawi achieve the 59% drop in maternal mortality between 1990 and 2010 are (a) the Millennium Development Goal

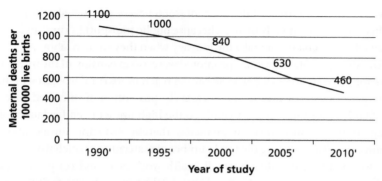

Fig. 5.1 Trends in maternal mortality ratio Malawi, 1990–2010.

Data from *Trends in Maternal Mortality: 1990 to 2010 WHO, UNICEF, UNFPA and The World Bank estimates*, copyright © World Health Organization 2012, available from <http://whqlibdoc.who.int/publications/2012/9789241503631_eng.pdf>.

initiative, which requires countries to report to the UN annually on progress made towards the attainment of the MDGs; this motivated programme managers, like myself, to strive to ensure annual reports showed progressive improvements. (b) The African Union's Campaign for the Accelerated Reduction of Maternal Mortality in Africa (CARMMA), launched in 2009 to address the challenges of maternal mortality on the continent, and Malawi was the third country on the continent to domesticate it. (c) The country's own launch of the Malawi Growth and Development Strategy in 2004, which identified health as a key strategy for socioeconomic development and improvement in maternal health as one of the priority areas for emphasis.[18] The document gave programme targets that were to be attained each year. The National Statistics Office produces annual Welfare Monitoring Survey reports which give levels of achievement.

Customs, social mores, and habits influencing heathcare-seeking behaviour and attitude to Western medicine

Low coverage for skilled attendant at childbirth was identified as a major factor for the high maternal mortality. The country was doing well for coverage of antenatal care but not so with institutional delivery for skilled attendant at childbirth. For over a decade, coverage for skilled attendance at childbirth stagnated at 55–56% (Malawi Demographic and Health Survey, 1992, 2000, 2004).

My assessment was that, while pregnant women were able to make the journeys to health facilities, mostly on foot, because public transport in rural areas is not available, they could not make the journey when they were in labour.

The strategic interventions I promoted were: (a) expansion of the infrastructure for basic emergency obstetric care to reach more rural women with basic emergency obstetric and neonatal care; (b) promotion of universal coverage for family planning services to address the high unmet need for family planning to reduce unwanted pregnancies, thereby reducing unsafe abortion deaths as well as reducing the total number of maternities, which would reduce the workload on the already small health workforce; and (c) promotion of birth preparedness to develop a culture of delivering in health facilities rather than with the traditional birth attendant. In addition, 'waiting homes' were to be attached to each Basic Emergency Obstetric and Neonatal Care (BEmONC) facility for mothers to stay there in the last fortnight of their pregnancies if they could not guarantee reaching the facility in time when labour commenced at home.

The role of traditional and opinion leaders in influencing behaviour in Africans, especially in rural areas

Being a low-resource country, Malawi has long realized that to achieve sustainable programme development there was need to implement task shifting as well as tap into both the human and non-human resources for the delivery of healthcare that existed outside the government structure, including those in the community.

Task shifting from physicians to non-physicians has been shown to be both safe and effective in countries that have organized and supported the extension of their maternal care in this way.[19-24] Since colonial days, non-physician practitioners, then referred to as assistant surgeons, worked where there were no doctors. These have since become clinical officers and medical assistants. Studies have shown that extra training and support can achieve task shifting and improve maternal and fetal mortality and morbidity in the areas where these schemes have been piloted. In Malawi more than 80% of the caesarean sections are performed by Clinical Officers, without whom caesarean section would be inaccessible to most women leading to even higher maternal mortality rates.[24]

In the light of shortage of midwives, childbirth services were for a long time shared with traditional birth attendants. Traditional birth attendants were more accessible as they lived in the communities with the pregnant women. With the support of WHO, a lot of investment was made in training TBAs to promote clean and safe delivery.

Community interventions

In reproductive health, the community mobilization strategy commenced when reduction of maternal mortality was identified as key for development.[25] My department conducted workshops for influential community leaders to sensitize them to the issues relating to maternal health. We identified traditional leaders as key actors and stakeholders. We then discussed with national safe motherhood stakeholders in the national technical working group on how to use the traditional leaders. Technical Working Groups are Sector Wide Approach (SWAp) structures, which every health programme has, consisting of programme managers and representatives of funding agencies. They and programme managers agree on implementation strategy and monitor resource allocation and utilization.

To address the issues identified I sought the support of USAID and UNFPA to take family planning services to the community using Community-Based Distributor Agents (CBDAs). It was noted that many women still did not use the contraceptive services taken to their communities earlier; the reason they gave was that they wanted the injectable contraceptives that were popular with women in urban areas. I decided, therefore, to take the injectable contraceptive to the community using trained but non-medical providers.

I did not seek permission from my boss, the Secretary for Health, as it is my belief that once you have been mandated to lead a programme, you have authority to do whatever you consider appropriate for the development of the programme, as long as you were convinced it would not cause any harm. At an annual programme review meeting attended by the Secretary for Health, all directors, and all other national and regional stakeholders and development partners, a fellow director publicly criticized me for endangering women's health by entrusting their health to non-medical professionals. I defended my decision by quoting the studies that have been conducted on the subject. My boss' reaction was to advise me to move cautiously. Several years on no harm has been reported, community-based delivery of medroxyprogesterone acetate has been institutionalized and the contraceptive prevalence rate has steadily risen, as seen in Fig. 5.2.

I knew the conditions from which the women were dying but needed to find out which women in particular were dying from these conditions. The answer was that it was women who gave birth or had an abortion outside the health facilities that were more likely to die from complications of pregnancy and

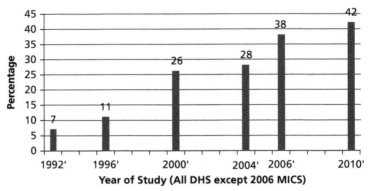

Fig. 5.2 Trends in contraceptive prevalence rate in Malawi.

Data from National Statistical Office [Malawi], *Malawi Demographic and Health Survey 1992*, National Statistical Office Zomba, Malawi and Macro International Inc. Calverton, Maryland USA, copyright © 1994; National Statistical Office [Malawi] and ORC Macro, *Malawi Demographic and Health Survey 2000*, National Statistical Office and ORC Macro, Zomba, Malawi and Calverton, Maryland, USA, copyright © 2000; National Statistical Office [Malawi] and ORC Macro, *Malawi Demographic and Health Survey 2004*, National Statistical Office and ORC Macro, Zomba, Malawi and Calverton, Maryland, USA, copyright © 2005; National Statistical Office [Malawi] and ORC Macro, *Malawi Demographic and Health Survey 2010*, National Statistical Office and ORC Macro, Zomba, Malawi and Calverton, Maryland, USA, copyright © 2011; and National Statistical Office [Malawi], *Malawi Multiple Indicator Cluster Survey 2006*, National Statistical Office and United Nations Children's Fund, Malawi, copyright © 2007.

childbirth. Women who delivered at health facilities did sometimes bleed after birth and experienced rises in blood pressure. They were, however, less likely to die compared to those who developed these complications outside the health facility because treatment was commenced earlier; whilst many who travel to the health facility after the complications had occurred either did not get to the health facility alive or reached the facility in too poor a condition to be saved. An analysis of 81 maternal death audit reports (2005) from various districts in the country showed that 85% of the deaths took place in rural areas, compared to 15% in urban areas.[26]

In 2007, my department also conducted a national study that confirmed what WHO had reported earlier to the effect that TBAs did not contribute significantly to reductions in maternal deaths and, therefore, it was not a good investment to continue to fund them. With the support of the Sexual and Reproductive Health Technical Working Group, I went along with the study findings and reassigned TBAs preventive roles and banned them from delivering the babies. What is the purpose of conducting a study if you were not going to accept the recommendations based on the findings of the study to improve patients' outcomes?

The decision to ban traditional birth attendants from conducting deliveries was not popular with many politicians and, of course, the traditional birth attendants themselves whose livelihood depended on it. The opposition from the Traditional Healers Association was fierce with their usual threats with witchcraft. I was, however, convinced that this was the right thing to do and all I needed was the support of the communities. A district health officer once called me to enquire as to why I had reversed the decision when he, like other district health officers had received a letter purported to have been signed by me indicating that the decision had been reversed. I found out that the circular letter was written by the Secretary of the Traditional Healers' Association.

Those who opposed the decision to stop TBAs from conducting deliveries believed that our health facilities were too distant for women to access and, therefore, they thought it unreasonable for me to make this decision. I did not develop penalties for anybody who did not deliver in the health facilities; in fact my idea was to monitor which areas of the country would show that women would not be able to access available services so that those areas could be priority areas for building basic emergency obstetric and neonatal care structures. The results indicated that when the TBA option was removed, women were able to make the journey to the health facilities.

Training and support to traditional leaders

My department organized workshops on the status of safe motherhood and the various strategies that MOH was promoting to tackle each one of the major factors for maternal and neonatal morbidity and mortality. The participants were traditional leaders and men champions that would inspire and help women and other men to lead healthier lives and become more involved in safe motherhood activities. They were to participate in organizing and leading activities. The traditional leaders turned out to be effective leaders who had knowledge of how to approach their people. Influential traditional chiefs and members of parliament were made guests of honour at our community mobilization meetings. These opinion leaders brought their ability to relate to their people to transform health and well-being in their communities. They empowered and motivated men to get involved in healthy social activities, and helped their subjects to enjoy healthier lives by raising awareness of health and healthy choices, removing barriers and creating supportive networks and environments.[27]

For a long time as a physician, however, I did not think community leaders with little formal education could support volunteerism or indeed comprehend the health strategy I was promoting to address maternal health in their communities. I was wrong; the response of the traditional leaders was most encouraging. I learned that traditional leaders had insight into what worked for them. They provided feedback on their views as to how we could help them best. At their prompting my department provided (a) bicycle ambulances at rural health centre level and proper ambulances and basic emergency obstetric and neonatal care facilities; (b) refurbished selected rural health facilities to increase delivery sites; and (c) provided feedback on maternal deaths that occurred in their areas, including reductions, since their involvement, and solicited their views for improvement. They quickly moved on to develop bye-laws that created penalties for men whose spouses gave birth in the communities instead of the local health facilities. The use of traditional authorities further has promoted local ownership of the community mobilization campaign in Malawi. This community mobilization intervention was supplemented by the messages that health surveillance attendants, the lowest cadre of health workers in the Ministry of Health, who work in the community and the Safe Motherhood Ambassador (and Vice President Joyce Banda) passed on through meetings at village, district and national levels.

With the support of the African Development Bank, my department accelerated the expansion of the infrastructure for basic emergency obstetric and neonatal care, and required all pregnant women to deliver in health facilities. The expansion of the infrastructure has unfortunately stalled by the fact that one can only build as many delivery-rooms as one can afford to place midwives there. I needed to have at least two skilled service providers at each health centre to be able to provide 24-hour cover.

Community mobilization

Malawi has a long history of community mobilization, especially for creating demand for child health preventive care services. In the area of safe motherhood, the initial personal contact community mobilization approach involved targeting men with the objective of getting them involved in safe motherhood to facilitate women to avail antenatal care services and deliver in health facilities. We called this birth-preparedness.

People in Malawi usually consulted the traditional healer before they availed health facilities; for pregnant women this meant care by the traditional birth attendant who hangs onto them for the rest of the pregnancy. In addition, women cannot visit a health facility without permission from their spouses or their in-laws; when labour starts there is too little time available for bureaucratic process.

I collaborated with Commissioner Bience Gawanas (who wrote Chapter 10) at the African Union Secretariat to produce the Continental Framework for Sexual and Reproductive Health in Africa, which was enthusiastically endorsed by the Conference of African Ministers of Health in Gaborone Botswana in 2005; the conference requested an implementation framework, which Commissioner Gawanas requested me to put together and was accepted by the Conference of African Ministers of Health in Maputo the following year and is commonly referred to as the Maputo Plan of Action for Sexual and Reproductive Health. Through this Commissioner Gawanas introduced the Campaign to Accelerate the Reduction of Maternal Mortality in Africa (CARMMA), which was launched in 2009.

At the launch of CARMMA in Malawi, my department installed the Vice-President (now President of Malawi) Joyce Banda, an energetic women's rights' activist, as the Safe Motherhood Ambassador for Malawi. This too was a very unpopular decision. In crisscrossing the country to mobilize the communities for safe motherhood, to great effect, she was too much in the limelight and was seen as a threat to other politicians. I was under pressure to reverse the decision but I did not go beyond just promising to do so, in writing. Vice-President Joyce Banda mobilized the business community to participate in Safe Motherhood and assisted my department to neutralize opposition from the Traditional Healers' Association whose membership included traditional birth attendants.

In the health facilities, service providers gave women who were accompanied by their spouses priority by serving them first. This policy remains so today. The result has not only increased antenatal care coverage, but skilled attendance at childbirth also increased to 75% in one year. Malawi has now attained the MDG5 target of having at least 80% of pregnant women deliver with a skilled attendance at childbirth.[28] The increased coverage for institutional delivery led to increased coverage for HIV services for newborns, thereby cutting down on vertical transmission of the HIV infection. Fig. 5.3 shows the increases in skilled attendance at childbirth.

As time went on the traditional leaders were given feedback on the impact of their activities, and exchange visits were sponsored for them to share ideas for improvements in maternal and neonatal health with traditional leaders in other districts. During the debriefing meetings they could see that the impact on maternal health was greatest where the leadership was strong. It was noted that the chiefs were encouraged by the direct outcomes of their efforts. The study tours also promoted networking for improvement in maternal health, which led to the cascading of the community mobilization activities.

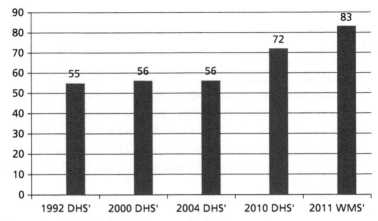

Fig. 5.3 Percentage skilled attendance at childbirth.

Data from National Statistical Office [Malawi], *Malawi Demographic and Health Survey 1992*, National Statistical Office Zomba, Malawi and Macro International Inc. Calverton, Maryland USA, copyright © 1994; National Statistical Office [Malawi] and ORC Macro, *Malawi Demographic and Health Survey 2000*, National Statistical Office and ORC Macro, Zomba, Malawi and Calverton, Maryland, USA, copyright © 2000; National Statistical Office [Malawi] and ORC Macro, *Malawi Demographic and Health Survey 2004*, National Statistical Office and ORC Macro, Zomba, Malawi and Calverton, Maryland, USA, copyright © 2005; National Statistical Office [Malawi] and ORC Macro, *Malawi Demographic and Health Survey 2010*, National Statistical Office and ORC Macro, Zomba, Malawi and Calverton, Maryland, USA, copyright © 2011; and National Statistical Office [Malawi], *Welfare Monitoring Survey 2011*, Government of Malawi, copyright © 2012.

Problems encountered

Among the problems encountered in the implementation of this policy was the fact that there were too few midwives to cope with the demand for services leading to minimal monitoring of patients in labour. The health workforce (doctors/nurse midwives/clinical officers/medical assistants) ratio was a mere 0.27/1000 population against the WHO defined threshold of at least 2.3 well-trained doctors, nurses, and midwives per 1000 people.[29] The increased demand for services resulted in crowding in the delivery rooms compromising on asepsis. Nonetheless it made me identify the problems and institute corrective measures.

The health system is grossly under-resourced: per capita expenditure is about US$12. In 2002 there were only 19 maternity beds for every 1000 deliveries and 3 delivery couches for every 1000 institutional deliveries. Healthcare resources are not evenly distributed around the country either. The healthcare infrastructure is not adequate; only 46% of the population is within a 5-km radius of a health facility, and only 20% of the population lives within 25 km of a hospital

(Essential Health Package document 2004). In rural areas the situation is worse as distribution of health personnel favours urban areas, and secondary and tertiary levels of care. Moreover of the 2928 nurse/midwives in the country, 1108 were in urban areas, 852 in semi-urban areas and only 972 in the rural areas where 80% of the population was based. In addition, 97% of clinical officers and 82% of nurses in the public sector are in urban areas.[30]

Way forward

Since she took over as President of Malawi, Mrs Joyce Banda has established a Presidential Initiative on Maternal Health and Safe Motherhood. The goal of the initiative is to reduce maternal and neonatal mortality and morbidity through community mobilization and empowerment towards quality health-care service delivery. She also recruited traditional chiefs as champions of this cause in recognition of the great contribution they were making to promote reproductive health and safe motherhood; she has made one of the traditional chiefs a chairperson of the initiative.

The Presidential Initiative prioritizes three main interventions: (a) community mobilization and training of village and regional chiefs, (b) construction of maternity waiting homes* at health centres, and (c) training of skilled community midwives. The plan is to construct an additional 150 waiting homes for expectant women, and expand electricity to hospitals and clinics across the country, and the training of 1000 community nurses to work in rural BEmONC sites by 2014.[31] The initiative has introduced a short midwifery course for school leavers to train as community midwives who would work in their home communities and deliver women at the local facilities. The initiative also focuses on increasing salaries and improving working conditions for nurses and midwives among other priorities to make the profession attractive.

Family planning remains an area of emphasis. The department has recently adopted a postpartum family planning policy, whereby women are offered contraceptives before they are discharged from the health facility after delivery. With a high coverage for institutional delivery, contraceptive prevalence rate is expected to soar. Here too the chiefs have taken on the task. At one national public meeting a chief castigated churches that discouraged their members from using contraceptive services. The chiefs' intervention is expected in view

---

* Blueprints for these structures were developed by the Ministry of Health, and take two forms: a 24-bed version or a slightly larger 32-bed structure. They are estimated to cost about $70 000 and $80 000 each, and it is expected that they will be funded by Malawi's private sector and external donor support.

of frequent newspaper reports of villagers killing each other in land disputes as land becomes scarce in a rapidly increasing population.

The issues on which to collaborate with the traditional leaders continue to expand as we evaluate our programme; they now include lifestyle changes among community members. I am currently working with them to push for abortion law reform that would make safe abortion more accessible and thereby reduce abortion-related deaths, to supplement the family planning service strategy.

At a meeting President Banda was briefing Traditional Chiefs on the Safe Motherhood programme, Senior Chief Lukwa remarked that the MDG5 target was not going to be met unless the restrictive abortion law was reformed to make safe abortion more accessible to women. Also, at one of the national safe motherhood meetings, Chairperson of the Presidential Initiative on Safe Motherhood, Senior Chief Kwataine, said that community leaders and their members in the country, including men, have a big role to ensure that women attend antenatal clinics, prepare for birth, and deliver at health facilities under the watch of skilled birth attendants.[32]

This is testimony that Malawi has found traditional leaders to be extremely helpful in the mobilization of communities against maternal deaths and the traditional leaders have come to own the initiative. This is on the principle that involving community leaders in planning can increase their commitment to the programme apart from increasing the resources available for the programme.

Key considerations for processes and policies: building consensus at the country level

Collaboration between program managers and community leaders is important for promotion of health in the community. Continuous assessment of the health needs of the community, and coming to an agreement with the community leaders on the strategy to alleviate their felt needs, promotes compliance.

Programmes should not be slow in moving from research to policy; it is the right of the people to benefit from science without delay. Even for controversial issues, such as screening of women for HIV to protect both the mother and baby, project managers should move on to policy changes quickly; the resulting positive impact will influence the conclusion of the debate. The debate on safe abortion remains fierce in the USA, but it is going on while women have access to unsafe abortion and not dying from complications of unsafe abortion, as is the case in Africa.

Consensus building with development partners on the direction of the programme is also very important. Despite being a low-resource country, Malawi has been able to lead in the introduction of Option B + PMTCT resulting in accelerated reduction in HIV-related morbidity and mortality. This said, programme managers should still have the final say on the direction the programme should take.

Conclusion

The collaboration of the Ministry of Health and traditional leaders to mobilize women for the maternal care service facilitated the proper use of time, and use of skills and the expertise of traditional leaders. The traditional leaders functioning as local volunteers have inspired and encouraged men to be involved in the promotion of women's health.

Community mobilization continues to gather momentum as traditional leaders continue to introduce more and more bye-laws, which include preventing men from marrying off their underage daughters but instead keeping them in school and embracing family planning services. The Department of Reproductive Health Services facilitates study tours of traditional leaders to well-performing constituencies thereby cascading community skills against maternal deaths in Malawi.

Traditional leaders not only provide leadership and organizational capacity at the community level, but also important communications' channels to the community. Gaining their participation helped the Ministry of Health to raise awareness of safe motherhood issues at the community level and to promote the use of information and services, as well as improve clients' understanding of the services being offered. Specific barriers to service access and use identified were addressed and service utilization increased. The result is a steady decline in maternal morbidity and mortality.

The Ministry of Health has now developed a health system that routinely identifies and builds on the community assets identified to promote healthcare improvement. The Reproductive Health Department as a result of this approach is now connected well to the community. Involvement of Traditional Authorities has facilitated local ownership and the sustainability of the health programmes.

References

1 Malawi Population and Housing Census, Zomba, Malawi, 2008.
2 Political Map of Malawi, Nation Online, http://www.mapsofworld.com.
3 Malawi HRH Census Report, Ministry of Health, Goverment of Malawi, April 2008.
4 Ministry of Health. RHU, Report of a Nationwide Assessment on Emergency Obstetric Care Services in Malawi, Lilongwe, July 2005.

5 **Olefile KM, Khondowe O, and M'Rithaa D.** Misoprostol for prevention and treatment of postpartum haemorrhage: A systematic review, *Curationis*, 2013, **36**(1), Art. #57, 10pp.

6 **Justus Hofmeyr G, et al.** Misoprostol to prevent and treat postpartum haemorrhage: a systematic review and meta-analysis of maternal deaths and dose-related effects. *Bulletin of the World Health Organization*, 2009, **87**: 666–77.

7 **Starrs A and Winikoff B.** Misoprostol for postpartum hemorrhage: moving from evidence to practice *International Journal of Gynecology and Obstetrics*, 2012, **116**: 1–3.

8 United Nations General Assembly, Resolution 2, Session 55, United Nations Declaration, 8 Sept 2000.

9 Malawi Demographic and Health Survey 2000. National Statistics Office, Zomba, Malawi.

10 Government of Malawi Ministry of Health. Quarterly HIV Program Report: HIV Testing and Counseling, Prevention of Mother to Child Transmission, and Antiretroviral Therapy (October–December 2011), Lilongwe, Government of Malawi, 2012.

11 Government of Malawi Ministry of Health. Quarterly HIV Program Report: HIV Testing and Counseling, Prevention of Mother to Child Transmission, and Antiretroviral Therapy (April–June 2011), Lilongwe, Government of Malawi, 2011(a).

12 CD4 are better known as helper T cells. The acronym CD4 refers to 'cluster of differentiation 4' of these white blood cells. These cells protect the body from infection.

13 WHO. *Antiretroviral drugs for treating pregnant women and preventing HIV infection in infants.* Recommendations for a public health approach (2010 version). Geneva, WHO, 2010.

14 Malawi Demographic and Health Survey, 2004. NSO Zomba.

15 Malawi Demographic and Health Survey, 2010. NSO Zomba.

16 Malawi Penal Code 243.

17 Malawi Health Sector Employee Census, 2007. Centre for Social Research, University of Malawi.

18 Malawi Growth and Development Strategy, 2004.

19 **Bergström S.** Who will do the caesareans when there is no doctor? Finding creative solutions to the human resource crisis. *Brit J Obst Gyn* 2005;**112**:1168–9.

20 **McCord C, et al.** The quality of emergency obstetrical surgery by assistant medical officers in Tanzanian district hospitals. *Health Affairs* 2009;**28**(5):W876–85.

21 **Mullan F and Frehywot S.** Non-physician clinicians in 47 sub-Saharan African countries. *Lancet* 2007;**370**:2158–63.

22 **Pereira C, et al.** Meeting the need for emergency obstetrical care in Mozambique: Work performance and work histories of medical doctors and assistant medical officers trained for surgery *Brit J Obst Gyn* 2007;**114**:1530–3.

23 **Chilopora GC, et al.** Postoperative outcome of caesarean sections and other major emergency obstetric surgery by clinical officers and medical officers in Malawi. *Human Resources for Health* 2007;**5**:17–23.

24 **Pereira C, et al.** A comparative study of caesarean deliveries by assistant medical officers and obstetricians in Mozambique. *Brit J Obst Gyn* 1996;**103**:508–12.

25 Malawi Growth and Development Strategy, Central 2004, Malawi Govt.

26 An analysis of maternal death audit (2005). Reproductive Health Dept, Ministry of Health, 2005.

27 'Community Mobilization and Participation'. Women and Child Development Department, Govt. of Orrissa, pp. 197–205.

28 Malawi Welfare Monitoring Survey, NSO, 2011.

29 HRH Census Report, Ministry of Health, Govt. of Malawi, April, 2008.

30 Government of Malawi. Situation analysis on human resource in the light of EHP implementation. June 2003, Lilongwe, Malawi.

31 Presidential Initiative on Maternal Health and Safe Motherhood, 2012.

32 **Crossette B.** A traditional chief slashes maternal death in Malawi. *Africa Health and Population, Women Issues*, Apr. 18, 2013.

Chapter 6

Epidemiology and health policy in Africa

Luis Sambo

Regional Director of the African Region of the World Health Organization

Luis Gomes Sambo is an Angolan medical doctor and specialist in public health who has been the Director of the African Region of the WHO since 2005. He was previously Angola's Vice Minister of Health before joining the World Health Organization where he has been WHO country representative and Director of Programme Management. In this chapter he describes the epidemiological challenges facing Africa, the way in which the wider determinants of health affect the population, and the wider international context within which health systems developed in recent years. He reveals a continent that is facing a disproportionately large share of the world's burden of disease with a tiny part of its resources. He also shows how Africans, supported by international partners, have tackled these problems with considerable success. As he describes clearly, however, some of the intractable public health challenges and underlying systems' issues remain serious challenges to be tackled in coming years. Dr Sambo concludes the chapter by sharing his thoughts on how health in Africa has changed in the last 10 years and his vision of the need for a more holistic health systems approach in the future.

The WHO African region

With more than 740 million people spanning 47 countries, the WHO African Region accounts for 12% of the world's population, which is growing by 2.5% annually. The African Region lags behind other regions in terms of health and human development. A powerful contributory factor for this is the very heavy burden of infectious disease, particularly the interrelated group of HIV/AIDS, tuberculosis, and malaria, and the rising trend of non-communicable diseases. The very high diseases burden increases the demand on often weak, under-funded, and overstretched health services and compromises the improvement of health. It has a particular impact on the most vulnerable segments of the population causing high infant and maternal mortality.

Poverty and poor quality of life are the main drivers of diseases and weakening of the social and economic fabric in Africa. Scientific knowledge and relevant technologies to address many of the health problems that affect African populations are available, but not accessible to all. Getting the right interventions to the right people at the right time, and at the right price, remains a challenge. Nevertheless, Africa is moving in the right direction. Political commitment is high, there is international solidarity, and people are increasingly aware of their rights to better living conditions and health.

This chapter reviews the position in Africa in three sections: the first deals with the way health systems and policy have developed over the last 60 years; the second looks at health status; whilst the third reviews the key determinants of health.

Health systems

The health status of the majority of Africa's population remains poor despite huge progress in health sciences and technology. If we look back ten years and take as reference the health Millennium Development Goals, we can see that health systems in sub-Saharan Africa were seriously deficient in achieving their goal of improving people's health.[1] Most of the SSA's population has only limited access to health services and some of those living in the most remote areas have no access at all. As a result progress in reducing diseases' burden and maternal and child mortality was not as good as anticipated. There were gaps in being able to deliver evidence-based interventions and, as a consequence, most countries won't reach the 2015 targets.

In maternal health in 2011, for example, only 74% of pregnant women attended an antenatal clinic; 48% had a skilled attendant at birth; unmet need for family planning services was 25%; while the contraceptive prevalence rate was 24%. It is a similar story elsewhere: measles immunization coverage among 1-year-olds in 2010 was 76%; 82% of children didn't sleep under mosquito nets; only 50% of pregnant women with HIV received anti-retroviral treatment to prevent mother to child transmission; while the detection rate for all forms of tuberculosis was 60%.[2,3] These coverage gaps compromise the progress towards the achievement of national and internationally agreed health goals such as those stemming from the Millennium Declaration. Weak health infrastructure, inefficiencies in resource management, inequities and gaps in provision of quality health care are key explanations for these problems, as well as slow progress in addressing other key health determinants. Moreover, health systems remain in a process of change as reforms are introduced and health managers have to deal with complex problems in a changing environment.

At the policy level, fundamental issues are often raised: first, the health sector is usually considered as non-productive and resource consuming, and therefore not prioritized in terms of resource allocation. Second, policy makers find it difficult to identify the best way to provide financial risk protection in poor resource settings in the overall context of weak economic performance and financial crisis (equity in health has a cost, and who should pay for it?). Third, reference is made to development assistance in health reform processes and outcomes: can global health initiatives deliver more effectively and more efficiently at local level? Could they strengthen and sustain national health systems capacities? The fourth issue relates to resources' management and accountability: could national health systems deliver more and spend the same or less? Are governments optimizing their domestic and foreign aid investments? The fifth issue relates to community participation: could local communities be more effectively and actively involved in the processes of designing solutions for their own future health? So, what are the health systems issues underlying these intractable challenges?

In sub-Saharan Africa, during the last 60 years, we can identify a whole series of trigger points for health policy reforms: the end of colonialism by the 1960s, which empowered the creation of national health services;[4] the structural adjustment programmes by the end of the 1970s[5] in which emerged the Health-For-All policy[6] and the Alma-Ata Declaration on primary health care; the onset of the HIV/AIDS pandemic in early 1980s;[7] the end of the Cold War and start of political democratization by the end of the 1980s;[8,9] and the expansion of market economies and globalization by the end of the 1990s;[10-12] and, finally, an increasing number of international health partners and global health initiatives including the Millennium Development Goals.[13,14]

During the first years of independence in the early 1960s and 1970s, the generally stable political environment and the favourable economic conditions made it possible for most countries to achieve considerable socio-economic development. In the health sector, the main achievements were related to the expansion of healthcare services to rural areas, the development of human resources for health, and improvements in controlling communicable diseases and preventing major epidemics.

The economic downturn in developed countries, which followed the oil shocks of 1973 and 1979, ultimately led to a profound world recession that left many of the African economies in difficulties. Huge national debts, among other factors, forced most of the countries to embark on economic reform measures that involved the development and implementation of structural adjustment programmes whose components included currency devaluation, cuts in government spending, and trade liberalization. The social sectors, particularly health and education, were hardest hit by the effects of economic decline and the way economic reforms were being implemented. Not only did the measures slow the pace of health development in most African countries, they also weakened their health systems to the point of near collapse. This was followed by increased levels of poverty, unemployment, lack of motivation of health professionals and brain-drain, and increased inequalities in access to healthcare and other health determinants.[15,16] The economic crisis deprived health systems of important inputs like human capital, financial capacity, and technologies at a time when both demand and costs were increasing. Increasing poverty levels led to worsening health in the majority of the population who had moved down the social ladder. However, while recognizing that structural adjustment programmes may have been coupled with austerity measures that undermined the fiscal capacity of African countries to invest in health services, the World Bank argued that such programmes cannot be invoked as a root cause of low or declining government spending on health.[17]

The emergence of the HIV/AIDS pandemic in the early 1980s further eroded the health status, the economic productivity, and human development in Africa.[18] The growing healthcare needs for people living with HIV/AIDS placed an unprecedented burden on African health systems during a period in which all countries of the continent were facing economic downturn and a number of man-made disasters.

By the end of the 1980s and early1990s, the end of the Cold War triggered a process of democratization in most African countries, increasing the participation of people in the political arena. At this time, the number of man-made disasters predominated, in particular political instability that led to increasing number of internal displacements of people and forcing some of them to become refugees. Starvation and diseases affected almost half of the population, particularly in Southern and the Horn of Africa. Malnutrition was associated to more than one-third of infant and child mortality in rural and urban districts. The World Bank in 1994 reported on the inadequate quality and quantity of food intake, which was causing growth failure, decreased immunity, learning disability, poor reproductive outcomes, and reduced productivity. With a population crippled by high infant and maternal mortality, persistent illness of its workforce, and low life-expectancy, no African country attained high level of economic and human development. This was rather aggravated by the severity of poverty that became a matter of public and international concern.

The end of the 1990s and beginning of the twenty-first century brought a flow of information and commodities (goods and services) and movement of people in medium and high-income African countries. Low-income countries did not enjoy most of the benefits of globalization due to weak economies and poor connectivity in information technology and communication.

In the year 2000, the Millennium Declaration brought a new international commitment for sustainable development in which health featured in three out of the eight Millennium Development Goals (MDGs) and shared in the others.[19] The MDGs created a framework of reference that pushed governments, international partners, and communities towards joint efforts aimed at reducing the burden of communicable diseases (MDG6); reducing by two-thirds the maternal mortality ratio (MDG5), and reducing the morbidity and mortality of children under 5 years old (MDG4). These were more realistic endeavours that to some extent replaced the goal of Health-for-All in the year 2000.

Healthcare delivery

In most African countries, healthcare delivery is organized within the context of National Health Services (NHS) and Ministries of Health are responsible for leadership, policy development, the definition of norms, regulation, monitoring, and evaluation. The public sector is fundamental, particularly in preventive care and in the control of endemic diseases and epidemics. Non-profit and NGOs (non-governmental organizations) institutions, together with the most peripheral health units of the NHS, play an important role in the delivery of essential healthcare. Communities and citizens are gradually becoming more aware of their rights and responsibilities, and are more interested in participating in community health initiatives and other determinants that might improve their health and well-being. Nevertheless, health systems are still predominantly centralized in terms of policy development, management of resources, and delivery of quality services. In addition the contributions of the private sector remains minimal in most countries, thus placing the financial burden of delivering healthcare almost entirely to national governments.

Health systems have undergone various generations of reforms in response to the changes described above, including the founding of national health services at the brink of the independencies and promotion of primary healthcare as a route to achieving Health for All.[20] A criticism of this route has been that it gave very little attention to people's *demand* for healthcare, and instead concentrated almost exclusively on people's perceived *needs*.[21,22] This gave way to universalism in health—a form of public intervention that has governments attempting to provide and finance everything for everybody. This philosophy dominated for about 20 years from early 1970s; it shaped the formation of well-established national health services that achieved temporary health successes following the independence of African countries. During this period, health sector reforms in African countries were driven by different motivations. Poor quality and inequities within health systems and services, demographic and epidemiological changes, increasing demand for services, political and ideological changes, economic factors such structural adjustment programmes were amongst the main factors behind health reforms. Improved access and coverage, improved quality of services, improved health status, improved efficiency, resource mobilization, and improved community participation were considered the major objectives of these reforms.

The reform agendas focused mainly on health systems' stewardship (policy formulation/update, decentralization, redefinition of roles and functions, including restructuring ministries of health, partners coordination, and intersectoral collaboration); organization and management of health services (definition of a minimum package of services, strengthening institutional capacity, integration of services, community participation, promotion of public-private mix); provision of quality of care (human resources development, access to essential medicines, and research); and financing (broadening the resource base, improved management of resources). The main constraints in reform implementation were mainly related to inadequate human resources, inadequate financial resources, political instability and civil strife, weak institutional capacity, and resistance to change among others.

Most of these reforms, inspired by the ideals of universalism, failed to recognize both resource constraints and the limits of governments. This was followed by a period of profound political and economic changes, which included the emergence of market-oriented economies, reduced State intervention, fewer government controls, and more decentralization. This new context generated a gradual shift to what WHO (1999) called the 'new' universalism. The 'new' universalism recognized governments' limits, but retained government responsibility for leadership, regulation, and finance of health systems. The new universalism welcomed diversity and recognized that services are to be provided for all but not all services can be provided. It foresaw that the most cost-effective services should be provided first. It welcomed private sector involvement but it entrusted the public sector with the fundamental responsibility of providing strategic orientation, stewardship, and financing care for all. This is the ideology that underpins the current health sector reforms in most of African countries, which include the endeavour of *universal health coverage* meaning coverage of essential health interventions for all, but not coverage for everything.

However, the gaps in human resources for health, health facilities, medical devices, essential medicines, and health financing have led to gaps in the coverage of essential health interventions, as I have already described. The most updated WHO estimates of human resources for health illustrate disparities in its distribution across the world. Out of a total of 8 652 107 physicians available globally, the African Region has the lowest share of 1.4%; of the 16 689 250 nursing and midwifery personnel available worldwide, only 2.8% were in the Region; of the global 1 227 822 reported dentistry personnel, 1.4%, were in the Region; and out of the 2 114 282 pharmaceutical personnel world-wide, only 1.6% were in African Region.[23] It is estimated that there is a shortage of at least 817 992 health workers in the African region.

According to the World Health Report 2006, out of the 57 countries identified as facing human resources for health (HRH) crisis (health workforce density ratio below 2.3 per 1000 population), 36 are in the African Region. Health workforce shortages have been attributed to inadequate institutional capacity for HRH management, low levels of national investment in HRH production, slow progress in educational reforms, skewed distribution of health workers, lack of incentives and ineffective retention strategies.

Despite having 25% of the global disease burden, African human resources for health constitute only 1.3% of the total global health workforce. To meet the current human resources for health shortfall, most African countries would have to increase the size of their workforce by 140%. During the last 20 years there has been deterioration in the institutional, human, and technological capacities of medical schools and nursing and midwifery schools in Africa.[24] This problem is compounded by an imbalanced skill mix, uneven geographical distribution, non-optimal use of existing personnel, poor work environments, and low remunerations among other issues. The 62nd session of the WHO Regional Committee for Africa adopted a road map for scaling up the human resources for health, which, when fully implemented, may go a long way in addressing the health workforce crisis.[25]

Healthcare comprises a continuum from home-based self-administered treatment, health post, health centre, district hospital, provincial hospital to highly specialized care in specialized/tertiary hospitals. Health posts, where they exist, constitute the first level of contact between national health system and communities. The majority of countries in the African region have less than 11 health posts per 100 000 population; less than 11 health centres per 100 000 population; less than one district hospital per 100 000 population; less than 0.20 provincial hospitals per 100 000 population; and less than 0.20 specialist/tertiary hospitals per 100 000 population.[26]

In spite of the fact that most countries publish an essential medicines' list; the availability of medicines at public health facilities is often poor. Shockingly, some 77% of countries had a local price for medicines that was over twice the international reference price; in about 53% of countries the local prices of selected generic medicines in the private health sector were more than fourfold higher than the international reference prices. WHO estimated that about half of those in need do not have access to essential medicines in Africa.[27]

Turning to health financing: in 2010, African Region's per capita total expenditure on health was US $89 compared to US $3373 in the Region of the Americas and US $2217 in the European Region. Even though Africa has the highest disease burden, it has a low per capita spending on health, partly due to its low gross domestic product but also due to health financing practices that are not guided by evidence.

More than 40 years ago, developed countries committed to allocate at least 0.7% of their gross national product (GNP) to Official Development Assistance (ODA); in 2008, only 5 of 24 members of the Development Assistance Committee (DAC) allocated at least 0.7% of their GNP; and the total DAC's average contribution was 0.31%. The current global financial crisis affecting some of the developed countries is compromising foreign aid to African countries, although Africa itself is growing and has new opportunities for health sector reforms.[28]

By end of 2010, 49% of African countries had not achieved the International Taskforce on Innovative Financing recommendation of spending at least US$44 per person per year on health[29] and 91.5% of countries had not met the Abuja target they had all agreed of allocating at least 15% of total government budget on health sector. Evidence shows that when out-of-pocket payments (OOPS) as a proportion of total health expenditure (THE) are below 15–20%, the incidence of financial catastrophe caused by out-of-pocket health expenses is negligible.[30] In 2009, OOPS made up over 20% of THE in 34 African region countries (76%); and more than 50% in 14 countries. With the current model of healthcare financing it will be very difficult for African countries to achieve universal health coverage and ultimately improve the poor indicators of health status.

Universal health coverage

Universal health coverage is the new goal for many African countries. The World Health Assembly defined universal health coverage in 2005 as 'access of all population to key promotive, preventive, curative and rehabilitative health interventions at an affordable cost, thereby achieving equity in access.'[31] It is an aspiration of the majority of African countries, and indeed around the world, and requires an appropriate financing strategy. It should imply equitable and efficient revenue collection, prepayment and pooling, and purchasing of cost-effective health packages. Universal healthcare coverage, according to WHO recommendations, is expected to address the range of services to be covered, the financial coverage that must ensure social protection, and the population to be covered.

Progress towards universal health coverage is described by leaders from Rwanda, Ghana, and South Africa later in the book from Chapter 16 onwards, so will not be covered further here. I will, however, turn to the Global Health Initiatives (GHIs), which are typically funds targeted at specific diseases or health conditions, intended to bring additional resources to health development efforts of countries. The Global Alliance for Vaccines and Immunization (GAVI Alliance), for example, is a global effort to strengthen childhood immunization programmes and bring a new generation of recently licensed vaccines into use in developing countries. The Global Fund to Fight AIDS, Tuberculosis and Malaria, directly contributes to the achievement of MDGs 4, 5, 6, and 8. The United States GHI seeks to achieve significant health improvements and foster sustainable effective, efficient, and country-led public health programmes that deliver essential healthcare whose first principle is to focus on women, girls and gender equality.[32]

The potential of GHIs to raise and disburse additional funds to support disease control and strengthen health systems provides a unique opportunity for many countries to fill critical funding gaps in addressing their health development priorities. During the last ten years, the international health partnership landscape has become overcrowded. The creation of UNAIDS, Global Fund to fight AIDS, Tuberculosis and Malaria, the Roll-Back Malaria Partnership, UNITAID, GAVI, PEPFAR, PMI, the US Global Health Initiative, the European Global Health Initiative, the Bill and Melinda Gates Foundation and their increasing role in global health, among many other international health initiatives and agencies, show the increasing importance of health in the context of development; and indicates the need of dialogue and alignment of global and local efforts.

To address some of these concerns, the 2005 Paris Declaration on Aid Effectiveness provides a framework through which donor and developing country partnerships can fully exploit their potential.[33,34] The principles endorsed in the Declaration have now been adopted by a number of global health partnerships. An African coordination mechanism was established entitled Harmonization for Health in Africa (WHO, UNICEF, UNFPA, UNAIDS, UNWOMEN, USAID, NORAD, JICA, French Cooperation, GFATM, GAVI Alliance, World Bank, African Development Bank and Roll Back Malaria Partnership), in which the regional heads of UN agencies, international financial institutions, and bilateral agencies convene regularly under WHO secretariat to harmonize their strategies and actions in support to country coordination mechanisms and governments.[35]

But how do African communities perceive health systems? A multi-country study on Community Perception of Health Systems in Africa conducted by a group of experts in Africa revealed that 90% of people named public sector health facilities as the main sources of healthcare. On people's rating of the responsiveness of the health services, more than two-thirds of the 10 932 respondents rated the services at public sector facilities as inadequate. The main reasons cited for the poor rating were: unavailability of drugs and equipment (39.1%); poor attitude of health providers (27.7%); and delays in the provision of care and long waiting time (13.1%). In contrast, the respondents who reported that the services were good attributed this mainly to health personnel responsiveness to users (42.7%), friendly environment (18.9%), and availability of medicines (14%).[36]

Achieving the highest possible level of health in Africa implies addressing current and emerging health problems. Progress towards achieving health MDGs is unequal throughout the world. Some parts of the world are doing better than others. In sub-Saharan Africa, for example, very little progress was made towards achieving MDGs 4, 5, and 6. Therefore, Africa has to tackle both the intractable public health problems and new ones. New public health threats are commonly associated with socio-economic and demographic factors (e.g. population growth rates, international trade, poverty prevalence, urban migration, international travel, social disruptions); individual and collective human behavioural (e.g. diet, illicit drug use, sexual practices, and outdoor recreation); environmental considerations (e.g. use of pesticide and antibiotics in crop and livestock management, changes in food processing, inadequate coverage of potable water and sanitation); and health system factors (such as health policies, human resources capacity, health financing, community involvement, and availability and access to new technologies) among others.

New public health threats of particular significance in the African region are emerging. The recent droughts in the Horn of Africa and the Sahel have resulted in environmental distress that impacted negatively on food security, nutrition, and the health of people. Urbanization in Africa is rapidly evolving with overcrowding, urban sprawl, and pollution, which may create appropriate environments for outbreaks, violence, and other negative effects on people's health. Changes in the interface between wild and urban ecosystems are creating interactions between animal and human health, and increasing the risk of zoonoses and new pathogens. We are also seeing the emergence of germs that are resistant to common antibiotics, such as resistant strains of pathogens related to AIDS, tuberculosis, and malaria. New public health risks create increased demands on health systems to detect and control their spread.

Health systems in Africa require strong leadership and regulation by states because they are subject to powerful social and economic forces and influences that pull them from their intended goals. African countries need health policies based on equity and underpinned by a primary health care approach. Health reforms should address more holistically the health system problems and bring about the vision of a new public health. Stakeholders should share the new public health vision and assign responsibilities that address a broader range of actors that generate creative solutions in different contexts and environments. Strides towards universal health coverage presuppose a more critical approach in health systems thinking.[37]

Health status

Life expectancy

Life expectancy at birth (LEb) reflects the overall mortality level of a population; it is the sum of mortality levels at all stage of life. Whilst there has been a modest increase in LEb throughout the Region—from 51 years in 1990 to 54 years in 2009—some African countries have experienced sharp falls since 1990, probably due to HIV/AIDS and other highly endemic diseases. However, during the same period, some countries have increased LEb. In the majority of the countries, estimated LEb for women is 56 years and 52 for men, compared to the global average of 69 years.[38] The underlying reasons are associated with the social determinants of health and the burden of diseases, which mean that the population of the African region is losing a full 15 years in comparison with the rest of the world.

Mortality

The overall *mortality rate* in the African Region increased from the 1990 estimates of 366:1000 to 383:1000 population in 2009. The main factors for this may include the overall population increase, the double burden of communicable and non-communicable diseases, epidemics, and natural and man-made disasters. These regional averages mask big variations in country performances. The male mortality rate was 420:1000 in 2009, compared with 347:1000 for women. There have been improvements since 1990 in both the mortality rates for children aged less than five and maternal mortality, although both remain considerably higher than in other regions.[39]

The mortality rate for under-fives reduced from 175 per 1000 live births in 1990 to 95:1000 in 2013. The 2013 global average was 51:1000.[40] The maternal mortality ratio dropped from 820:100 000 live births in 1990 to 480:100 000 in 2010, reflecting some progress, but remains unacceptably high and reflects indirectly the low performance of health systems. A woman living in sub-Saharan Africa still has a 1 in 16 risk of dying due to pregnancy or childbirth. Globally, the maternal mortality ratio reduced from 400:100 000 live births in 1990 to 210:100 000 in 2010.[41] Africa is very unlikely to meet the MDG target for reduction in maternal mortality by 2015.

Burden of disease

Between 1990 and 2012, HIV/AIDS, malaria, and tuberculosis have been the leading cause of morbidity in the African Region. HIV/AIDS has had a devastating impact both on individuals and on health services, and co-infection with other pathogens has aggravated the pattern of other diseases such as malaria and tuberculosis, and increased the risk of maternal and child mortality. These facts, associated with high illiteracy rates and poverty, explain why the African Region leads the world in many aspects of morbidity and mortality. At present, non-communicable diseases account for 22% of the burden of disease. Most countries have combined communicable–maternal–nutritional disease burden rates of over 60% of total Disability Affected Life Years (DALYs).[42] This increases the demand on health services and requires greater infrastructure capacity and financing. This double burden of disease means that Africa needs to rollback communicable diseases and at the same time prevent the advance of lifestyle-related chronic diseases.

HIV/AIDS

The incidence of HIV infection and HIV/AIDS-related deaths is decreasing, partly due to the unprecedented scaling-up of care and treatment, and partly because of better information and communication. However, the most recent estimates put the number of people living with HIV as 33.5 million and more than two-thirds live in sub-Saharan Africa. It has 82% of the women infected with HIV globally; more than 90% of the children infected with HIV; and has an estimated 1.2 million deaths yearly associated with HIV/AIDS.[43] The burden of HIV/AIDS is not uniform across Africa, with Southern Africa having the largest number of people living with HIV/AIDS worldwide. Available data suggest that HIV prevalence in East Africa is stabilizing or declining, although some studies indicate a possible rise in high-risk groups.[44] There is a growing possibility that the most at-risk population groups, such as commercial sex workers, men having sex with men, and intravenous drug-users, are fuelling the epidemic.

Turning to treatment, anti-retroviral coverage has improved from 40 000 people or less than 10% of the infected population in 2001 to 7.5 million or 63% in 2012. Mortality associated with HIV/AIDS has declined from 219 per 100 000 habitants in 2005 to 139:100 000 in 2010.[45] New evidence has demonstrated that starting ART at a CD4 cell count of ≤500 cells/mm³ rather than ≤350 cells/mm³, has the potential to reduce HIV-related morbidity, mortality, and onward transmission of the virus. This has resulted in the WHO publishing new guidelines in 2013, which, if implemented, would mean an additional 53% or 6.6 million people in sub-Saharan Africa becoming eligible for further investments in health services in order to increase access and realize the full benefits of the scientific breakthrough. Whilst treatment of pregnant women to interrupt mother-to-child transmission has increased by 23% since 2008, nearly 40% of all HIV-positive pregnant women still do not have access to anti-retroviral therapy (ARTs).[46]

Tuberculosis

Africa is estimated to carry 27% of the global burden of tuberculosis (TB). In 2012, TB incidence in Africa was 255:100 000.[47] Prevalence has also greatly increased, with rates standing at 303:100 000 in 2010. Multi-drug resistant TB (MDR-TB) and extensively drug resistant TB (XDR-TB) add to the threat of the TB epidemic and draw attention to the need for adequate approaches and resources to prevent infections, improve diagnostic capacity, increase treatment, and maintain infection control in health facilities and communities. The number of MDR-TB cases notified by countries globally increased from 2445 in 2005 to 18 146 in 2012. During the same period, XDR-TB cases increased with 1501 cases reported in Southern Africa. The true extent of drug-resistant TB in Africa is not yet known because the Region has limited laboratory capacity to identify and monitor treatment. A related complication is limited access to second-line anti-TB medicines, partly due to the high cost and short shelf-life of some of these medicines. Of the 33 countries that have reported MDR-TB cases, only 20 are known to have a structured MDR-TB treatment programme.

In 2012, 13% of people who developed TB worldwide were HIV positive, with 75% of them being in Africa. On average, 37% of new TB patients in the Region are co-infected with HIV, compared with 8% globally. TB-related death rates in countries with high HIV prevalence have risen to as much as 20% during the past 10 years.[48] Co-infection increasingly causes TB to occur in younger and hence more economically productive members of society, especially girls and young women aged between 15 and 24 years.

Malaria and neglected tropical diseases

Africa is also the Region most severely affected by malaria. It accounted for about 80% (163 million) of the total number of cases notified worldwide and 90% of the deaths associated with malaria in 2012. On average, malaria accounts for 25%–45% of outpatient clinic attendance, and between 20% and 45% of hospital admissions. Furthermore, it is estimated that malaria represents 14% of mortality of children aged less than under five and is a major contributor to maternal mortality, reducing progress towards MDGs 4 and 5. The most commonly used interventions for prevention and treatment include use of: insecticide-treated nets for vector control, indoor residual spraying, intermittent preventive treatment of malaria in pregnancy, and artemisinin-based combination therapy.[49] While use of insecticide-treated nets is cost-effective and uptake is increasing, use by children and pregnant women is less than the 80% target.[50,51] Indoor residual spraying has increased, rapidly protecting up to 58 million people in 40 countries by the end of 2012.[52]

Thirty-four countries are now implementing malaria control and intermittent preventive treatment in pregnancy on a countrywide basis, and artemisinin-based control therapy is the treatment of choice in 42 of 43 countries.[53] However, only 16% of children with malaria are currently being treated with it. Use of artemisinin monotherapy continues in some countries, with risks of emerging resistance to artemisinin combination therapy. The proportion of suspected malaria cases tested in public facilities has increase dramatically in the past years from 37% in 2010 to 61% in 2012.[54,55] Financing for malaria control has greatly increased; however, better surveillance and reporting are needed to be able to target the money better and track the effectiveness of interventions.

There has been strong leadership in the fight against malaria. Globally leadership has come from the WHO, which created Roll Back Malaria in 1998, followed by Kofi Annan and the UN, which established it as a target in the MDGs. African Heads of State and Government signed the Abuja Declaration and Plan of Action in 2010, with the commitment to halve malaria for Africa's people by 2010. Subsequently the UN Secretary General put forward a bold vision aimed at stopping malaria deaths in 2008, and in 2009 African Ministers of Health adopted a WHO Regional Committee Resolution on '*Accelerated Malaria Control, Towards Elimination*' which called, among other actions, for the integration of malaria control interventions in poverty reduction strategies and development plans.[56] Also in 2009, Mr Jakaya Kikwete, President of Tanzania and past chairman of the African Union, launched the Africa Leaders' Malaria Alliance at the United Nations General Assembly with the purpose of ensuring efficient procurement, distribution, and utilization of malaria control tools; sharing of good practices; and ensuring that malaria remains high in the global and Africa's development agendas. As part of all these efforts, about US$3.9 billion per year has been dedicated by the international community to fight malaria over the period 2012–13.

These efforts and strong leadership from heads of state and community leaders have led to excellent results in eight countries (Botswana, Cabo Verde, Eritrea, Namibia, Rwanda, Sao Tomé e Príncipe, South Africa, and Swaziland) that reduced the morbidity due to malaria by 75% or more in 2012.[57] Others have not yet done so.

Approximately 1 billion people are at risk from one or more neglected tropical diseases (NTDs) worldwide of which approximately 50% are in Africa. These diseases are most prevalent among poor and under-served communities, particularly in tropical and sub-tropical areas, resulting in heavy morbidity often associated with deformity, disability, and mortality. In addition, the chronic nature of many NTDs perpetuates the cycle of poverty illness. The major NTDs occurring in Africa are guinea worm disease, leprosy, lymphatic filariasis, onchocerciasis, human African trypanosomiasis, and schistosomiasis. There are also soil-transmitted helminthiasis (STH), buruli ulcer, hookworm-ancylostomiasis, noma, yaws and other endemic treponematoses, leishmaniasis, trachoma, endemic zoonoses, and the recently identified nodding disease. Although NTDs may be of public health significance in the communities in which they are endemic, they are often not considered priorities and hence are neglected at national and international levels. Nevertheless, the incapacitation of NTD patients, as well as the impact on agricultural productivity, contributes enormously to poverty over generations. In terms of DALYs and deaths, of the 29% of the global burden attributable to infectious and parasitic diseases, NTDs account for 25% of DALYs and 10% of the deaths. In economic terms, the price of the neglect is too high, as NTDs continue to fuel, in part, the current cycle of poverty, ill health and under-development in the African Region.[58]

However, the African Region registered some significant achievements. For example, cumulative number of patients cured with multi-drug therapy, a combination of Rifampicin, Dapson and Clofazimin raised from 625 480 in 2000 to 1 120 489 and contributed to drop leprosy prevalence from 57 516 cases in 2000 to 19 670 cases in 2012, bringing the prevalence rate from 0.92 to 0.23 cases per 10 000 inhabitants. The annual incidence of guinea worm disease decreased from 20 581 cases in 2007 to 1028 cases in 2012 representing 95% reduction; while four countries (Chad, Ethiopia, Mali, and South Sudan) are still grappling to achieve the goal of eradication. The African Programme for Onchocerciasis Control (APOC) is a successful private–public partnership for disease control launched by WHO in 1974, which has broken the transmission of the disease and prevented more than 200 000 cases of blindness. It is the subject of Chapter 9 written by the former APOC Director, Dr Uche Amazigo. The success stories of leprosy, guinea worm disease, and onchocerciasis could be taken as models to inspire broader global and local undertakings to control and eliminate NTDs.

The 2012 London Declaration on NTDs, the WHO Global Plan to Combat Neglected Tropical Diseases 2008–15, and the WHO African Region NTDs Action Plan are three important milestones towards this endeavour.

Vaccine-preventable diseases

Immunization is a safe and cost-effective means for tackling pneumonia and diarrhoeal diseases, which contribute significantly to morbidity and mortality among children in Africa. There is a long history of immunization in Africa dating back to the immunization programme against smallpox in 1966, which became the Expanded Programme on Immunization (EPI) in 1974 covering diphtheria, whooping cough, tetanus, poliomyelitis, tuberculosis, and measles. This landmark programme was followed by the adoption in 1977 of the goal of Universal Childhood Immunization (UCI), which endeavoured to achieve 80% coverage for the six basic EPI vaccines by 1990. At the end of 1990, sub-Saharan Africa reported an increase of coverage from 5% in 1980 to 57%. In the meantime, the 1988 global poliomyelitis eradication initiative[59] led to the development of national expanded programmes of immunization (EPI) with special focus and resources dedicated to polio. This was remarkably successful, resulting in a 99% reduction of polio cases globally from an estimated 350 000 in more than 125 endemic countries, to 650 reported cases in 2011 with only 3 endemic countries, Afghanistan, Nigeria, and Pakistan.

The creation of the Global Alliance for Vaccines and Immunization (GAVI) in 2000, mobilized additional funds to increase the number of antigens provided in the EPI to 14 in some countries. The Measles Partnership efforts from 2001 to 2009 contributed to vaccinate more than 425 million children; reducing the number of cases by 92% and the number of measles deaths by 90%. However, in 2009 the number of cases increased, mainly because governments could not sustain the initial partnerships efforts.[60] In 2011, the ministers of health of African countries adopted a strategy aimed at measles elimination by 2020.[61]

Reaching Every District (RED), launched in 2002, helped in increasing and sustaining high levels of routine immunization:[62] by the end of 2013, about 80% of children in the Africa region have received the 3rd dose of DTP vaccine (DTP3). Another important recent development was the conjugate meningococcal *meningitis A* vaccine (MenAfriVac™), developed in 2009 for countries in the African meningitis belt through a partnership between WHO and the Programme for Appropriate Technology in Health (PATH).[63] Meningococcal meningitis caused by various serogroups of *Neisseria meningitidis* was associated with high case fatality rates, even where adequate medical services were available. However, the new vaccine prequalified by WHO in early 2010 was successfully introduced in hyper-endemic countries in Sahel. More than 100 million people have been vaccinated, resulting in a considerable reduction of meningitis epidemics, with an absence of meningitis A among people vaccinated.

New vaccines are being introduced for invasive pneumococcal disease, a main causes of deaths in children under five, and for rotaviruses, the most common cause of severe diarrhoeal disease and mortality among young children. Yellow fever is endemic in 31 African countries, with 22 at particularly high risk of outbreaks;[64,65] it remains a serious public health issue, despite the availability of a vaccine for 60 years. Other prevalent vaccine-preventable diseases in Africa include cancers caused by the human papilloma virus.

In May 2012, the WHA adopted the Global Vaccine Action Plan (GVAP) as part of the Decade of Vaccines.[66] It includes a focus on strengthening systems and creating synergies with other public health programmes, so as to use the capacity of national health services to provide universal access to vaccines and immunization.

Non-communicable diseases

Cardiovascular diseases, cancer, diabetes mellitus, mental health problems, chronic respiratory disease, violence, injuries and disabilities, and genetic disorders are significant public health problems and absorb substantial amounts of human and financial resources.[67] In Africa in 1990, NCDs accounted for 28% of morbidity and 35% of mortality. These figures are projected to rise over the coming years.[68] NCDs require national strategies based on prevention, surveillance, and case-management. African countries need to address behavioural and metabolic risk factors and promote other actions that contribute to reducing morbidity, disability, and premature deaths, and improving the quality of life.[69]

Lifestyle changes and urbanization are potential drivers of cancer. Survival rates for cancer in the African Region are low, due to problems with diagnosis capacity, late presentation, and unavailability of appropriate treatment. The cardiovascular disease (CVD) burden is also a public health challenge in Africa. Many chronic respiratory diseases are important killers. Mental and neurological disorders, including depression and epilepsy, are also major contributors to morbidity and premature mortality in Africa. The economic impact of NCDs goes beyond the costs to health services.[70] Indirect costs, such as lost productivity, can match or exceed the direct costs; moreover, a large part of the cost of care falls on patients and families. People now die from chronic diseases at dramatically younger ages; but because NCDs are not always understood as development issues, and underestimated as diseases with profound economic effects, many governments take insufficient interest in their prevention and control.

Epidemics and pandemics

Countries in the African Region experience recurring epidemics of communicable diseases that have significant impact on health and economic development. In 2011 a total 103 public health events were reported from 33 out of 47 countries. Some of the epidemic-prone diseases, such as viral haemorrhagic fevers caused by Marburg and Ebola viruse,s have demonstrated the potential to spread internationally. Meningococcal meningitis and cholera are the major epidemic-prone diseases with seasonal occurrence and are often associated with high rates of morbidity and mortality. Between 2001 and 2010, the reported cases of meningitis in affected countries were 453 315, including 48 594 deaths.[71] During the same 10-year period, 1 407 808 cases and 34 025 deaths of cholera were reported in Africa.[72] Other recently emerging epidemic-prone diseases, such as dengue and chikungunya, are becoming increasingly frequent. In 2009 and 2010, Africa experienced more than five dengue outbreaks; during the same period, it suffered the largest outbreak of dengue haemorrhagic fever, due to type 3 dengue, with over 21 000 cases reported in Cape Verde alone.

Traumas, injuries, and violence

Injuries account for 5.8 million or 10% of the world's deaths annually, with Africa having the highest rates.[73] The three leading causes globally are road traffic accidents (23%), suicide (15%), and homicide (11%).[74] In 2004, violence accounted for 35% of all injury deaths in Africa with a death rate of 37:100 000; suicide was the second leading cause with a rate of 13: 100 000 population, and deaths directly due to collective violence occurred at a rate of 5.5: 100 000 population.[75] The African Region also has the highest fatality rate for road traffic accidents, at 24: 100 000 population.[76] Adopting and enforcing legislation aimed at reducing drink-driving and speeding, and increasing seat-belt and motorcycle helmet use, if effectively implemented, will contribute towards reducing the injury burden.

Maternal health

Maternal mortality decreased, as we saw earlier, but the progress is not sufficient to achieve MDG 5. The lifetime risk of maternal death is 1 in 26 in Africa, as opposed to 1 in 7300 in developed regions.[77] Most deaths occur from preventable causes during or immediately after childbirth. WHO estimates that 34% of maternal deaths globally are due to haemorrhage, 19% hypertension, 9% abortion, and 9% sepsis. In sub-Saharan Africa, maternal under-nutrition, severe anaemia, tuberculosis, malaria, and HIV/AIDS increase the risk of maternal death at birth, and are associated with at least 20% of maternal mortality. Access to skilled birth attendance and emergency obstetric care coverage has also been very low because of weak health systems not geared towards women's health needs. For far too long, African women have suffered significant health disadvantages throughout the course of their lives—bearing the burden of unnecessarily high maternal mortality, HIV infection, and other largely preventable diseases. Despite progress, the current situation demands radical change.

The WHO Regional Office for Africa published a major report '*Addressing the Challenge of Women's Health in Africa*' in 2012 prepared by a panel of experts from across Africa under the leadership of Mrs Ellen Johnson Sirleaf, President of the Republic of Liberia.[78] The document shows that African women account for more 50% of deaths of women worldwide due to communicable diseases, maternal and perinatal conditions, and nutritional deficiencies; which are aggravated by the heavier burden of HIV/AIDS and gender-based violence affecting more women than men. The report illustrates how socio-cultural and economic aspects influence women's health and calls for rethinking of policies, health systems, and connections between women's health and socio-economic development. Implementing its recommendations will help to improve significantly the lives of women and boost prosperity across Africa by ensuring that their economic and social contribution can reach its full potential.

The 15th Assembly of the Heads of State and Government of the African Union meeting in Kampala in 2010 debated 'Maternal, New-born and Child Health and Development'. It attributed the high maternal mortality ratios to weak leadership and governance and challenges related to poverty, illiteracy, poor transport and communications networks, armed conflicts and domestic violence, inadequate domestic and international funding, competing priorities, inadequate level of skilled birth attendants, and limited coverage of ante-natal and delivery care. There was consensus on the urgent need to speed up actions for strengthening health systems to improve coverage of maternal, newborn, and child health services, and to address the broad determinants that can sustain improvements in health and development.[79]

Neonatal and child health

Under-five mortality (U5MR) has continued to decrease in Africa from 159 per 1000 live births in 2000 to 95:1000 in 2013. Infant mortality rate (IMR) decreased from 105 per1000 live births in 1990 to 63:1000 in 2013. However, nearly 34% of U5MR and 51% of IMR are attributed to neonatal mortality, suggesting there is an insufficient attention to healthcare needs of newborns during their first month.[80] Africa has the highest newborn mortality rate in the world, estimated at 45:1000 live births. Every year, one million babies in sub-Saharan

Africa are stillborn, of which at least 300 000 die during labour. A further 1.2 million babies die in their first month of life, with up to half these deaths occurring on the first day.[81] The major causes of neonatal deaths are: preterm births (29%); infections, including pneumonia/septicaemia (28%); birth asphyxia and trauma (27%); neonatal tetanus (2%); congenital abnormalities (7%); and diarrhoeal diseases (2%).

More than 80% of childhood deaths in Africa are caused by diarrhoea, pneumonia, malaria, measles, and HIV/AIDS. Diarrhoea is the leading cause of death in children under five, with 748 000 annual deaths. Only 37% of African children with diarrhoea receive the recommended treatment of low-osmolarity oral rehydration salts (ORS)—and trend data suggest that little progress has been made since 2000.[82,83] As we have seen in earlier sections, children are affected by malaria, HIV/AIDS, and pneumonia and other vaccine preventable diseases but progress is slow in all these areas.

African children make up one-quarter of the estimated 148 million underweight children globally. Although underweight prevalence has decreased slightly in Africa, the absolute number of underweight children has increased by 8 million. More than one-third of children under five in Africa are stunted.[84] Only nine African countries are on track to reach MDG Target 1 of halving hunger and malnutrition by 2015. Vitamin and mineral deficiency afflict one-third of sub-Saharan Africa's population, affecting minds, bodies, energies, and the economic prospects of nations.[85] The issue of vitamin and mineral deficiency in sub-Saharan Africa could, in principle, be resolved within a few years, and at an affordable cost. Cost-effective strategies do exist, but stakeholders at all levels, need to work together to apply related knowledge and tools. Africa bears 43% of deaths attributed to childhood and maternal under-nutrition: 47% were attributed to underweight, 4% to iron deficiency, 13% to vitamin A deficiency, 12% to zinc deficiency, and 23% to sub-optimal breastfeeding.[86]

Health determinants and risk factors

Health determinants

In this section we identify some of the main social and environmental factors that affect the health status of Africans. Health status has a direct effect on economic growth due to the way it affects the structure of the population, in particular those of working age. Changes in population size and distribution have an influence on health services' organization and health status; whilst health problems, conditions or injuries will in turn influence demographic patterns. The numbers of refugees and internally displaced people, alongside rapid population growth and the widespread migration of people from rural to urban areas, are re-shaping the structure of the population.

Increasing urbanization and the state-centred model of development and centralized administrative and political systems, have characterized the way countries have developed since independence. Colonial constraints on the development of secondary cities and small towns were continued in the years after independence, with continued neglect of peasant agriculture, general shortage of credit, poor infrastructure, and heavy handed government regulation.[87] Lack of planning for the growing urbanization has led to the illegal, anarchic, and informal development of cities and compromised the extension of water, electricity, solid waste collection and sanitation services, and road networks.[88] In 1950 only 14.5% of the population of sub-Saharan Africa lived in cities—in 1990 the percentage had risen to 34% and is expected to reach 50% in 2020; whilst the total population is expected to double by 2036.

Other important health determinants are related to environmental risks such as indoor air pollution, climate change, hazardous working conditions, and inadequate hygiene and sanitation conditions. WHO has estimated that around a quarter of the global disease burden is associated with environmental risk factors.[89] Climate change, particularly drought, is affecting agriculture in certain areas with all its attendant consequences of food insecurity, hunger, starvation, malnutrition, and disease. In some countries economic growth is leading to air pollution and urban transportation is becoming a health hazard; whilst sea pollution is becoming a problem in oil-producing countries.[90,91] Food security, nutrition, and food safety are also important determinants of health that are not adequately tackled in sub-Saharan Africa.[92]

Economic growth is creating new opportunities for investment in the health sector and other social sectors which, if managed appropriately, can improve health and reduce inequity.[93] In terms of education, for example, the literacy rate among adults aged 15 years and above was 63% in 2011.[94] Another example is the fact that sub-Saharan African countries invest very little in research and development; available data show that the proportion of GDP spent on R&D varies from 0% to 0.9%.

Risk factors for health

Some of the risk factors for poor health have been touched on in earlier sections: the big increases in non-communicable diseases, in addition to the long-standing burden of infectious disease,[95] can be attributed to population ageing, rapid urbanization, and globalization. The common modifiable risk factors underlying this pattern are: tobacco use, harmful use of alcohol, inadequate patterns of food consumption, and inadequate physical activity. These risks contribute to problems such as cardiovascular diseases, diabetes, cancer, injuries and trauma, mental illnesses, amongst others. The presence of multiple risks in the same individual are not uncommon; surveys conducted in some countries have found three or more risk factors in up to 35% of respondents.[96] Only a small number of countries have alcohol control policies or advertising regulation in place, and very few have any in-depth understanding of the nature and extent of drug use. Health services and interventions for those affected are few.

Tobacco use remains a leading cause of preventable deaths globally. It kills nearly 6 million people annually, and causes hundreds of billions of dollars of economic loss globally each year. The average prevalence of smoking any tobacco product among adults over 15 in the region was 17% for males and 3% for females in 2009. However, young people are more affected with the average prevalence of tobacco use among 13–15-year-olds being 20% for males and 13% for females.[97] In addition, about 48% of youth in the region are exposed to second-hand tobacco smoke in public places, thus increasing the susceptibility to respiratory diseases. In response to these problems, 41 of the 46 countries of the African Region had ratified or acceded to the WHO Framework Convention on Tobacco Control by the end of 2013.

The burden of diseases associated with excess of alcohol consumption is increasing in the Region. Alcohol is the third leading global risk factor for disease and disability, with 4% of all deaths worldwide attributable to alcohol. Harmful use of alcohol has acute consequences, including road traffic accidents and violence, particularly against children and intimate partners, child neglect and abuse, absenteeism in the work place among others. Alcohol is further associated with cancers, cardiovascular diseases, liver diseases, neuropsychiatric disorders, traumas, weight gain and obesity; and these may lead to disability and death. According to the most recent estimate by WHO, in the African Region, 30% of the population drink alcohol regularly. Overall adult per capita consumption of pure alcohol is 6.2 litres. The statistics show that men drink more than women—3.0 litres for women and 9.5 litres for men on average. Meanwhile, among people who drink alcohol, the average per capita consumption stands at 19.2 litres (ranging from 1.1 to 37 litres). Therefore, the two characteristics of alcohol consumption in Africa are the high level of abstention (averaging 70%), and the high volume consumed per drinker. Consequently, we can assume that increasing the level of abstention and reducing the volume of consumption would reduce the harm associated with alcohol.[98]

The 60th session of WHO Regional Committee for Africa adopted a strategy that aims to contribute to the prevention and reduction of harmful use of alcohol and related problems in the Region. Some of the priority interventions recommended in the strategy include development of alcohol control policies, legislation, and regulations; leadership, coordination, and partners' mobilization; awareness and community action; information-based public education; improvement of health sector response; strategic information, surveillance, and research; enforcing drink-driving legislation and countermeasures; regulating alcohol marketing; addressing accessibility, availability, and affordability of alcohol; addressing illegal and informal production of alcohol; and allocation of resources to implement these interventions.[99] Harmful use of alcohol is responsible for about 2% of the disease burden in sub-Saharan Africa, with wide variations between sub-groups of the population. Alcohol use is responsible for 12% of all deaths among young men aged 12–29.

Unhealthy diet is a major risk factor for non-communicable diseases.[100,101] In many countries of the Region, stunting and underweight among children as a result of food shortages and inappropriate feeding patterns remain issues of public health concern. However, overweight and obesity are on the increase, especially in urban areas. Due to lifestyle changes, people are moving away from traditional foods to diets rich in fats, sugars, and salt, but low in fruits and vegetables. Data gathered from STEPS surveys in the African region over the past 10 years show rates of obesity ranging from 1 to 31% among adults with higher percentages among females.[102] Physical inactivity is another equally important risk factor that needs to be addressed, given the high rates of urbanization. Within countries, high rates of physical inactivity are seen among women and children, in particular. WHO recommends that adults undertake 150 minutes per week of physical activity, for NCD prevention and maintenance of health.

Drug-use disorders are associated with increased risk for other diseases and health conditions, including HIV/AIDS, tuberculosis, hepatitis, suicides, overdose deaths, and cardiovascular diseases. It is estimated that 12.4% of the 1 778 500 of people who inject drugs in sub-Saharan Africa are HIV positive.[103] Significant increases in the availability of illicit drugs have been recorded in coastal areas both in west and east African countries. The prevention and treatment of drug dependence are essential to the reduction of demand for illicit drugs and prevention of drug-related harm. Globally, 7 606 083 deaths were attributed to addictive substances (tobacco use, alcohol use, illicit drug use); out of which 6% occurred in Africa.[104] HIV/AIDS prevalence continues to be high among young people. Risky sexual behaviours continue to be a strong risk factor for HIV infection, particularly among youth, with particular emphasis on women. A number of other infections result from risky sexual behaviour such as human papilloma viral infection, syphilis, gonorrhoea, and chlamydia, which are entirely attributable to unsafe sex.

Emergencies and disasters

Natural hazards, such as floods, cyclones, droughts, and disease outbreaks, are common in the region as too, sadly, are man-made disasters, such as civil strife and armed conflicts. Both compromise the provision of healthcare and damage the health status of populations. Civil strife and armed conflicts are responsible for about 50% of internally displaced persons (IDPs) in the world and 50% of the world's 14 million refugees. Most IDPs and refugees face insecurity and stress, violence, including gender-based violence and sexual abuse, lack of food, potable water, shelter, and sanitation facilities, which directly expose them, and increase their vulnerability, to outbreaks of epidemics. They are particularly susceptible to psychosomatic complaints and psychological disturbances, owing to the disruption of their emotional, cultural, and economic environments, and to the feeling of being caught in an impasse.[105] To prepare and respond to the health consequences of disasters, the Regional Director of WHO for Africa initiated a proposal adopted by the ministers of health to create the African Public Health Emergency Fund,[106,107] which was further endorsed by the Heads of State Summit of the African Union.

Conclusion

During the last 10 years, African countries have made important progress in improving the performance of health services. The healthcare coverage and health status of people improved as a result of government-driven health reforms with the support of the international community, particularly in least developed countries. Health policies and strategic plans have been updated but the implementation became problematic because of inadequate budget and financial capacity and inefficiencies in resource management.

Heads of state and governments have expressed genuine concerns and interest in improving the health status of their people. Whenever called to exercise their personal leadership to advance public health agendas, such as fighting HIV/AIDS, eradication of poliomyelitis, eradication of guinea-worm disease, even health financing and universal healthcare initiatives, the heads of state, and in some cases first ladies, got involved and galvanized the energy of a large part of the society towards the implementation of related public health interventions. It was found that sometimes, heads of state were not in possession of the right and updated evidence for decision-making, demonstrating information gaps on health matters.

On the other hand, the political power of ministers of health, in general was not strong enough for them to influence through their leadership, the required changes in health-related sectors in charge of managing key determinants of health. There is a need to strengthen the leadership skills and roles of ministers of health, as well as their time in office, giving them enough time to initiate and sustain successful reforms that are further consolidated by their successors. The economic downturn and global financial crisis hampered domestic investments in health and created, particularly in low-income economies, an excessive dependency from donors/partners on priority programmes such as HIV/AIDS, malaria, tuberculosis, and immunization; therefore compromising efforts to achieve sustainability.

Furthermore, resource allocation within the health sector has tended to favour the central level of national health services, restricting the capacity at local level; also, curative services absorb most of resources if we compare with disease prevention, health promotion and rehabilitative services. These concerns call for evidence-based health financing strategies. Increasing disease burden and unhealthy environments create a very high demand in terms of health infrastructure, particularly medicines, vaccines, diagnostics, and other health technologies, most of it not produced in Africa. The high diseases burden, the persistent health inequities, the escalating costs of healthcare associated with poverty of the majority of people, and poor economic performance mean that most individuals cannot access—and governments cannot afford to provide—quality health services. Therefore, innovative health-financing models are required to initiate and sustain the endeavours of universal health coverage. With the advent of political democracy and growing decentralization of government functions to local level, with economic growth and increasing number of trained professionals in various health-related categories; the health sector in Africa has new opportunities.

I am persuaded that the intractable issues that compromise the technical performance of health systems call for more suitable philosophy, theory, and more effective methodologies. Some of these issues are related with consensus building, inter-sectoral collaboration, partner's coordination, accommodating stakeholders different interests and aspirations, housing tensions between different health professional groups, dealing with uncertainty, enhancing community participation, dealing with politics, and articulating global, national and local systems, just to mention a few.

However, health sector reforms in Africa have been fundamentally supply driven and underpinned by the positivist paradigm that puts emphasis on what is observable and measurable, tending to ignore what is not measurable in a scientific and objective manner. For example, health needs are identified through epidemiological and demographic data, while healthcare delivery is governed by norms that mostly don't consider equity or people's views; decision-making should be based on all these concerns. However, it is important to recognize that the positivist paradigm has greatly contributed to advances in health sciences, in particular on health technology and innovation that have improved the viability and performance of health systems.

Nevertheless, in my opinion, health systems are too complex to be understood on the basis of a single paradigm. The high number of important variables and the myriad of interactions of health system components in a permanent process of change and interaction with its environment, make it highly complex. The primary health care approach and the new public health theory are major developments that could further cross-fertilize with the interpretive school of thought and critical systems heuristics. I think that, in general, health system thinking is missing vital insights and creativity that could be provided by a more in-depth consideration of alternative paradigms and related methodologies towards a more critical approach.[108]

It is time for Africa to take up its responsibilities and move towards effective implementation of health policies and plans, optimizing existing resources and increasing investments in health; while relying on international solidarity to fill the gaps, particularly in low-income countries. Poverty, economic inequities, international financial crisis, environmental degradation, intensified global market exchanges, cross-border exchanges, and new lifestyles affect global and local epidemiology profiles and feed endless processes of health sector reforms. Africa is coming from a long socio-economic and health systems history. There is progress—a little—but progress. The world is going through fundamental processes of changes that create new opportunities and new public health threats. With the current trend of decline in fertility and mortality rates, sub-Saharan Africa may soon face a demographic transition with change in the age structure in which youth with good health and education level will become an important leverage to expand economic opportunities. Important factors are currently converging in Africa offering an unprecedented opportunity to yield more benefits from the existing potential for economic and social development.

Governments should generate and use strong evidence to guide policy and investments in health. Reforms should be inclusive, led by governments and embrace negotiated views and diversity of stakeholders, including communities and the private sector; they are expected to leverage the weak components of health systems and improve health outcomes. Health leaders and managers should keep their eyes on moving heath targets. Africa has to speed-up and pave the way for greater successes in health and development.

References

1 WHO/AFRO. *Monitoring the Implementation of the Health Millennium Development Goals*; document AFR/RC61/9. 2013.

2 WHO/AFRO. *Health Situation Analysis in the African Region. Atlas of Health Statistics.* 2012.

3 WHO. *World Health Statistics.* 2013.

4 WHO/AFRO. *Development of Basic Health Services*; WHO Regional Committee for Africa resolution AFR/RC18/R4. 1968.

5 **Loewenson R.** Structural adjustment and health policy in Africa. *International Journal of Health Services* 1993; **23**(4):717–730.

6 WHO. *The Declaration of Health-for-All (HFA).* World Health Assembly, 1977.

7 **Illife J.** *The African AIDS Epidemic: A History.* Ohio University Press, 2006.

8 **Bratton M, van de Walle N.** *Democratic Experiments in Africa: Regime Transitions in Comparative Perspective.* Cambridge University Press, 1997.

9 **Olsen G.** Europe and the promotion of democracy in post-cold war Africa: how serious is Europe and for what reason? *African Affairs* 1998; **97**(388):343–67.

10 **Sachs J.** International economics: unlocking the mysteries of globalization. *Foreign Policy* 1998; **110**: 97–111.

11 **Fidler DP.** The globalization of public health: the first 100 years of international health diplomacy. *Bulletin of the World Health Organization* 2001; **79**: 842–9.

12 **Yach D, Bettcher D.** The globalization of public health, II: The convergence of self-interest and altruism. *American Journal of Public Health* 1998; **88**(5):738–44.

13 **Biesma RG, et al.** The effects of global health initiatives on country health systems: a review of the evidence from HIV/AIDS control. *Health Policy and Planning* 2009; **24**:239–52.

14 WHO/AFRO. *Optimizing Global Health Initiatives to Strengthen National Health Systems*; document AFR/RC62/15. 2012.

15 **Kanji N, Manji F.** From development to sustained crisis: Structural adjustment, equity and health. *Social Science & Medicine* 1991; **33**(9): 985–93.

16 **Sanders D, Sambo A.** AIDS in Africa: the implications of economic recession and structural adjustment. *Health Policy and Planning* 1991; **6**(2):157–65.

17 World Bank. *Better Health in Africa: Experience and Lessons Learned*; World Bank; 1994.

18 **Dixon S, McDonald S, Roberts J.** The impact of HIV and AIDS on Africa's economic development. *BMJ* 2002; **324**: 232–4.

19 United Nations. *The United Nations Millennium Declaration*; General Assembly Resolution A/55/2. 2000.

20 **Sambo LG, Lambo E.** Health sector reform in Sub-Saharan Africa: A synthesis of country experiences. *East African Medical Journal* 2003; **80**(6 Suppl): S1–S20.

21 WHO/AFRO. *Health Systems in Africa: Community Perceptions and Perspectives*; the report of a multi-country report. 2012.

22 **Travis P, et al.** Overcoming health-systems constraints to achieve the Millennium Development Goals. *The Lancet* 2004; **364**(9445): 1555–6.

23 WHO. *World Health Statistics 2012*, 2012.

24 **Fitzhugh Mullan F, et al.** Medical schools in sub-Saharan Africa. *The Lancet* 2011; **377**(9771): 1113–21.

25 WHO/AFRO. *Road map for scaling up the human resources for health for improved health services delivery in the African Region 2012–2025*; document AFR/RC62/7. 2012.

26 WHO. *Global Health Observatory*. 2013.

27 WHO. *World Health Statistics*. 2013.

28 WHO. *Global Health Observatory*. 2013.

29 WHO. *World Health Statistics*. 2013.

30 **Sambo LG, Kirigia JM, Ki-Zerbo G.** Health financing in Africa: overview of a dialogue among high level policy makers. *BMC Proceedings* 2011, **5**(Suppl 5): S2. <http://www.biomedcentral.com/1753-6561/5/S5/S2>.

31 WHO. *Sustainable Health Financing, Universal Coverage and Social Health Insurance*; World Health Assembly resolution WHA58.**33**, 2005.

32 The United States Government.*Global Health Initiative*; strategy document; 2011. <http://www.pepfar.gov/documents/organization/136504.pdf>.

33 OECD. *The Paris Declaration on Aid Effectiveness*. 2005.

34 OECD. *The Accra Agenda for Action*. 2008.

35 Harmonization for Health in Africa. *An Action Framework*. 2006. <http://www.who.int/healthsystems/HSS_HIS_HHA_action_framework.pdf>.

36 WHO/AFRO. *Health Systems in Africa: Community Perceptions and Perspectives*; the report of a multi-country report. 2012.

37 **Sambo LG.** *Health Systems Thinking: The Need for a More Critical Approach*. Doctor of Philosophy Thesis: The University of Hull. 2009.

38 WHO/AFRO. Health situation analysis in the African Region; *Atlas of Health Statistics*. 2012.

39 WHO/AFRO. Health situation analysis in the African Region; *Atlas of Health Statistics*. 2012.

40 Commission on Social Determinants of Health. *Closing the Gap in a Generation: Health Equity Through Action on the Social Determinants of Health*. 2008.

41 WHO. *Trends in Maternal Mortality: 1990 to 2010*. 2012.

42 **Murray CJ, et al.** Disability-adjusted life years for 291 diseases and injuries in 21 regions, 1990–2010: a systematic analysis for the global burden of disease study 2010. *The Lancet* 2012; **380**: 2197–223.

43 UNAIDS Global Report. UNAIDS report on the global epidemics. 2013.

44 **Opio A, et al.** Trends in HIV-related behaviours and knowledge in Uganda, 1989–2005: evidence of a shift toward more risk-taking behaviors. *Journal of Acquired Immune Deficiency Syndromes* 2008; **49**: 320–6.

45 UNAIDS Global Report. UNAIDS report on the global epidemics. 2013.

46 UNAIDS Global Report. UNAIDS report on the global epidemics. 2013.

47 WHO. Global tuberculosis report. 2013.

48 WHO. Global tuberculosis report. 2013.

49 RBM. *Counting Malaria Out*. WHO, April 2009.

50 WHO. *Insecticide-Treated Mosquito Nets*: a WHO Position Statement. 2007.

51 WHO. *World Malaria Report*. 2012.

52 WHO. *World Malaria Report*. 2012.

53 WHO. *World Malaria Report*. 2012.

54 WHO. *World Malaria Report*. 2012.

55 **Zarocostas J.** Malaria treatment should begin with parasitological diagnosis where possible, says WHO. *British Medical Journal* 2010; **340**: c1402.

56 WHO/AFRO. *Accelerated Malaria Control: Towards Elimination in the African Region*; 2009.

57 **Sambo LG, Ki-Zerbo G, Kirigia JM.** Malaria control in the African Region: perceptions and viewpoints on proceedings of the Africa Leaders Malaria Alliance (ALMA). *BMC Proceedings* 2011; **5**(Suppl 5): S3.

58 **Conteh L, Engels T, Molyneux DH.** Socioeconomic aspects of neglected tropical diseases. *The Lancet* 2010; **375**(9710): 239–47.

59 WHO. *Global eradication of poliomyelitis by the year 2000*. World Health Assembly resolution WHA41.28; 1988.

60 Global Polio Eradication Initiative. 2013. <http://www.polioeradication.org/Aboutus/History.aspx>.

61 WHO/AFRO. *Measles Elimination by 2020—A Strategy for the African Region*; document AFR/RC61/8; 2011.

62 WHO. *Global Immunization Vision and Strategy 2006–2015*. Geneva, WHO and UNICEF, 2005.

63 **Frasch CE, Preziosi M-P, Marc LaForce FM.** Development of a group A meningococcal conjugate vaccine, MenAfriVacTM. *Human Vaccines & Immunotherapeutics* 2012; **8**(6): 715–24.

64 WHO/AFRO. African Health Observatory. 2013. <http://www.aho.afro.who.int/profiles_information/index.php/AFRO:Yellow_fever_control>.

65 **Garske T, et al.** *Yellow Fever Burden Estimation: Summary*. WHO, 2013.

66 WHO. *Global Vaccine Action Plan*. 2012.

67 WHO/AFRO. *The Brazzaville Declaration on NCDs Prevention and Control in the WHO African Region*. 2011.

68 WHO. *Global Burden of Disease*; 2004 update. 2008.

69 WHO/AFRO. *Consideration and Endorsement of the Brazzaville Declaration on Non-Communicable Diseases*. WHO Regional Committee resolution AFR/RC62/R7, 2012.

70 WHO. *2008–2013 Action Plan for the Global Strategy for the Prevention and Control of Non-communicable Diseases*. 2008.

71 WHO Global Health Observatory data repository, 2013. <http://apps.who.int/gho/data>.

72 WHO Global Health Observatory data repository, 2013. <http://apps.who.int/gho/data>.

73 WHO. *Global Burden of Disease*; 2004 update; 2008.

74 WHO. *Global Burden of Disease*; 2004 update. 2008.

75 WHO/AFRO. *Report on Violence and Health in Africa*. 2010.

76 WHO/AFRO. *Report on Violence and Health in Africa*. 2010.

77 **Black RE, et al.** Maternal and child undernutrition: global and regional exposures and health consequences. *The Lancet* 2008, **(371)**9608: 243–60.

78 WHO/AFRO. *Addressing the Challenge of Women's Health in Africa: Report of the Commission on Women's Health in the African Region.* 2012.

79 **Sambo LG, Kirigia JM, Ki-Zerbo G.** Perceptions and viewpoints on proceedings of the Fifteenth Assembly of Heads of State and Government of the African Union Debate on Maternal, Newborn and Child Health and Development, 25–27 July 2010, Kampala, Uganda. *BMC Proceedings* 2011; 5(Suppl 5):S1. URL: <http://www.biomedcentral.com/1753-6561/5/S5/S1>.

80 United Nations Children's Fund. *Levels & Trends in Child Mortality.* Report 2013 Estimates, 2013.

81 The Partnership for Maternal, Newborn & Child Health. *Opportunities for Africa's Newborns: Practical Data, Policy and Programmatic Support for Newborn Care in Africa.* WHO, 2006.

82 WHO/UNICEF. *Joint Statement: Clinical Management of Acute Diarrhoea.* 2004. <http://whqlibdoc.who.int/hq/2004/WHO_FCH_CAH_04.7.pdf>.

83 WHO. *WHO Vaccine-Preventable Diseases: Monitoring System.* 2009 Global Summary; document. WHO/IVB/2009. 2009.

84 WHO. *World Health Statistics 2009*; 2009.

85 UNICEF. *Vitamin and Mineral Deficiency in Sub-Saharan Africa. A Partnership Drive to End Hidden Hunger in sub-Saharan Africa*; report 66, 2004. <http://www.unicef.org/videoaudio/PDFs/africa_dar.pdf>.

86 WHO. *Global Health Risks: Mortality and Burden of Disease Attributable to Selected Major Risks.* 2009.

87 **Rakodi C.** *The Urban Challenge in Africa: Growth and Management of Its Large Cities.* The UN University Press; 1997, pp. 628.

88 **Rakodi C.** *The Urban Challenge in Africa: Growth and Management of Its Large Cities.* The UN University Press; 1997, pp. 628.

89 WHO. *The World Health Report 1999—Making a Difference.* 2009.

90 WHO. *Preventing Disease Through Healthy Environments: Towards an Estimate of the Environmental Burden of Disease.* 2006.

91 WHO & UNEP. *Traditional and Current Environmental Risks to Human Health. First Inter-ministerial Conference on Health and Environment in Africa.* 2008.

92 **Sambo LG.** Editorial: Policy responses to food insecurity in Africa. *African of Food Agriculture, Nutrition and Development* 2012, **12**(4).

93 **Sambo LG.** Poverty, inequity and public health in the African Region. *Ethos Gubernamental* 2007; **IV**: 135–54.

94 UNDP. Human Development Report 2013. *The Rise of the South: Human Progress in a Diverse World.* 2013.

95 WHO. *Global Strategy on Diet, Physical Activity and Health.* Fifty-seventh World Health Assembly Resolution WHA57.17; 2004.

96 WHO. *The WHO Framework Convention on Tobacco Control (FCTC).* 2003.

97 WHO. *World Health Statistics.* 2013.

98 **Rehm J, et al.** Global burden of disease and injury and economic cost attributable to alcohol use and alcohol-use disorders. *The Lancet* 2009; **373**: 2223–33.

99 WHO/AFRO. *Reduction of Harmful Use of Alcohol: a Strategy for the WHO African Region*; document AFR/RC60/4; 2010.

100 WHO/AFRO. *Health Promotion: Strategy for the African Region*; document AFR/
   RC62/9; 2012.

101 **Sambo LG.** Africa's priorities to achieve its goal for the development of better health.
   In: Ilona Kickbusch, John Kirton, James Orbinski (editors): *Global Health 2012*. London: Newsdesk Media; 2012, pp. 24–5.

102 WHO/AFRO. *STEPS Survey on Chronic Disease Risk Factors*; 2013. <http://www.afro.
   who.int/en/clusters-a-programmes/hpr/health-risk-factors/diseases-surveillance/
   surveillance-country-profiles/step-survey-on-noncommunicable-disease-risk-factors.
   html>.

103 **Mathers BM, et al.** Global epidemiology of injecting drug use and HIV among people
   who inject drugs: a systematic review. *The Lancet* 2008; **372**: 1733–45.

104 WHO. *Global Health Risks: Mortality and Burden of Disease Attributable to Selected
   Major Risks*. 2009.

105 WHO/AFRO. *Disaster Risk Management: a Strategy for the Health Sector in the African Region*; documents AFR/RC62/6 & AFR/RC62/R1. 2012.

106 WHO/AFRO. *Framework Document for the African Public Health Emergency Fund
   (APHEF)*. Sixty-first session of WHO Regional Committee for Africa; document: AFR/
   RC61/4. 2011.

107 WHO/AFRO. *The African Public Health Emergency Fund (APHEF)*. Progress report of
   the Regional Director, 2013.

108 **Sambo LG.** *Health Systems Thinking: The Need for a More Critical Approach*. Doctor of
   Philosophy Thesis, University of Hull. 2009.

Part 3

All the resources of the community

Chapter 7

Introduction to Part 3: All the resources of the community

Francis Omaswa and Nigel Crisp

This chapter describes how many African health leaders have been very effective in using the resources of their community in their efforts to improve health. They have improvised and innovated: pressing sometimes very unlikely equipment, facilities, and people into service. This Part of the book opens with two accounts, one from Kenya (Chapter 8) and one from Nigeria (Chapter 9), of how two leaders have developed new approaches to tackling disease through building on the strengths of local communities. They are followed by Chapter 10 'Politics, economics, and society' written by former African Union (AU) Commissioner Bience Gawanas, which describes the wider political, economic, and social context and the work of the AU.

Ubuntu

Many African health leaders have been very effective in using the resources of their community in their efforts to improve health. In part, this can simply be seen as a response to the lack of resources available to them: necessity has been the mother of invention. This is also to do, however, with distinctively African attitudes to community and the extended family. The sense of *ubuntu—I am who I am because of you*—and the traditions of hospitality and clan bonds are markedly different from both Western and Eastern societies. The community and these community bonds are more obviously resources that are available to be used.

Communities in Africa and elsewhere can and do provide resources to be used in improving health. However, it is important to remember that their impact is not always helpful. Traditional beliefs and behaviours can be rigid and stifling whilst some attitudes, particularly to women, can be harmful to health and wellbeing. Authors in this book describe how they have worked very positively alongside traditional leaders and healers: Chisale Mhango, for example, described in Chapter 5 how he influenced traditional leaders to encourage pregnant women to seek antenatal care and get trained help when they delivered, whilst Hannah Faal in Chapter 13 used older village women to help identify eye problems. They and others, however, have also tried to change and, where necessary, confront old beliefs and practices. Couching, to take just one example, which is a very long-standing and widespread practice of treating cataracts by knocking the lens out of the eye with a piece of wood, is both ineffective and dangerous.

The place for traditional healers and traditional medicine in twenty-first century African health and healthcare is still unresolved and contested. Many African health leaders are mindful of the disastrous consequences of the then health minister in South Africa trying to justify her wholly inadequate response to HIV/AIDS as being based on 'African science'. President Obama's famous response that 'there is no *African* science but only science' says all that needs to be said.[1] There are, however, many local examples where efforts have been made to integrate helpful insights and practices into health systems and to discard the others. Catherine Odora-Hoppers in Chapter 15 sets out wider and deeper issues about indigenous knowledge systems ranging from the patenting of herbal remedies to the conceptualization of what is meant by health.

History and economics have, of course, played a major part in throwing Africans back on the resources of the community. As Professor Gottlieb Monekosso describes in Chapter 14, during both colonialism and post-colonialism it was only the elite, whether foreign or African, who had access to organized health services. Others were excluded. Even today, most people's first port of call in a health emergency is their family or a traditional healer and most healthcare is paid for in cash.[2]

We must be careful not to over-generalize about a continent of many countries that is changing so fast. Migration to cities, economic growth, and conflict have changed and are changing Africa. Communities break up and traditions are lost. This is the changing context that Commissioner Gawanas describes and that she and others argue is in need of new and better governance structures and behaviours.

Looking forward, Africa needs more resources for health and greater access to scientific knowledge and technological know-how. However, its tradition of building on the resources of the community has a great deal to teach the more developed countries of the world. As Nigel Crisp has argued elsewhere, the growing global epidemic of non-communicable diseases demands a new approach and much can be learned from the African experience.[3]

This introduction is followed by accounts from two African leaders about how they have confronted major public health issues on a national or wider scale and in doing so developed new ideas that have great resonance elsewhere.

Dr Miriam Were's (Chapter 8) account of developing community health, community workers, and community governance started in the 1970s and has influenced developments in her own country and beyond. Dr Uche Amazigo's (Chapter 9) story of developing community directed treatment to tackle river blindness should lead in the next few years to the elimination of the disease from Africa, as well as providing a means to offer treatment for other diseases.

References

1 **Foster D.** *After Mandela: the Struggle for Freedom in Post-Apartheid South Africa.* Liveright Publishing Corportaion, 2012, p. 417.
2 See Dr Luis Sambo writing in Chapter **6** of this volume.
3 **Crisp N.** *Turning the World Upside Down—the Search for Global Health in the 21st Century.* CRC Press, 2010.

Chapter 8

Community health, community workers, and community governance

Miriam Khamadi Were

Member of the UN's Independent Expert Review Group on Women's and Children's Health; formerly Chair of Kenya's National AIDS Control Council

Professor Miriam Were is a distinguished Kenyan doctor who has spent a life-time promoting health in Kenya, whether country-wide as the National Aids Champion or in pioneering community health-worker programmes at the most local level. Her achievements have been recognized nationally and glob-ally with the Hideyo Noguchi Prize and other awards. In this chapter she describes how as a medical student she realized that improving the environ-ment and the health of people in local communities was the foundation for improving the health of the nation as a whole. She describes the importance of creating new community norms of behaviour that promote health and hygiene and prevent disease. She also shows how it is possible to empower communi-ties, contrary to most professional opinion, and integrate locally based com-munity workers into a national system. As she says: 'In Africa if it doesn't happen in the communities, it doesn't happen. And if it happens in communi-ties it happens in the nation.' Her systematic approach to promoting commu-nity programmes was amongst the first in Africa—long before this became common practice—and led the way for wider developments elsewhere. Even today, almost 40 years after her first pioneering work, she believes there is still much more to be done to ensure that Africa stops just copying other countries and concentrates on 'tailoring her approach to identifying her problems and tailoring solutions to those problems'.

Introduction to the importance of the community

In my studies in the five-year programme (1968–73) at the Faculty of Medicine of the University of Nairobi, the 3rd year was devoted to lectures in the whole range of medicine and surgery as practiced in a hospital setting, with Grand Rounds making part of the teaching set up. In the 4th year, one of the rotations we went through was to spend a term of 12 weeks in the Department of Community Health, along with rotations in paediatrics and obstetrics/gynaecology.

I was one of a group of students who were attached to a Health Centre in Machakos District. We worked in the Health Centre to which we were assigned and carried out community diagnosis in the catchment population of the Centre. We also went to areas near Lake Victoria to study the impact of malaria and leprosy on people's wellbeing and spent a few days at the leprosy hospital at Alupe. During these excursions we saw that many households lived 10 or more miles from health facilities. At that time it had already been shown that facilities more than 5 miles from a household were of little relevance or use to them.[1] By the end of the 12th week in the community health rotation, it was clear to me that the health of people in communities in Kenya needed improvement if the health status of the nation was to improve.

During my 5th year, I was curious as to how much of the illness we saw in the communities poured into the Kenyatta National (teaching and referral) Hospital. The supervised study I carried out showed that over 80% of admissions were from preventable causes, with over 50% having an oral–faecal connection. Furthermore, during my leave in the period of my internship, I carried out a study in the population within 5 miles of a hospital in my home area of Western Province on 'Health problems amenable to public health action'. Findings from the study pointed out that most of the health problems reported by the people and in hospital admissions were preventable. Even more revealing was the finding that many of the people who lived close to the hospital did not use the hospital.

'Why?' I asked them. 'We are not welcome there', some said. So they only brought relatives to hospital as a last resort when everything else had failed and the relatives were close to death. It was no wonder that many deaths in the hospital occurred within 24 hours, with over 70% occurring within 48 hours. This gave the hospital the name of 'The place where you go to die'. So it was generally known in the area that if you wanted to live, you kept off hospital premises! It was clear that the rather impersonal environment in Western-style health facilities was abhorred by the people. They preferred the traditional practitioners for their greater personal attention and the interest they took in each client and the client's social environment. It so happened that the study was undertaken soon after a measles epidemic, so we saw how diseases preventable by immunization and diarrhoea caused death in the villages. Most households had two or three fresh mounds in their compound, where they had buried their dead young children.

My study of medicine came after I had a BA from the USA in the combined fields of biology, chemistry, and physics and, subsequently, a postgraduate Diploma in Education from Makerere University, which enabled me to teach at high school. One of the reasons pushing me to study medicine was that I was bothered by the number of sick young people I was teaching. Given these prior qualifications and my performance in my medical studies, I was recruited to join the teaching staff in the Faculty of Medicine, Department of Community Health in October 1974 after a period of only a little more than a year as a Medical Officer in Kenya's Ministry of Health. Armed with the evidence I had accumulated on the importance of what happened in the community and the health of our people, I was eager to share the evidence with colleagues in the Faculty of Medicine.

'At least', I proposed, 'the Faculty of Medicine should spearhead two programmes in the country: one for widespread childhood immunization and another for the construction and use of latrines.' One Professor responded, 'The immunization problem we could do something about. But you can forget the one of latrines.' Another exclaimed, 'Latrines! You want us to discuss the construction and use of latrines in a Faculty of Medicine Board Meeting?' 'Yes!' I replied. 'Many of the cases being treated at this hospital and elsewhere have links to human waste disposal.' He shook his head and walked off.

The issue of latrine construction and use continued to be treated as a joke. Once I went to a gathering of my colleagues and one of my senior colleagues called out, 'Here comes the Professor of Latrines!' I responded with, 'Thank you, Sir, for the honour'.

The group looked at me as if I was completely crazy. The title was intended to embarrass me and here I was seeing it as an honour! The situation seemed to need an explanation. So I said, 'If being called Professor of Latrines resulted in all our people having and using latrines, it would be a great honour to me for it would drastically reduce the cases that come to health facilities and the cost of health services in this country.' One of my former teachers said, 'If you hadn't received the honour of having been the Best all Round Graduating Medical Student of your class, I would have dismissed you as a half-baked doctor.' He went on to state that in academic medicine, topics that were worthy of discussion were such as how to distinguish various heart murmurs and their diagnosis.

Even though I didn't say so, I was saying inwardly that I, too, was interested in these murmurs. But so long as the lines at health facilities were full of the 'dramatic diseases' of malaria with convulsing children, diarrhoea, and vomiting cases, what chance was there that a child or adult with a 'silent disease' like heart disease or a cancer or kidney failure could ever be attended to? Later on I was asked what, as an academician, my area of research was going to be. I replied,

'People's participation in their own healthcare.' 'You can't be serious', someone said. 'Yes, I am' I replied and there was a chuckle all round.

In 1975 I went to the School of Public Health of Johns Hopkins University for public health qualifications. For my Doctor of Public Health dissertation, I chose that title and it was enthusiastically received by the Department of International Health where I was based. When I returned to Kenya to teach and carry out field work on this title, all of a sudden, there was positive attention to my work. I guess once an academically outstanding university such as Johns Hopkins thought the title was all right, then it became all right for my senior colleagues. This saddened me a bit because I thought, and still do think, that our focus in academics and elsewhere should be how best to solve the problems facing our people in order to improve the quality of life in our countries.

When Kenya's Ministry of Health saw the reports coming out of this work the project became designated as the National Pilot Project in Community-Based Healthcare. It formed the basis of Kenya's presentation at the International Conference on Primary Care held at Alma Ata in 1978 and the Department of Community Health of the Faculty of Medicine of the University of Nairobi won the 1978 UNICEF Maurice Pate Award on account of this project. This project was the basis of my book *Organisation and Management of Community-Based Healthcare.*[2]

Factors that support the community approach to healthcare

Over and above matters of distance and socio-cultural disconnect between people in their communities and health facilities, other factors underscore the importance of the community approach. These include the need to pass on information through community mobilizations. Often, there are efforts to give health education talks to people waiting for services at health facilities. People come to health facilities when they are unwell or are bringing someone who is unwell and whom they are worried about. We found that people are not in a state of mind to receive general information on health-promotion and disease-prevention. This is best done during community mobilization events such as community dialogue days when community health personnel can discuss health problems identified by the community, as well as those brought up by community health personnel. This way, the people get to understand the source of the health problems and what can be done to prevent them: such as the importance of improving hygiene and the construction and use of latrines to control diarrheal diseases.

Through this approach, health-promoting and disease-preventing community norms develop in the communities, which in traditional settings are much stronger than an individual acquiring a new norm by him or herself. Since communicable disease are still responsible for a lot of the morbidity and mortality in Africa, development of positive norms in communities can result in major positive changes in the health of communities, as has been the case in Kenya, Uganda, Ethiopia, and elsewhere. Examples from this project of positive changes within a 3-year period are shown in the tables: Table 8.1 shows the increase in health promoting and disease prevention measures; Table 8.2 the impact on the population; and Table 8.3 the increased uptake of antenatal care through community mobilization.

Table 8.1 Increased health-promoting measures in the home and environment[3]

Action Area	Mean Percentage Positive		
	October 1977	April 1979	January 1980
Dishrack presence and use	1	96	88
Latrine use	1	95	91
Grass cut within 16m of house	15	90	85 +
Home free from potholes and stagnant water	14	84	85 +
Cleaned up water source	12	77	81 +

Reproduced from Were MK. *Organisation and Management of Community-Based Health Care,* p.95, UNICEF. Copyright 1982, by permission of the author.

Table 8.2 Latrine use and worm infestation[4]

	1977	1978	1979
Percent of households using latrines	1	96	91
Percentage positive with*			
Intestinal worm ova	80	64	6
Sample size	245	241	250

*Children up to 12 years of age.

Reproduced from Were MK. *Organisation and Management of Community-Based Health Care,* p.101, UNICEF. Copyright 1982, by permission of the author.

Table 8.3 Increased uptake of antenatal care (% of population)[5]

Year	ANC with CHW	ANC at Clinic
1977	Not applicable	14
1979	10	42
1980	48	35

Reproduced from Were MK. *Organisation and Management of Community-Based Health Care,* p.96, UNICEF. Copyright 1982, by permission of the author.

These activities were used as rallying points for the mobilization and motivation of entire communities' involvement in health activities. Facilitation was provided to communities on how to use existing community structures and create new ones towards improving their own health through (a) health promotion, (b) disease prevention, and (c) first-line curative services at the community level. Once mobilized, motivated, and organized, community members were able to request services from government sectors; services they had come to see as favours rather than their right! It was also shown that an improved and clean home environment set the ball rolling for better health practices. How else can this be done except in the community?

Isn't it a shame that diseases spread by the faecal–oral route continue to be responsible for such a high percentage of the disease burden? Yet it was established long ago that motivating communities to build and use latrines, followed by periodic de-worming campaigns, would remove this as a source of disease? How can this be done in Africa except in a community context?

The need for family planning services was raised in the context of the negative consequences from short birth intervals on the mother and offspring. The mean percentage of women using contraceptives in the communities moved from 8% to 34% of the target groups between 1979 and 1980, even though family planning services were not provided at the community level. When community-based distribution was later added to Kenya's family planning services under the GTZ-Kenya collaboration, contraceptive prevalence rates shot to over 60% (see Table 8.4).

These tables from the Kakamega project illustrate that for over 30 years, it has been clear that we could change health status and reduce disease burden through active community involvement. At last in the Strategic Plan 2006–2010, Kenya formally included the Community level as Level 1 in the National Health System. Better late than never! Every country in the continent should ensure that community health services reach every single community and village in Africa. These kinds of changes can drastically reduce the damage from current major causes of illness and death in sub-Saharan Africa.

Table 8.4 Increased immunization rates (% of population)[6]

	1977(1703)*	1979(1905)	1980(1785)
Child Welfare Clinic attendance	26	12	41
With polio immunization	8	16	29
With BCG immunization	10	38	48
With smallpox immunization	12	26	47

*Number of children observed in brackets.

Reproduced from Were MK. *Organisation and Management of Community-Based Health Care*, p.97, UNICEF. Copyright 1982, by permission of the author.

Now, of course, non-communicable diseases are emerging everywhere in Africa and leading to the double burden of both communicable and non-communicable diseases. Even for the prevention and/or management of non-communicable diseases such as diabetes, cardio-vascular diseases, and others, lifestyle matters are of great importance and so positive community norms can have major positive health outcomes in communities and nations.

Empowering communities is also of fundamental importance. As community health personnel interact with communities, it is critical that they do so through facilitating processes for development of leadership and acquisition of knowledge and skills in communities that result in empowered people in communities. This way the people themselves can carry on the community health activities and extend them to the entire spectrum of sustainable development, with the potential to support the sustainable development of nations. In particular, communities tend to expand their involvement into issues such as the availability of clean water, agriculture, and food production, education as well as gender dynamics. All these are well-known social determinants of health and disease.

In Africa if it doesn't happen in the communities, it doesn't happen. And when it happens in the communities, it happens in the nation. It is essential that well-articulated policies and strategies are subjected to the process of being implemented in communities with effective facilitation to bring about empowerment of people and positive community norms through people's participation. When we work and succeed at the community level with a focus on people's empowerment towards improving the quality of their lives, we touch the core of social transformation towards vibrant communities and vibrant nations. It is worth repeating that if it doesn't happen in the community, it doesn't happen. If it happens in communities it happens in the nation, for vibrant communities result in vibrant nations and, indeed, with great potential for resulting in an entirely *vibrant Africa*.

The health workforce at the community level

When I started on community-based healthcare projects in Kenya in the 1970s, I was not aware of any other undertakings in Africa in which people in their communities were being organized to become partners with ministries of health in their healthcare and development. Therefore, we worked on processes from scratch. I worked with a team who were trained and competent on facilitating roles in group discussion. Mrs Fanice Khanili was the leader of this team.

The first issue for discussion was what was to constitute a 'community'. Was it to be the most peripheral level of the government's administrative structure?

Was it to be along blood-lineage groups? Was it to be along faith-based groups? After a long discussion, the groups adopted an approach that decided on people living in a geographical area under the traditionally selected headman or *Liguru* in the local language. In the project sites we had selected, it turned out that there were to be 92 communities to work with. The facilitating team took turns working with each community. After each discussion session, the team and community members would agree on the issue to be tackled at the next meeting so that both the facilitating team and the community people would do some 'homework' in preparation for the next time they met, usually after two weeks.

Prior to carrying out this work, it had been said that people do not always identify health problems as their priority. So the initial discussions focused on communities identifying their priority problems. Maybe because malaria, measles, and whooping cough epidemics, as well as intestinal worms, were major concerns in the area, it turned out that the priority problems identified were all health-related. By forming tallies of identified problems, the health problems ranked as the most serious included malaria, diarrhoea, measles and whooping cough, intestinal worms, pregnancy-related problems, child birth problem, general body/joints problems, homestead/environmental/water-related challenges, short birth intervals, and special needs of school-age children.

Once the top-priority health problems had been identified, the next meetings would go through a process like this:

'Who is to solve these problems?'
    'The government' was always the first response.
    'Who in government should do it?' they would be asked.
    'Doctors! We want doctors to come solve these problems.'
    'How many communities are there in the country?' they would be asked.
    'There are very many communities' was the response.
    'And how many doctors are there in the country?'

Through this process the people realized that even if it was a good idea, there were not enough doctors, nurses, or other professional health-workers to have a group in each community. 'Then we just wait to die!' one depressed elder said.

'But what is the nature of the problems?' the people were asked.

That question led to reviewing problem by problem in terms of how it was caused, whether or not it could be prevented, and the point at which it could be best prevented. If the problem was not prevented, where would one get treatment? Were treatments simple or complicated? Through this process, the people came to realize that there was a lot that they could do for themselves.

'Train one of us to lead us in how we ourselves solve these problems', most groups requested.

And that is how we came to agree on the need for a Village or Community Health Worker (V/CHW) and worked out the details of how they were to be trained. At the same time, it was recognized that all steps on all problems could not be solved within the community. One of the tasks for homework by both groups was to make a list on what needs to be done on each identified health problem and review the list under three categories:

♦ Issues we can deal with ourselves within the community.

♦ Issues on which we need help from other levels of the health sector.

♦ Issues on which we need help from other sectors, e.g. a bridge to facilitate transfer of a woman in obstructed labour to a health centre or hospital.

Through this process, the community began to explore ways for finding solutions to all types of problems, including how the V/CHW was to be supported and the links the community needed to have with the nearest health facility. Work in these communities went on from 1977 to 1982. Some of the positive changes observed in these communities have been referred to above.

Many other activities took place around this time, including the Alma Ata Declaration[7] of 1978, the Saradidi Project under the leadership of Dr Dan Kaseje,[8] and AMREF, the African Medical and Research Foundation[9] was expanding its work in community-based healthcare. But all in all, these remained isolated events that did not reach a critical mass to change the health indices in the country and Kenya's Ministry of Health seemed to ignore the importance of putting this approach into the formal health sector. Even when the Ministry of Health articulated a Health Policy Framework for the period 1994–2004, with substantial inputs into health facilities and training, there was no provision for a community health strategy.

It was expected that the focus on improving services at health facilities would positively affect health indices, even though the majority of the population lived far from health facilities. The findings from an independent evaluation under the leadership of the World Bank in 2004 pointed out that rather than improve, the health indices had worsened.[10] Analysis of the factors contributing to this dismal state of affairs included the observation that the community element had more or less been ignored. Therefore, Kenya's next National Health Strategic Plan, 2006–10 included a community health strategy. Implementation of this community health strategy has been on-going to date, with revisions from the lessons that were being learnt and with substantial inputs from International Partners, including JICA, USAID, and UNICEF.

It is to be noted that the term 'community health worker' (CHW) tends to be used to apply to various cadres with health-related duties at the community level. Different countries may have different names by which these community health workers are known.

Since the adoption of the Declaration of Alma Ata by the World Health Assembly in 1979, a number of African ministries of health established policies and programmes in which health services have been brought close to the people, as is the case in Ghana. Other countries have established training programmes for health workers, which include mobilizing communities to actively participate in their own healthcare and development. Ethiopia, Malawi, South Africa, and Zambia are examples of countries where this is happening. In most of the countries where this is taking place, there is a designated group of cadres who provide healthcare at the community level. This may include a health professional such as a nurse being assigned to provide health services to communities as is the case in Ghana. In Malawi, health surveillance assistants have been key in promoting health in communities. In Zambia, community health assistants are being trained to carry this out. In Ethiopia, health extension workers have been trained for these tasks and each works with village health volunteers in promoting health in communities. Here I use Kenya as an example of a community level health workforce.

Kenya's four-cadre community health workforce

In Kenya the Community Health Unit (CHU), through which community health services are provided, applies to what is known in the government administrative setup as a sub-location. On average, the CHU has a population of about 5000 in about 1000 households. However, the numbers are adjusted to fit the local situation, depending on whether we are dealing with sparsely populated rural areas or densely populated urban slums.

The Kenyan community level health workforce has both technical and governance structures. The technical cadres are: community health extension workers, community midwives, and community health volunteers. The governance structure is the community health committee. The numbers required by 2017 and their roles are as follows.

Community Health Extension Workers (CHEWs)

The projected population of Kenya for the year 2017 is 46 465 827 million, which is an equivalent of 9294 community units health with a population of 5000 people in each unit. Each unit will have five CHEWs (one midwife + four general CHEWs) making a total of 46 470 CHEWs. These CHEWs are salaried staff, recruited and posted to their own communities. Currently 2100 CHEWs are working in Kenya with a further 2900 being trained in the current financial year. Many more will be needed by 2017.[11]

The roles of CHEWs are: sensitizing communities for uptake of quality health services; managing common ailments and minor injuries at community level;

carrying out basic diagnostic tests, such as malaria, pregnancy, and HIV tests at household level; following up community members and tracing defaulters to ensure compliance with health interventions, such as immunization, tuberculosis treatment, malaria control, anti-retroviral treatment, malnutrition, and antenatal care; conducting community health diagnosis and recommending suitable interventions; referring health cases to appropriate health facilities; coordinating community health activities, workers, and committees; monitoring, evaluating, and preparing community health reports; facilitating planning activities at community level; mobilizing the community and other stakeholders; advocating and mobilizing resources for community health activities; and facilitating, training, and developing community health volunteers/workers and members of community health committees.

Community Health Volunteers (CHVs)

Each CHEW is to be supported by two CHVs, making a total of 92 940 CHVs spread across the country. These volunteers have basic training to augment the services offered by CHEWs. They are mainly involved in community mobilization and sensitization, linking CHEWs to households, being birth companions to mothers going to deliver at facilities and any other tasks as requested by CHEWs. They are also involved in health education and raising awareness of health matters in the community.

Community Health Midwives (CHMWs)

This is a new cadre included in the community health workforce due to continuing high maternal mortality in Kenya. This cadre is specifically to address reproductive health matters at the community level with the aim of reversing the high maternal mortality and neonatal rates in Kenya. One midwife is to offer services in every community health unit making a total of 9294 midwives by 2017. This is a salaried position.

The key responsibility of the midwife is to keep track of those in their last month of pregnancy and ensure that they deliver at a health facility followed by family planning advice. Being a Community-based health worker, the midwife also serves as a link between level I and the formal health system in data collection and service provision for mothers and children.

Governance structure: Community Health Committees (CHC)

Each community unit has one Community Health Committee (CHC), making a total of 9294 committees by 2017. Each committee has 9 to 13 members; one being the Senior CHEW who functions as the technical advisor to the committee and also its Secretary. The roles of CHCs are to provide leadership and governance oversight in the implementation of health and health-related matters in the community, prepare and present the community annual work plan, network with other sectors and development stakeholders towards improving the health status in the community, provide management oversight of the community health workforce as well as financial management. CHC members are not on the Health Ministry's payroll.

For harmonious functioning of these cadres, it is crucial that there is clarity on the following issues:

1 The terms of services, e.g. salaried or not.

2 The selection criteria, such as level of literacy and personal characteristics.

3 Representation from all areas in the community, particularly in the cases of CHVs and CHCs. It should be ensured that there are some women and one youth representative in the CHC.

4 Stakeholder consultation on roles and responsibility of each cadre and agreement reached among the key stakeholders.

5 A curriculum developed for each cadre, tailored to the competencies required to carry out the roles and responsibilities. A training manual is also needed that provides overall guidance on the approach to training, within which local flexibility can be exercised

It is of note that in the Kenya Health Policy Framework 2013–30, the CHC is recognized within the overall governance framework, which runs from local communities through to the national level. This formal recognition of the CHC points to the realization that health services at the community level are now part of the national health system; indeed, the foundation of the national health system.

Strategic links to the health system as a whole

However well the functions at the community level take place, community health services cannot be 'stand-alone'. They function best within a continuity established in the overall national health system.

The nearest health facility to a community was designated as the link health facility to the community. If a community was close to two health facilities, the community was asked which facility they would prefer to be linked to. Occasionally one facility is linked to more than one community. These links are important because:

- The chairmen of CHCs linked to the facility are members of the facility management committee.

- When the CHC—with facilitation from the CHEWs—prepares the community annual work plan, it is in consultation of the facility management committee.

- It is to the link facility management committee that the CHC forwards its annual work plan for onward forwarding to the district/sub-county management team.
- Referrals are made from communities to the link facilities and vice versa.
- Supervision of the community level is by the sub-county health management team.

Governance links and referral linkages are both very important. The more streamlined the referral process is, the more smoothly the functions at each level perform, and the greater the satisfaction of patients. The process of referral is greatly facilitated when a member of the community health workforce is an employee of the ministry of health. In the Kenyan setting, the presence of the CHEW in the community easily links with the CHEW-level workers at the link health facility for each community. It is also useful for the CHVs to be brought to the link health facility in order for them to be familiar with the set-ups either during the training of the CHVs or on a familiarizations visit. It is useful for the health personnel to see the volunteer CHVs to take note that they are made of flesh and blood like themselves rather than thinking of them as visitors from another planet! It is useful to have a referral form that is agreed upon by the CHEWs working at the community level and the health personnel at the facility level. It is also useful to have an arrangement whereby those being referred go to a particular place, rather than starting off on the line of those to be seen for the first time.

It is to be noted that only two or three CHUs have some kind of building in which the people may sit in to carry out some functions. Yet this should not be only for two or three, but for every community health facility in view of the duties performed at the community level. For one, those in the facilities or district/sub-county level carry out supervisory visits to the CHUs. The presence of a Community Health Resource Centre facilitates this interaction as there is a place to inspect how certain functions are carried out and for providing feedback. Moreover, it is a responsibility of the CHEWs to compile data collected by CHVs for use at community dialogue days in the community, as well as preparing data for forwarding to the district level. As electronic communication becomes routine, the CHEWs should be doing this on a computer situated in the Community Resource Centre and electronically transfer the data to the district level.

Another function at the community level is that of meetings of various kinds, such as meetings of the CHEWs alone or with CHVs. Then there are the routine meetings of the CHC, especially as it prepares the community annual work plan. It is a nuisance to try and do this under a tree, due to the wind and rain and the difficulty of writing on paper on one's lap! Moreover, such a centre would be useful for holding refresher training courses for the CHVs and for holding community meetings.

What is envisaged for a Community Health Unit Resource Centre is a simple structure with one large room and two or three smaller ones, of which one would be a store for records. As communities get medical kits to use in the community, this also would be the base for keeping such kits. In the three places where such a resource centre is present, the value of the community health unit resource centre is very clear and it should be part of the planning in establishing all community health units.

Leadership and governance nationally and locally

The slogan 'Getting rid of ignorance, poverty and disease' rang across the African continent as each country attained political independence in the late 1950s and in the 1960s and after. There were vigorous beginnings in a number of countries. But in most countries, these efforts became derailed. One of the challenges was lack of appreciation of just how complex the issues of governance were, if progress was to be achieved to ensure improvement in the lives of the people in these three major enemies of development.

The next problem was a preoccupation with continuing the governance processes of the colonial masters, 'So we can show them that we can do what they used to do'. Yet the goal of governance in post-independent Africa was to have been improvement of the quality of life of all the citizens, which was not necessarily the goal of the colonial masters. So how would 'doing as they did' help to improve the quality of life of all the people since post-independent Africa continued the focus on what was happening in urban areas? How could this result in national development when less than 10% of the people lived in these centres in the immediate post-independent era? Other than keeping an eye on security matters in post-independent Africa, rural areas were left to fend for themselves 'as they had always done', i.e. continuing in ignorance, poverty, and disease.

The third problem was that a virulent social virus became prevalent in Africa. This was the virus of the ruling class doing everything to live in the circumstances in which the colonial masters had lived in isolation from all their people. To do this, they used the national resources for personal aggrandizement, living far above the means of the nations. So even what came into countries to support development was trapped into these grandiose personal schemes. In the process, many institutionalized corruption and dishonesty without any sense of embarrassment of the ignorance, poverty, and disease in which the rest of the people became increasingly trapped. As the elites joined the ruling class, less and less of the national resources, and even official development assistance, went to benefit the people.

Some of the grandiose schemes that the elites pushed for were 'white elephant' hospitals that would consume most of the health budget to which most of the population had no access. The focus was on having a grandiose place in which to work, no matter how few people benefited. By the time I was graduating from medical school in 1973, the preoccupation was to be a doctor competent to function in London, Paris, New York, and anywhere in the world. Even though this was not bad in itself, the elites in the medical field pushed into the background the fact that some of the problems we had were not the same as those in Britain or France; such as the issue of contaminating water sources and ground with open defecation in the bushes around where we live. The current elites need to recognize that our challenges are at least different and we can not only ape solutions from elsewhere where they have different problems. We have to find new solutions for our problems.

Why am I going into all this at this point? It is because even at this time there are some leaders in Africa's health sector who still want to only have a hospital or facility focus, even in those countries where the majority of the people are still in communities languishing in ignorance, poverty, and disease 50 years after political independence. It is time that Africa tailored her approaches to identifying her problems and tailoring solutions to those problems!

In the health sector, this includes recognizing that over and above providing health services, there is need to provide opportunities for creating new health-supportive community norms. We must seriously take note of the home, the household, and the community level where health is made and where health can be promoted and many diseases prevented. We must leverage the potential of the people to be involved in establishing the basis for healthy lives. This means that health at the community must be seen for what it really is: the foundation of the National Health System. The more we are successful at the community level on matters such as safe water for household use, adequate food, and supportive gender relationships, to name a few, the more we shall be in a position to reduce the crowding in our health facilities. The more communities grasp their power in terms of maintaining healthy status, the more effectively they will be able to tackle the lifestyle-related diseases that are now becoming prevalent among our people. And these changes can bring about robust national changes because, even while our countries are still in low economic status, we *can* reduce morbidity and mortality, as has been done elsewhere. When we do this, we contribute to having productive populations that can contribute to economic development.

Conclusion

Everywhere in Africa, people are becoming aware of their human rights. And in some constitutions, such as the one of Kenya of 2010, people's right to health is clearly spelt out. A time is coming; indeed, it is already here, when the ruling class and the elites will no longer have the choice of ignoring the majority of the people, while they live like Princes and Princesses of Europe. Therefore, effective healthcare from the community level is no longer a matter of scattering a few community health workers here and there, who seem to be floating in space with no anchor in the national health system.

What must be done is to have community health workers anchored in the national health system within a national governance framework that ensures their success. On this hinges the success of the entire health system that will significantly contribute to keeping the people of Africa in good health status and thus enabling them to become economically productive, so that Africa becomes a worthy global partner in matters of controlling morbidity and mortality, rather than the underdog that we are with only about 12% of the global population, yet providing 51% of child deaths and 51% of maternal deaths, and with the far greater weight of HIV/AIDS than any place in the world. It has been shown on parts of the continent that we can do it.

So let's do it. If health development does not happen in African communities, it will not happen in African nations. And if health development happens in African communities, it will happen in the nations resulting in a robust and vibrant continent whose daughters and sons can take their place in the development of the world as a partner among equals.

References

1 *Medical Care in Developing Countries*; a Symposium from Makerere edited by Maurice King, 1967.
2 **Were MK.** *Organisation and Management of Community-Based Health Care.* UNICEF 1982.
3 **Were MK.** *Organisation and Management of Community-Based Health Care.* UNICEF 1982, p. 95.
4 **Were MK.** *Organisation and Management of Community-Based Health Care.* UNICEF 1982, p. 101.
5 **Were MK.** *Organisation and Management of Community-Based Health Care.* UNICEF 1982, p. 96.
6 **Were MK.** *Organisation and Management of Community-Based Health Care*; UNICEF 1982, p 97.
7 Report of the International Conference on Primary Health Care—Alma Ata, USSR, 6–12 September 1978.
8 **Owino Kaseje DC and Sempebwa EKN.** An integrated rural health project in Saradidi, Kenya, 1989.
9 **Kibua TN, Muia DM and Keraka M.** *Efficacy of Community-Based Health Care in Kenya: An Evaluation of AMREF's 30 Years in Kibwezi*; AMREF Discussion Paper Series, 2009.
10 Ministry of Health, Kenya. *Reversing the Trends, The Second National Health Sector Strategic Plan of Kenya*, NHSSP II—2005–2010.
11 These figures are all from a Community Health Services Unit Working document 2013, Ministry of Health, Kenya, which the author participated in writing.

Chapter 9

The development of community directed treatment for tackling river blindness

Uche Amazigo

Formerly Director of the African Programme for Onchocerciasis
Control (APOC)

Dr Uche Amazigo is a Nigerian scientist who from 1996 to 2011 had the responsibility, first, as the scientific lead and later as director, to develop, implement,
and scale-up community-directed treatment across sub-Saharan Africa on
behalf of the African Programme for Onchocerciasis Control (APOC). Onchocerciasis or 'river blindness' is a devastating blinding disease that has afflicted
some of the most remote villages in Africa but can be prevented by prophylactic
treatment with ivermectin. This chapter tells the story of how African researchers developed a way of engaging rural communities themselves in delivering
and monitoring the treatment—with spectacular results. It is, as Dr Amazigo
says, 'the first programme . . . to achieve a true partnership with the rural poor
to address a regional public health issue on an unprecedented scale'. Dr Amazigo describes the difficulties they faced in bringing together all the participants,
aligning organizational and national interests, working in post-conflict situations, and developing the network of villages and community distributors. The
chapter shows how she and her colleagues succeeded through a rigorous and
energetic approach—she herself travelled extensively—and through supporting the local people. As one told her 'The problem in the field is not at the community level, it is somewhere else. The communities have the disease. They
appreciate the programme.'

The results are impressive. More than half a million community distributors
have delivered more than 600 million treatments to prevent blindness and
thereby saved an estimated 2.5 million disability adjusted life years by 2012. The
programme has also delivered 61 million treatments for other diseases. It is a
tribute to the many partners involved, from the researchers and community
distributors to local and international NGOs, donors and to Merck, which has
supplied ivermectin free since 1987.

The scourge of river blindness

Onchocerciasis, also known as river blindness, is the world's fourth leading cause of blindness. In the past approximately 120 million people were at risk of infection in 30 endemic African countries. The disease affects the poorest populations and plagues victims with maddening itching, skin disease, physical unsightly scars, de-pigmentation, impaired vision, and, ultimately, irreversible blindness.[1]

The development of a drug called ivermectin (Mectizan*) in the 1980s was the first time there was a safe and effective drug that could improve symptoms and decrease the chances of disease transmission. In 1987, the manufacturer Merck pledged to provide the drug free of charge for as long as needed to overcome river blindness as a public health problem. However, the availability of ivermectin would prove to be only half the solution. The biggest challenge was to determine a simple and effective delivery system of getting ivermectin to communities in river blindness stricken villages. The peripheral health facilities were understaffed and ill-equipped to treat common illnesses.

The solution: the development of CDTI

The community-directed treatment with ivermectin (CDTI) system became the novel idea that would revolutionize the management of onchocerciasis in endemic countries. It was born out of a necessity to enable access to ivermectin in endemic villages in sub-Saharan Africa, where villagers sometimes must trek up to 15 kilometres to access the nearest health facilities.[2]

Research and clinical trials had shown that one dose of ivermectin could relieve the disabling symptoms of the disease and kill up to 95% of the tiny worms (offspring of the adult worm) but the drug was considered at that time to have limited effect on the transmission of the parasite. Therefore, annual treatment to all endemic populations had to be continued for an indefinite period to ensure sustained control of the disease.[3] To achieve uninterrupted annual treatment in remote villages of Africa was very doubtful unless we had an effective and low cost/affordable control strategy. These challenges were so daunting that in the early 1990s the elimination of transmission of onchocerciasis was a 'far-fetched dream'.

Prior to CDTI, the Onchocerciasis Control Programme (OCP), established in 1974 by WHO, had from 1988 pioneered mass distribution of ivermectin using mobile teams. OCP virtually stopped the transmission of the disease in 11 West African countries but there were 19 countries in East, West, and Central Africa that needed control activities. The focus then was on blindness, the most devastating consequence of onchocerciasis. For this reason, and because of lack of resources, it was difficult to justify an extension of control to outside the savannah belt of West Africa, as the strain of parasite prevalent in East and most parts of Central Africa exacts its toll in the destruction of skin and is less blinding. Moreover, the stigma and disability due to onchocercal skin rashes and itching were difficult to quantify. The alternative vector control strategy of OCP was not considered feasible or cost-effective in APOC countries, given the size and thick forests that cover the river basins, except in a few places. By 1995, research studies provided evidence on the social consequences of skin diseases and unrelenting itching,[4-6] and labour losses due to itching, which ran into the millions of person-years every year,[7] justifying the expansion of control.

In 1995, the African Programme for Onchocerciasis Control (APOC) was created to extend ivermectin treatment to the 19 Central, Eastern, and Southern African countries where hundreds of at risk communities remained in great need of control activities.

CDTI development: the power of investing in research

The OCP began the search for simple and effective methods of ivermectin delivery that were sustainable in the context of the socio-economic constraints of the endemic African countries. The mobile treatment introduced by OCP was relatively expensive and had limited coverage.[8] The existing community based ivermectin treatment programmes were unable to scale up or increase treatment to more than 1.5 million people annually. The search was for a delivery system that would enable the inclusion of populations in high need communities in 19 African endemic countries with or without functional health systems.[9]

In 1994, the newly created Task Force on Onchocerciasis Operational Research (OOR) and the OCP began a series of meetings in search of a simple and sustainable strategy of delivery of ivermectin. It advertised for a multi-country study in African countries and called for proposals from a multidisciplinary group of medical, public health, and social scientists. From many applications, the task force invited African researchers and others from Europe and North America to a protocol development workshop that was held in Bamako, Mali in June 1994.

The teams submitted final research proposals from which the task force selected eight multi-disciplinary teams from five countries, Cameroon, Nigeria, Ghana, Uganda, and Mali, to participate in the study. The research questions for the study were simple and novel: 'Can communities design and implement ivermectin distribution?'; 'Which was the most effective distribution system, one designed for the community or a distribution system designed by the community?'

The main study began in mid-1995. A special feature of this study was the task force's close monitoring of the research team's activities in the field and the careful documentation of community perception and perspectives. Task force members, two per group, visited the research teams during the field work; interacted with community leaders and members to document community views about a new strategy that would delegate authority to the community to make decisions on health matters and community willingness to play a major role in the design of annual mass ivermectin distribution; community perspectives on compliance to treatment and support to community selected distributors.

The researchers, all of whom were Africans, decided on structural community participation and focused on six key components of the CDTI approach. The key components were: the characteristics of the distributors; mode of distribution of the drug; method of procurement and collection of the drug from a central collection point; referral of adverse events; supervision; and channel of communication within the community. In the report of the study, the manager of the task force and CDTI research, Dr Hans Remme, wrote: 'Trust, honesty and reliability were the main criteria used by communities for selection of Community Drug Distributors'.[10]

The multi-country study results showed coverage rates were higher in programmes designed by communities, and the community directed approach was feasible and effective in different geographical and cultural settings in Africa. The result of the study was approved by the technical consultative committee (TCC) of APOC in September 1997. In December of the same year, the governing body of APOC, the joint action forum (JAF) adopted CDTI as APOC's principal control strategy.

The results: the CDTI success story

The CDTI strategy put communities at the heart of disease management in ways that no public health programme had done before. The premise was simple: it empowered the communities to take full responsibility for ivermectin delivery, by their own decisions as to how, when, and by whom the ivermectin treatment should be administered. The community directed distributors (CDDs) would go from household to household and from village to village delivering ivermectin on an unpaid voluntary basis. In the rural isolated populations or conflict-torn countries where health systems were always weak and under-resourced, CDTI proved to be one of Africa's most successful programme in reducing onchocercal disease at low cost. Within four years of community directorship (1997–2000), the number of persons who received ivermectin treatment increased from 1.5 million to 20.4 million.[11]

I had the privilege of oversight responsibility in APOC to turn the concept of CDTI into an innovative practice, on a large scale and with proven results during 1996–2011. From 1996 to 2005, most of my country visits focused on capacity building: training of health personnel, at national, district, and front-line health facility levels; on community ownership or demonstration trainings for the NGDO staff and health workers. As the scientist to the programme, chief of sustainable drug distribution unit, and later director in 2005, I would visit on average 16 remote villages per year in the endemic countries, always accompanied by national onchocerciasis control team members. We travelled the motorable routes in 4-wheel drive vehicles trekking the rest of 1–3 kilometres until we reached the 'forgotten' villages. In all cases, the villages we trekked to turned out to have the worst cases of onchocerciasis—blindness as I witnessed in Gashaka village in Taraba state, unsightly skin lesions in Uganda, Sudan, CAR, Tanzania, and Cameroon.

'This is the first health team ever to come to our village' was a common statement by community leaders and members of the worst 'oncho communities', as these were infamously called during my over 20 years (1990–2011) walking through dangerous tracks with the natives, national control teams, and NGDO partners to find the affected villages and victims of onchocerciasis.

Following her visits to onchocerciasis endemic communities in Uganda, Hannah Brown wrote: 'After a brief exchange with the long serving nurse-cum-midwife, Dr Byamungu explains that the health centre staff want to know if this time he is accompanied by the programme's personable director, Uche Amazigo, whose innumerable visits to APOC's project sites—from Uganda's bustling west to remote mountain villages in Cameroon are just one of the reasons her programme has been lauded as the most successful public health effort in Africa.'[12]

The passion and dedication of rural communities and ivermectin distributors who worked at the forefront of the CDTI strategy often inspired me to advocate this approach among the scientific community, donors, and civil society groups. I had Agnes, my role model in Etteh, Nigeria, who became a CDD as soon as her skin lesions improved. In the southwest Province of Cameroon, a CDD who had served his community for 10 years expressed his intention to continue to serve. He cultivates tobacco and during the distribution period, dedicates time distributing ivermectin and making referrals of peers who experience side-effects. He treks 7 kilometres to collect ivermectin from the health facility.

His contribution reminded me about a statement by a member of health staff during a workshop in the early days of CDTI development: 'The problem in the field is not at the community level, it is somewhere else. The communities have the disease. They appreciate the programme.'[13] Over 1.2 million community members in 15 countries have volunteered as CDDs in 142 338 communities. Some CDDs have served for more than 10 years without external cash incentives; two CDDs lost their lives while distributing ivermectin in Sudan.

Lessons learnt: CDTI in practice; challenges and opportunities

Implementing and scaling-up of CDTI in countries

The control of river blindness now had a new weapon, a delivery strategy that seemed powerful enough to address the problem of access of the poor to a public health intervention tool. The next challenge for APOC was to implement CDTI in hundreds of remote villages, where there are no roads, no doctors, no health facilities, but where ivermectin is in high need. This task was assigned to me from inception of the strategy under the guidance of the Technical Consultative Committee (TCC) of APOC, a committee of experts in epidemiology, parasitology, medicine, ophthalmology, entomology, and public health established by the JAF in December 1995.

In 1996, the TCC and APOC management began by designing the guidelines for countries to develop national plans and project proposals in order to access ivermectin and the APOC Trust Fund. The TCC held two annual meetings in Ouagadougou, Burkina Faso. By September 1997, a guideline was ready after long and sometimes tumultuous debates on technical, medical, public health, and political issues. Issues addressed were: which countries should be provided financial and technical assistance to start the new CDTI?; what are the roles and responsibilities of the different players in CDTI?; how can we tackle all the issues of procurement and supply chain of ivermectin from the port of entry in a country to the peripheral health facilities?; plus feasibility of community ownership, sustainability of the new strategy, and capacity building of the implementation teams in countries.

The interpretation and decision on what level of disease prevalence merited intervention, the classification of endemic foci as hyper, meso, and hypo, as well as the cut-off point that determines a focus, as needing mass-distribution of ivermectin or clinic-based treatment were debated at length.

The debates though professionally handled by these experts, occasionally pointed to personal or a partner's 'hidden agendas'. Oladele Kale, the Nigerian-born public health specialist, skilfully managed heated debates, and at times struggled to keep the partnership from disintegration. Meeting reports prepared by Daniel Etyaale and myself were skilfully edited by Kale and Yankum Dadzie, first Director of APOC to minimize tension in subsequent deliberations.

Another challenge for the TCC and management was the demand of administrative fees for field operations in countries. To maximize the use of donor funds for CDTI, the World Bank and the WHO had waived all administrative fees, so 100% of donor funds could be used for CDTI and the salaries for four (lean) staff at the programme secretariat in Ouagadougou, Burkina Faso.

Among the implementing partners (communities, NGDOs, MoH), a few NGDOs demanded that the trust fund should cover the overhead costs of their support to the MoHs and communities. The TCC agreed in its deliberations for some costs to be covered from donor funds. However, the partnership was seriously challenged when some NGDOs initially asked for overhead costs of more than 25% of the annual current cost of a CDTI project. How much would be left to support affected communities in the implementation of mass drug distribution? The TCC, NGDOs, and the APOC management struggled to deal with this challenge. After extremely difficult sessions, with the majority of the NGDOs insisting on a lower overhead cost, the NGDOs agreed to receive 7.5% of the approved annual budget of a project. Interestingly, two European-based NGDOs (CBM and Sightsavers) offered their 7.5% to support CDTI and mentor a local NGDO (MITOSATH).

To set up countries' CDTI delivery and distribution systems, the TCC and management provided an annual application process for requesting financial support from WHO/APOC to release APOC trust funds administered by the World Bank. The ministries of health and their development partners' international NGOs submitted the applications. The TCC reviewed, approved, modified, or rejected annual budgets of CDTI projects and by 1998 prepared guidelines for estimation of the cost of treatment.

A next major task was how to support countries to scale up the CDTI systems. A lesson from the OCP was the epidemiological mapping of onchocerciasis prevalence in endemic areas.[14] The OOR task force, building on previous work in OCP and Cameroon, developed a system—the Rapid Epidemiological Mapping of Onchocerciasis (REMO)—which made it possible for national control programmes with APOC support to delineate over 11 600 hypo-, meso-, and hyper-endemic villages in 19 countries by 2008. As a result, beneficiary countries and the number of CDTI projects being implemented scaled up much more rapidly than otherwise would have been possible. However, the extreme shortage of infrastructure and human resources in onchocerciasis endemic areas were constraints to the completion of the REMO in countries like CAR, Chad, Liberia, and Sudan until 2010.

The book *Charting the Lion's Stare: the Story of River Blindness Mapping in Africa,* narrates the experiences of African scientists and national teams on REMO missions: '. . . the team members have coped with danger that many people would shy from but it is these experiences for which they get no recognition.'[15]

Despite these challenges, the uptake of CDTI across endemic communities was fast. The transfer of ownership to poor people became popular also, partly because of the effectiveness of the 'wonder drug' as ivermectin was called by rural poor in several of the endemic countries. The community directorship, the CDTI system, proved to be a feasible and effective way of reaching the endemic populations.

From 1997 when CDTI was launched, the number of persons who received ivermectin treatment increased rapidly. Three years after the adoption of CDTI as APOC's control strategy, the Mid-term (Phase I) External Evaluation Team in its report, dated September 2000, emphasized as overall achievements of the programme the launching of the CDTI as 'a timely and innovative strategy for fighting a widespread scourge'; the generation of enthusiasm and commitment on a wide scale; the importance of APOC field operations having positively influenced the health services of the participating countries.[16]

The establishment of CDTI was done through projects. Each CDTI project covered a limited geographic area in an endemic country, such as a number of adjacent health districts. This project approach spearheaded by Dr Azodogo Sekétéli, APOC director 1999–2005, allows for a phased introduction of CDTI in a country, focusing support to the early phases of CDTI development and applying the lessons learned to the rest of the country. Each CDTI project should be self-sustainable within a period of about 5 years after the cessation of APOC support.

By December 1997, four CDTI projects had been set up in Nigeria and Uganda, while 69% of the CBIT projects established by the NGDOs had been changed to CDTI and expanded in scope by 2000. Additionally, there were a total of 109 CDTI projects in 16 countries (Box 9.1) by 2011. The scaling-up of CDTI would not have succeeded without the dedication of NGDOs in blindness prevention's support to endemic countries in implementation and capacity building of communities.

Problems in the development of CDTI

Several problems were experienced in the development of CDTI. In the first three years, health personnel were reluctant to allow the communities to exercise authority and control over decisions and the resources of CDTI. Other challenges were the re-orientation of the attitude of implementers to consider ownership of CDTI at different levels; understanding the right way and right messages in approaching communities; de-emphasizing CDTI as a means of accruing per diems and allowances; training CDDs with special emphasis on

---

Box 9.1 CDTI in conflict and post-conflict countries 1999–2009[17]

+ 40 out of the total 108 CDTI projects are operating in 7 fragile countries: Angola, Burundi, CAR, Chad, DRC, Liberia, Southern Sudan.

+ 25 million persons treated in 2009 representing 38% total people reached through APOC.

+ <63 000 rural communities involved.

+ <10 000 CDDs distributing ivermectin, albendazole, vitamin A, and anti malarials.

+ <12 000 ministry health staff trained.

Data from World Health Organization (WHO) and African Programme for Onchocerciasis Control (APOC), *The World Health Organization Year 2009 Progress Report: 1st September 2008–31st August 2009*. Copyright © African Programme for Onchocerciasis Control (WHO/APOC) 2009.

---

individual and communities' long-term compliance to treatments (i.e. beyond the period of the 'feeling of well-being'). We struggled with these challenges. Re-orientation of attitude of health workers at national, regional, district, and health facility levels seemed the most difficult in my personal experiences.

Implementing and managing CDTI in conflict countries

Political instability also threatened the expansion of CDTI. By 1997 when the strategy was adopted by APOC, almost 50% of endemic countries were in conflict. The changing structures of endemic communities, which are of central importance in the implementation of a CDTI system, and the displacement of trained distributors of ivemectin and health workers as a result of conflict, posed challenges. Interestingly, the challenge was in some countries South Sudan, DRC and CAR that had both blinding and skin disease.

To establish CDTI in a conflict-ridden country, a thorough scan of the financial and human investments required were first carried out. This notwithstanding, we failed in the first attempts to establish CDTI in DRC, South Sudan, Liberia, and CAR. In some countries, CDTI was re-launched up to three times. The failure, as documented later in a partner's meeting, was mainly driven by two factors: sudden and incessant displacement of target populations and their distributors of ivermectin, and collapse of health infrastructure. The UN travel restrictions on WHO/APOC staff made it even more difficult to re-launch CDTI in conflict countries.

We were confronted with these issues in 1997 in the national onchocerciasis workshop in Khartoum, which I co-facilitated, and at subsequent workshops. At the pre-meeting in Khartoum, the Sudanese working for the Government of Sudan and those of Operation Life Line Sudan (OLS) had 'agreed to a close cooperation and collaboration to guarantee continuous distribution of ivermectin irrespective of the governing authority at the time.'[18] They agreed that for CDTI to be successful, health workers on both sides of the war should work under the umbrella of the Sudan NOTF. Over 20 Sudanese from the South were able to attend the first workshop in Khartoum in September 1997 and treatment in the south during the war reached 750 000 persons per year. By 2000, when CDTI was established in Chad, it became less difficult to present the system and evidence that the rural communities in sub-Saharan Africa, no matter how economically and socially poor, can play a major role in achieving favourable health outcomes. The secret is flexibility in process. For example, the communities in fragile South Sudan had helped to complete the REMO mapping of 5701 communities to delineate areas for mass drug administration by 2009; 12 000 CDDs had been trained and, with the support of APOC, CBM, Malaria Consortium, and RTI, the CDDs were treating over 3 million people annually. The success of the programme in these countries is shown by the figures in Box 9.2.

Motivation and cash incentives

Community financing of ivermectin distribution was another programme challenge we had to deal with in some countries. In Uganda, for example, mass ivermectin distribution to endemic populations had begun before the creation of APOC and the introduction of the CDTI strategy.[19] Following the adoption of CDTI, existing CBTI and mobile treatment projects began the 'painful' transition from a community based to a community directed approach. It was 'painful' for ivermectin distributors who had been receiving stipends from external partners. The CDTI strategy emphasizes non-payment of distributors by outside agencies. It was challenging, as CDD performance reduced due to non-payment of stipends they had been used to, thus resulting in fluctuating treatment coverage rates.

The management team, in particular those working directly with me, felt trapped in a dead-end of materialistic culture. We received letters from national programmes about queries from health workers and ivermectin distributors. Health workers in Uganda and CDDs demanded cash incentives and threatened a face-off. I flew to Uganda and in the company of the National Coordinator, Dr Ndyomugyenyi, and the Uganda NGDO chair, Dr Katabarwa, we travelled to the Masindi district, on my arrival in Entebbe.

On arrival in one of the villages in Masindi, a group of ivermectin distributors confronted us with their requests for cash remuneration, gumboots, raincoats, and plastic bags to safeguard treatment registers during rainy seasons. I had no contacts with Ouagadougou to seek approval and on my discretion approved that plastic bags, raincoats, and gumboots be given to CDDs working in very remote locations. Non-payment of cash incentive is an intrinsic part of the CDTI philosophy and strategy, thus non-negotiable. Given the levels of poverty prevalent in the communities, it would have been insensitive to inform CDDs they will not receive cash incentives without further explanation. The trio had to make an on the spot decision on how to address this challenge.

Seated on the grass with community leaders and members of about 80 people, we role-played the responsibilities of each partner in the 'APOC family business'. Each one of us, representing Merck, the World Bank and donors, MoHs and NGOs, shared with the attentive community the responsibilities and financing we commit to ensure that ivermectin reaches Masindi district and peripheral health posts and train CDDs. Amazingly, after we informed them about how much other partners are contributing to prevent them and their future generations from going blind, community leaders and members agreed to find financial and non-monetary remuneration for their CDDs. Our method and message to the community on that day was adopted by other countries and is to this day used in resolving the issue of payment of external monetary incentives.

We had no scientific evidence to show that provision of financial incentives to CDD can be sustained by governments or that it will improve treatment coverage rates. Any modification to CDTI in the field was science-based. To advocate for a standardized policy on incentives among agencies supporting community based health interventions, I initiated operational research and, with the help of Hans Remme, set up a multi-country study team to examine the benefits of external monetary incentives. The findings of the study were contrary to payment of cash incentives to ivermectin distributors, as that would lead to unsustainable and expensive CDTI.[20] Uncoordinated policies on external monetary incentives to community resource persons remains today an unaddressed issue that negatively impacts on delivery systems in Africa.

The challenge of engaging women distributors

As CDTI systems developed and got scaled up, we met another deadlock in communities where, due to religion, women in seclusion could not be treated. Decision-making in communities on the selection of distributors tends to follow socio-cultural hierarchies based upon patriarchy and gerontocracy. Only 21% of CDDs are women; they received less support than their male counterparts but were willing to continue as CDDs.[21] Interestingly, data of 6069 household survey respondents in three countries, Cameroon, Nigeria, and Tanzania, showed women CDDs performed as well or better than men in ivermectin distribution. We had consultations with several members of TCC and national onchocerciasis control country teams. Guided by their wisdom, Lydia Clemmons and I worked on strategies that would increase the participation of women as CDDs. During the same period, the studies of Katabarwa in Uganda convinced countries and partners on the usefulness of our approach, which significantly increased the number of female CDDs in some endemic countries.[22]

There was serious concern about the sustainability of CDTI after the cessation of the APOC trust fund, which the Onchocerciasis Unit of the World Bank had efficiently managed for almost a decade. I was encouraged by discussions with WAHO, and later with Mamoun Homeida, APOC technical staff, and Oladele Akogun, to initiate and in 2007 to launch the introduction of a curriculum and training module on community-directed interventions (CDI) in the faculties of Medicine and Health Sciences in 14 Universities in Africa.[23]

Breaking the barriers: CDTI as a vehicle for other health interventions

Though CDTI was slow in being scaled up, in post-conflict countries it led to novel ideas for other health interventions. Two innovative approaches by the Northern Sudan programme, then led by Mamoun Homeida, increased treatment coverage in displaced camps in Abu Hamad. First, the use of soldiers trained in CDTI to deliver ivermectin to communities cut off from the main population increased awareness and demand for ivermectin and greater appreciation by partners of the strength of CDTI to address the challenges of accessibility. Second, other health interventions (vitamin A supplementation, iodine, and cataract surgery) were delivered through CDTI.

The idea to use CDTI to deliver other interventions was discussed during our joint field mission to North Gondar in Ethiopia with Pamela Drameh, then coordinator of the NGDO Coalition. The Sudan CDTI was the first to demonstrate the value of 'add-on' now called 'integration' of other health interventions to ivermectin delivery in 1998. The Carter Centre supported CDTI project in Nassarawa State in Nigeria was next and on a large scale: 'Because APOC integrates into Africa's primary health care system, it has become a model for distributing other interventions. Particularly exciting is the observation that CDTI greatly enhances the efficiency of other health interventions . . . by piggybacking onto CDTI, anti-malarial bed net distribution increased nine fold'.[24]

The Role for CDTI in weak health systems in Africa

The evaluation and monitoring reports showed that the status and viability of the health systems and financial support of governments for CDTI varied significantly from country to country and from district to district within the same country. The pace of integration was promising in Uganda and Tanzania with decentralized health systems.

For sustainability, mass drug administration should be integrated into health systems but most countries' health systems were weak or non-functional in onchocerciasis endemic districts. Integration into weak systems would jeopardize the success of CDTI. The systematic neglect of peripheral health facilities and scarce resources of health delivery services were of great concern to the partners. 'We know that ivermectin is effective, that the community is not the problem. The inability of the health system in the region to assume fully its responsibilities as a partner, is our concern' a Ministry of Health staff member shouted out of frustration during the workshop on CDTI in Kenya in 1998.[25]

Because the concern about health systems in Africa remained for a longer period than expected, a similar concern was expressed in 2000, after 5 years of CDTI development.

To mitigate failure of CDTI due to weak health systems, frequent multi-country meetings and deliberations of national onchocerciasis coordinators, NGDOs organized by the APOC management exerted peer pressure on countries' decision-makers and their professional staff to deliver results. In country meetings, there was regular reference to the political and logistic difficulties in achieving sustainability of CDTI projects through integration into weak PHC systems. Country health personnel argued that the beneficiary districts are often short of resources, even where there is political will. The annual meeting of the governing body, a unique forum of health ministers of endemic countries, donors, and representatives of the NGDO coalition, was instrumental in addressing sustainability issues.

An unusual voice in international partnership

CDTI is the first programme strategy in sub-Saharan Africa that administratively and technically created a true partnership with the rural poor to address a regional public health issue, on an unprecedented scale. Until 1995, when APOC was launched, communities were not considered a lead partner in implementing the control of onchocerciasis. By officially adopting CDTI as its principal control strategy in December 1997, the APOC partnership structure was modified to include the affected communities as a major contributor in disease control. The NGDOs played a key role. This turning point in the partnership structure, the philosophy of APOC—giving authority to the poor to make decisions and implement their decisions—is one of the undisputed reasons for the success of APOC.

At every opportunity, we thought of ways to encourage ownership of the CDTI at all levels and with all partners, including the donors, not just the community. The national task forces began to identify with CDTI as their programme, refraining gradually from taking undue advantage of the projects through the drawing of per diems and allowances. This transition took much of the first four years of the development of CDTI.

During country visits, with the support of the international NGDOs, I was able in most instances to convince NGDOs' country staff and MoH personnel that approaching the communities to introduce CDTI does not require giving an impression of overt wealth, e.g. moving with a large convoy of 4-wheel vehicles. Doing so tells the community, the team has funds from the World Bank and WHO to share; and the introduction of a community directed programme is killed at that first visit to the community. The APOC training manual and video in CDTI, well-crafted by Andy Crump and APOC management, has been instrumental in scaling up CDTI.[26]

Between 1996 and 2005 I received incredible support from several NGDOs and other colleagues, in particular, Yankum Dadzie, Boakye Boatin, Jeff Watson, Josephine Namboze, Moses Katabrawa, Jonathan Jiya, Richard Ndyomugyenyi Rose Befidi, Mamoun Homeida, Hans Remme, Bruce Benton, Ok Pannenborg, Patricia Mensah, Pamela Drameh, and Elizabeth Elhassan of Sightsavers, and a host of other giants. We searched for methods to increase the empowerment of endemic communities in governance, planning, and managing CDTI.

How to achieve success in community-based programmes

A comprehensive analysis in 2001 of over 14 900 household interviews in 26 CDTI projects showed that 29% of 669 communities experienced shortages in the supply of Mectizan®, and there is a significant inverse relationship between shortage and treatment coverage ($P = 0.005$). In the same year, a visit to Tanzania with colleagues from the NGDO Coalition and the World Bank was quite revealing. We visited the Ulanga and Kilombero districts in the Morogoro region. In a meeting with over 60 community members, village and district leaders in the Kilombero district, the community was quite vocal and blamed the national coordinating team and district health workers for bringing ivermectin when most community members had left for their farms located several kilometres from the village. As a result of late arrival of the drugs, treatment coverage was low for two years.

Box 9.2 Achievements of CDTI by 2011

♦ 89% of APOC ivermectin ultimate treatment goal (90 million) was reached.

♦ More than 603 million treatments provided by communities 1997–2011 (cumulative).

♦ 61 million treatments/commodities were delivered for other health interventions by the network of community volunteers.

♦ The number of sites in which elimination of onchocerciasis was assessed increased 3-fold between 2009 and 2012.

Data from African Programme for Onchocerciasis Control, *The World Health Organization Year 2012 Progress Report: 1st September 2011–31st August 2012.* © Copyright African Programme for Onchocerciasis Control (WHO/APOC), 2012. All rights reserved, available from <http://www.who.int/apoc/publications/ENAPOCPR2012_ProgressReport2012.pdf>.

During the many visits to communities and health posts, I learnt how resilient and determined resource-poor communities are to defeat river blindness; but their efforts were sometimes undermined by the lack of training and retraining of those they selected as distributors and the late arrival of ivermectin to their collection points. Treatment coverage rates increased when communities received ivermectin at the time they decided for distribution and with regular retraining. The level of involvement of communities in CDTI programmes varied from country to country and improved through community meetings, which I was privileged to include in almost all missions, having learnt from early days at Nsukka, Nigeria before joining WHO, that valuable knowledge will be gained from listening to rural people.

I was pleased when in 1999 Dr Sekétéli approved the invitation of a community leader to speak to the Joint Action Forum, the governing body of APOC. The community leader's message was an appreciation of their having ultimate ownership, and being seen as visible stakeholder in the control of a disease. The success was real as shown by Box 9.2.

Conclusion

Onchocerciasis used to be an important public health and socio-economic problem in Africa. Over 37 million people were infected, with millions suffering from severe and unsightly skin lesions, unrelenting itching, low vision, and blindness. Investments in CDTI provided the rural poor with access to the tools and specialized knowledge they lacked, and they have exceeded our expectations of them. Through their efforts and steadfast support of NGDOs, governments, and donors, the epidemiological situation has changed dramatically; the battle against onchocerciasis has a tool, ivermectin, and a new weapon; there has been evidence of zero infection in several foci and elimination of this scourge is feasible in the foreseeable future.[27] The ability to stop transmission of river blindness in sub-Saharan Africa with weak health systems in remote areas, using a single dose of ivermectin once a year, with distribution planned and managed by trained community selected persons, is nothing short of a miracle.

CDTI is time-consuming but a strategy that allows rural Africans to design and implement delivery of interventions and services based upon long-standing cultural practices. The current trend for 'quick results and a quick fix', which undermines capacity development and the creation of partnership in which end-users can live in greater dignity, is unfortunate.

The WHO estimates that 80 million people were treated in the 19 APOC countries with ivermectin by CDTI strategy in 2011 alone, resulting in the prevention of approximately 54 000 cases of blindness each year. The annual cost of APOC operations, taking into account the free ivermectin, is approximately $0.58 per person treated. A recent modelling of the health impact of APOC estimated that between 1995 and 2010, APOC prevented 7 million years' worth of healthy life from being lost due to onchocerciasis, at a cost of US$257 million and will double this health impact between 2011 and 2015, at a cost of about US$221 million.

This makes APOC one of the most cost-efficient, large-scale public health programmes in the world, thanks to CDTI. APOC has been widely acclaimed as one of the most successful programmes in public health in Africa but the challenges at the beginning of CDTI were daunting.

Lessons

There are lessons both for the Sustainable Development Goals (SDGs) post-2015 and health providers in the Africa region. While the MGDs did not sufficiently focus on reaching the very poorest and most excluded people, CDTI focus was exclusively on the poorest populations in sub-Saharan Africa. CDTI provides lessons on successful community participation in health system's governance, partnership, financing, management, accountability, and delivery. The partners in CDTI set up and institutionalized systems for the promotion of community voices in governance and equity, built trust, and established rigorous community participation monitoring systems. The investments in research capacity building and utilization were instrumental to the success of CDTI. More than 95% of the researchers and implementers of CDTI were Africans.

CDTI system protects communities from political interference in decision-making processes; provides the poor access to break the cycle of extreme poverty; established a network of over 1.2 million trained community resources' persons in 16 countries, which if harnessed could improve access of the poor to other public health interventions. Under-utilization of this workforce will be a huge waste of donors and governments' investments in capacity development for community health strengthening, and undermine the global agenda on task-shifting.

Acknowledgements

I wish to thank the management of APOC, in particular the current Director, Dr Roungou, for granting me access to APOC's latest data; Mr Honorat Zoure, Mr Chukwu Okoronkwo, and Ms Patricia Mensah for their assistance with documentation; Professor M. Homeida and Dr B. Boatin for their valuable comments and suggestions on the manuscript. The success of community-directed treatment is the result of the contributions of many individuals —the poor, scientists from Africa and other parts of the world, ministries of health, civil society, donors, WHO, TDR, and the World Bank. The experiences in this chapter are my own perspective of the story of the development of CDTI. Thus, the errors are mine.

References

1 WHO. *Onchocerciasis and its Control*; report of a WHO Expert Committee on Onchocerciasis Control. Technical Report Series No. **852**, 1–104 Geneva, 1995.

2 **Amazigo UV, et al.** Community-driven interventions can revolutionise control of neglected tropical diseases. *Trends in Parasitology* 2012; **28** (6):231–8.

3 **Remme J, et al.** Large scale ivermectin distribution and its epidemiological consequences. *Acta Leiden* 1990; **59**:177–91.

4 **Amazigo UV, Obikeze DS.** *Socio-Cultural Factors Associated With Prevalence and Intensity of Onchocerciasis and Onchodermatitis Among Adolescent Girls in Rural Nigeria.* 1991, SER/TDR Project Report, WHO.

5 **Amazigo UV.** Onchocerciasis and women's reproductive health: indigenous and biomedical concepts. *Tropical Doctor* 1993; **23**:149–51.

6 The Pan-African Study Group on Onchocercal Skin Disease. *The Importance of Onchocercal Skin Disease*; report of a WHO/TDR/OOR sponsored multi-country study Applied Field Research Reports No. 1. TDR/AFR/RP/95.1 1995.

7 **Kim A, et al.** *Health and Labor Productivity: the Economic Impact of Onchocercal Skin Disease*; World Bank; 1997. Policy Research Working Paper 1836.

8 **Boatin BA, et al.** The impact of Mectizan on the transmission of onchocerciasis. *Annals of Tropical Medicine and Parasitology* 1998; **92** (Suppl. 1):S46–60.

9 WHO. *African Programme for Onchocerciasis Control.* Programme Document for Phase **1**. (1996–2001).

10 WHO. *Community-Directed Treatment with Ivermectin: Report of a Multi-country Study*. TDR/AFT/RP/**96**.1, 1996.

11 **Amazigo UV, et al.** Community-driven interventions can revolutionise control of neglected tropical diseases. *Trends in Parasitology*, June 2012, **28** (6), 231–8.

12 **Brown H.** *Engaging the Community: An Interview with Uche Amazigo*. PLOS Neglected Tropical Diseases. 10.1371/journal.pntd.0000268), 2008.

13 WHO/APOC. International Workshop on the Philosophy of the African Programme for Onchocerciasis Control (APOC), Concept and Harmonization of Community-Directed Treatment with Ivermectin (CDTI) projects implementation, Enugu, Nigeria (21–25 April 1997).

14 **De Sole G, Giese J, Keita FM, Remme J.** Detailed epidemiological mapping of three onchocerciasis foci in West Africa. *Acta Tropica* 1990;**48**: 203–1.

15 WHO/APOC. *Charting the Lion's Stare: the Story of River Blindness Mapping in Africa*; 1997, WHO/APOC/MG/09.2.

16 WHO. Report of the mid-term (Phase I) external evaluation of APOC. Document WHOAPOC/CS/00.3, 2010.

17 WHO-APOC. *African Programme for Onchocerciasis Control Annual Progress Report September 2008–August 2009*, Ouagadougou, 2009.

18 WHO/APOC. Workshop on the Philosophy of the African Programme for Onchocerciasis Control (APOC), Concept and Harmonization of Community-Directed Treatment with Ivermectin (CDTI) projects implementation, Khartoum, Sudan (1–6 September 1997).

19 **Meredith SE, Cross C, Amazigo UV.** Empowering communities in combating river blindness and the role of NGOs: case studies from Cameroon, Mali, Nigeria, and Uganda. *Health Research Policy and Systems* 2012;**10**:16.

20 WHO, APOC. *External Monetary Incentive Policies for Community Volunteers: Analysis Report of a Multi-Country Study*. 2008.

21 **Clemmons L, et al.** Gender issues in the community-directed treatment with ivermectin (CDTI) of the African Programme for Onchocerciasis Control (APOC). *Annals of Tropical Medicine & Parasitology* 2002;**96** (Suppl.1): S59–S74.

22 **Katabarwa MN, Habomugisha P, Ndyomugyenyi R, and Agunyo S.** Involvement and performance of women in community-directed treatment with ivermectin for onchocerciasis control in Rukungiri District, Uganda. *Annals of Tropical Medicine & Parasitology* 2001; **95** (5):485–94.

23 WHO. *Curriculum and Training Module on the Community-directed Intervention (CDI) Strategy for Faculties of Medicine and Health Sciences*, 2010, 1st edition. WHO/APOC/MG/10.1.

24 **Hotez PJ.** *Forgotten People and Forgotten Diseases: the Neglected Tropical Diseases and their Impact on Global Health and Development*. ASM Press, 2008.

25 WHO/APOC. International Workshop on the Philosophy of the African Programme for Onchocerciasis Control (APOC), Concept and Harmonization of Community-Directed Treatment with Ivermectin (CDTI) projects implementation, Nairobi, 20–25 April 1998.

26 **Tekle Eh AH, et al.** Impact of long-term treatment of onchocerciasis with ivermectin in Kaduna state, Nigeria: first evidence of the potential for elimination in the operational

area of the African Programme for Onchocerciasis Control. *Parasites & Vectors* 2012;5:28.

27 **Coffeng LE, et al.** *African Programme for Onchocerciasis Control 1995–2015: Model-Estimated Health Impact and Cost. PLoS Negl Trop Dis* 2013; 7(1): e2032. doi: 10.1371/journal.pntd.0002032.

Chapter 10

Politics, economics, and society

Bience Gawanas

Special Adviser to the Minister of Health and Social Services in
Namibia; formerly African Union Commissioner for Social Affairs

Advocate Bience Gawanas is a Namibian lawyer who was the Ombudswoman
of Namibia from 1996 before becoming the African Union Commissioner for
Social Affairs in 2003. She is currently the Special Advisor to the Minister of
Health and Social Services in Namibia. In this chapter she describes the way in
which African organizations have developed their leadership roles, saying in
conclusion that 'Africa has set for itself a strategic direction as far as health matters are concerned. It has spoken loud and clear for all to hear. What is needed
now is the support to be aligned to the implementation of these policies and
frameworks at national level.' The first section of the chapter deals with the
socio-economic and political context, arguing that 'health reforms and interventions must take into account the history of the anti-colonial struggles, the
underdevelopment of Africa and the independence of Africa'. It describes the
way health is interconnected with all other aspects of life and the disproportionate burden that women bear. The second section documents the deliberations and decision-making of the African Union and associated bodies,
demonstrating how it has enabled African leaders to work cooperatively to
exercise their leadership roles.

The African Union

From 2003 until 2012, I served as Commissioner of Social Affairs for the African Union tasked with protecting and defending the dignity and humanity of
the marginalized, excluded, vulnerable, and displaced; and upholding social
justice for all. The Department of Social Affairs (DSA), which I headed, has
been committed to carry forth this mandate with all responsibility.

It is widely acknowledged that the goal of a health programme is to achieve
well-being, social justice, and equity, and the convening of the 4th Session of the
African Union Conference of Ministers of Health under the theme 'Strengthening Health Systems for Equity' strengthens this position. Similarly, the Report

of the Commission on Social Determinants for Health[1] (CSDH) 2008 contains overarching recommendations to close the equity gap in a generation by improving daily living conditions, tackling inequitable distribution of power, money, and resources, measuring and understanding the problem, and assessing the impact of action. It is also stated 'that achieving various global health and development targets without ensuring equitable distribution across populations and within populations is of limited value.'[2]

In the final analysis, health issues are human rights' issues based on the principles and values of social justice and equity. In this regard, health interventions must take into account the need to address the wider issues of poverty, inequalities, and social exclusion.

The DSA developed policies, plans of action, declarations, and participated in continental, global, and national platforms to give Africa a voice in the area of human and social development. In particular, it worked to support Africa's governments to delineate their priorities and to ensure that the world's donors align their support around these priorities where possible, not just to follow their own agendas. We engaged with sectoral ministers and sought the counsel and guidance of the African Union Assembly of Heads of State and Government. We followed up on the implementation of these policy instruments and reported progress.

One of the highlights in my career as Commissioner for Social Affairs was the convening and supporting of the African Union Conferences of Ministers of Health every two years, helping thereby to shape the continental health agenda. During my tenure, four AU Conferences of Ministers of Health and special sessions were held, as well as Special/Extraordinary Summits on health issues. During the ministerial meetings, debates were heated but most times led to consensus on major decisions and policy instruments. These ministerial meetings were held under various themes and major policy instruments were adopted, notably the Africa Health Strategy, Policy Framework on Sexual and Reproductive Health and Rights and the Maputo Plan, African Regional Nutrition Strategy and the Pharmaceutical Manufacturing Plan for Africa. I have often been asked what Africa's health priorities were and my answer was look at the decisions taken and the policy instruments adopted and help us implement these.

Given the above, I have no doubt that African health ministers and heads of state and government provided the leadership in setting the health agenda for Africa, particularly in leading the fight against HIV/AIDS[3] and putting health on the development agenda. It created the political space within which member states, partners, and stakeholders can pursue health goals and actions. It is imperative, therefore, that interventions and support be harmonized and coordinated around continental and regional plans and strategies.

We cannot discuss health in Africa without reference to the situation of women because the health status of a country is measured by the extent to which women enjoy equal rights, in particular their sexual and reproductive health and rights.

This chapter is divided into two sections: 'Socio-economic and political context' describes the political, economic, and social context of African countries with all their diversity of experience, culture, and ethnicity, as well as their common history of colonialism, and post-colonial development. It will further look at governance issues including decision and policy making at the global (UN and other multilateral institutions), continental (AU and Regional Economic Communities (RECs)) and the national level (AU Member States), and the role of multiple actors. It will also highlight specific issues or challenges. The second section 'The African Union response to these issues' will discuss the response of the AU and its member states to health challenges on the continent, including a list of the AU Conferences of Ministers of Health and AU Special Summits on health.

The chapter will also take into account my insights gained as Commissioner for Social Affairs[4] helping to set the health policy agenda and working with African Union health ministers, experts, UN agencies, Civil Society Organizations, etc.

Socio-economic and political context

At independence, African countries had to deal with the legacy of colonialism, exploitation, and abject poverty, including the inheritance of a lopsided healthcare system. For example, in Namibia, the healthcare system was divided along racial and ethnic lines, and this necessitated the creation of one integrated healthcare system for all Namibians at independence. It also had to expand the services to rural areas, which had limited access to healthcare services. In order to improve the impact of colonialism and underdevelopment, countries drew up development plans and programmes. This was also coupled with policy reforms such as the structural adjustment programmes introduced by Bretton Woods Institutions (the World Bank and the International Monetary Fund) for the purpose of bringing about economic growth and recovery. Regrettably, these policy reforms were based on a narrow quantitative concern for economic growth and macro-economic stability. There was little or no concern for questions of equity, livelihoods, and human security.

The situation in Africa is described in the Social Policy Framework,[5] which noted that the tragic waste of human potential in Africa is caused by many factors, including a high disease burden (most of which is preventable); a lack of basic infrastructure and social services, such as roads, potable water, and sanitation; inadequate healthcare and services; poor access to basic education and training; high illiteracy rates; gender inequality; youth marginalization; and political instability in a number of countries. The population dynamics that include high infant and child morbidity and mortality rates, high maternal mortality, high prevalence of HIV/AIDS, and low life-expectancy also have serious implications for socio-economic development in Africa. The continent's situation is further aggravated by external factors such as debilitating debt, unfavourable terms of trade, and declining Foreign Direct Investment (FDI) flows.

It is against that background that we maintain that health reforms and interventions must take into account the history of the anti-colonial struggles, the underdevelopment of Africa, and the independence of Africa. The very establishment of the African Union[6] is a signal of Africa's quest for unity, development, and integration of the continent to ensure human and social development. But the dire situation of people on the continent, especially women and the rural poor, bears testimony to the challenges of fighting poverty, disease, and growing inequalities in the countries.

Despite the fact that Africa is endowed with a wealth of natural resources, it also has the poorest of people. Statistics show that the average growth rate in Africa has been increasing over the years and yet such economic benefits have not translated into a better standard of living for the people. This has left huge populations without access to basic healthcare and has increased inequalities. Thus according to the Commission on Social Determinants of Health there is a need to deal with fundamental structures of societies, including who controls power and resources.

In general, social development and hence health was seen as a drag on economic development, which has become the dominant development paradigm and created a false dichotomy between social development and economic development. But as Mkandawire (2004)[7] argues 'this approach undermines the intrinsic value of social policy and development, and the fact that issues of equity and improved livelihoods are important development goals in their own right'. Therefore, whilst most countries have macro-economic policies, the same cannot be said of social policies. Largely because of this dominant development paradigm, countries place greater emphasis on macro-economic policies rather than social policies and hence there is relatively low expenditure and investment in social development.

Africa has a disproportionately large burden from communicable and non-communicable diseases, which continues to undermine socio-economic development. However, women suffer the most. According to the findings of the Commission on Women's Health[8]: 'women bear an unacceptably huge burden of disease and death'. It explains that the state of maternal health in Africa is dismal, with the Region accounting for more than half of all maternal deaths worldwide, each year; and, sadly, the situation is not improving significantly. Although MDG 5 targets a 75% reduction of global maternal mortality between 1990 and 2015, requiring an average annual reduction of 5.5%, the actual annual average reduction in the African Region from 1990 to 2010 was 2.7%. More than half of maternal deaths occur within 24 to 48 hours after delivery due to complications ranging from postpartum haemorrhage to sepsis and hypertensive disorders. Some African mothers simply bleed to death after delivery because no skilled healthcare professional is present to help. It is estimated that about a quarter of maternal deaths could be prevented through emergency obstetric care. The situation is even more tragic considering that maternal mortality is largely preventable, as evidenced by the global disparity in maternal health outcomes. Indeed, in Europe maternal mortality is a rare event, occurring in only 20 out of 100 000 live births, compared to 480 per 100 000 in the African Region, the highest ratio of all the regions in the world.

While HIV/AIDS and maternal mortality continue to predominate in the morbidity and mortality statistics of the Region, other problems loom. In their advanced ages, African women suffer increasingly from non-communicable diseases (NCDs), notably cardiovascular diseases, cancers, diabetes, and chronic respiratory diseases. The report notes that NCD prevalence rates are generally not recorded by the health services in Africa, but the few studies undertaken suggest that they are high and even increasing. According to WHO, if nothing is done to address the issue of NCDs, they will represent at least 50% of mortality in the African Region by 2020.

I agree, therefore, that even though AIDS, tuberculosis, and malaria pose the greatest challenges, they should not overshadow the severe burden of other communicable and non-communicable diseases, as well as maternal and child mortality.

Africa's heavy burden of disease is coupled with challenges such as the poor state of or weak health systems, shortages of human resources, poor infrastructure, poor quality of public health facilities and patient care; bureaucratic delays; poor availability of medicines; slow pace of implementation and poor use of research/evidence in programme and policy intervention design. It is, therefore, clear that some countries in Africa are still not on track to meet the health MDG targets, particularly 4 and 5.[9]

Addressing Africa's heavy burden of disease will require investing in health systems and the need for collective efforts by African governments and the international community because diseases know no borders. This will also enable Africa to attain some of the global health commitments, such as the MDGs.

Much has been written and said about the lack of political will and political commitment to health issues but it is my contention that it is not a question of the lack of political will but rather the lack of implementation and the active participation of all stakeholders in the design of policies and plans. Africa is aware of the issues surrounding poor health and service delivery systems on the continent and has shown substantial political will to address these challenges, as illustrated by the significant number of commitments, decisions, declarations, strategies, programmes, and plans of action adopted at various levels of the AU leadership over the years. I wish, in particular, to refer to the AU Conferences of Ministers of Health, which provided an opportunity for the ministers and partners to share experiences on how to improve the health situation in Africa and chart the way forward.

In comparison to the past evidenced by conflicts and coups, many African countries have gone through elections that have ushered in democratic governance. This has created a space for people to be more aware of their rights to demand quality and equitable health services and there is rising expectation that government will deliver such services. However, rising costs of health competing alongside other priorities depends on the availability of resources, which means that most countries cannot deliver quality health services to people, especially those in need of such services in the rural areas.

Equally, creating better health for all is not the sole responsibility of health ministries but involves all other sectors. As was pointed out in the Report of the Commission on Social Determinants of Health cited earlier, other sectors also determine the health status of people. Thus, insufficient investment in social determinants of health and preventive action, such as clean water, improved sanitation, sustainable use of environment, and improved nutrition, which can contribute to or account for as much as between 10% and 40% of ill health in most countries and aggravate mortality especially for infants, children and adults affected by other health conditions.

One cannot write about the socio-economic and political context in Africa without reference to the situation of women. Despite legal instruments both at global and continental levels[10] guaranteeing equal rights and opportunities to all, the situation, particularly the health status, of women and girls has not improved. According to the Report of the Commission on Women's Health, women's health is the foundation for social and economic development in the African Region. Women's health is recognized as a human rights' issue and should be promoted and defended as such. Women in Africa represent slightly over 50% of the continent's human resources and so women's health has huge implications for the Region's development. The Report focused in particular on the unacceptably high level of maternal mortality in sub-Saharan Africa and calls for a fundamental rethinking of approaches to improving women's health informed by an understanding of the socio-cultural determinants that are so important in shaping it.

Women still occupy a low status in many African societies and gender inequality has rendered women and girls most vulnerable to violence against women and diseases, such as HIV/AIDS, which accounted for the high rates in maternal mortality.

A related issue is that of harmful social and cultural practices[11] resulting from the deeply entrenched patriarchal views and beliefs about the role and position of women and girls in many African societies and communities. The differentiation in roles and expectations between boys and girls, relegating girls to an inferior position, starts from birth and continues throughout their whole life. Harmful traditional practices and their impact on health, therefore, cannot be addressed without raising the questions of human rights and gender discrimination, which is at the root of such practices.

Governance

The current debate on the post-2015 development agenda, raised questions around how institutional arrangements for collective action have not kept pace with the magnitude of development challenges, the lack of equitable representation, especially for developing countries, and how coordinated groups such as the G20 have emerged in part response to the ineffectiveness of the global governance. Coupled to this is the question as to who defines Africa's health priorities and needs, and sets the health agenda. Whilst partnerships are important to mobilize resources for equitable and quality healthcare services, the issue of African ownership and leadership, as well as coordination and harmonization, remain.

Globally, the health agenda[12] is set by multilateral institutions such as UN, IMF, World Bank, plus institutions such as the Global Fund, Gates Foundation, PEPFAR, Global Commissions and taskforces, and civil society actors. The World Health Organization (WHO) as the primary UN agency is leading the global health agenda and was the first UN agency to establish a Cooperation Agreement with the former OAU in 1969. During the last two decades the WHO has been the most ardent supporter of OAU/AU health programmes, be it at country or continental levels.

However, an issue that raises concern is the African health ministers' membership of various organizations such as the AU, RECs, UN, etc. The AU health ministers' conferences are attended by all-African States except Morocco, which is not an AU Member State. On the other hand, WHO is divided[13] into the

Africa Regional Committee and the Eastern Mediterranean Regional Committee. At times decisions taken at these WHO regional meetings are at variance to those of the AU, even though all purport to set the health agenda for Africa. During the World Health Assembly, these groups meet in three separate meetings convened by AU and the two WHO Regional Committees, respectively, and each group will have to defend positions adopted at these meetings. Fortunately, ministers of health have upheld decisions that they have taken at the AU. WHO might have to reconsider these regional divisions, especially for Africa, as it also impacts on African integration and unity. For example, the AU and ECA convene the Ministers of Finance and Economic Development in one conference rather than in separate conferences as in the past and this might be a model to consider.

There also exist numerous commissions and task forces, which make recommendations including how to meet the health challenges globally and particularly in Africa. The problem is, however, those bodies at times do not acknowledge the on-going efforts on the continent leading to duplication of efforts and resources.

Continentally, the African Union is the prime organization. It works with RECs and member states to develop continental policies, programmes, and structures and, therefore, sets the health agenda for Africa. As stated in the section 'The African Union response to these issues', the AU Conference of Ministers of Health and Assembly has adopted decisions that have a far-reaching impact for African people. Since 1996, the DSA has promoted the establishment of Social Affairs and Health Desks in all Regional Economic Communities, as these Regional Groupings tended to focus efforts only on economic issues. The role of the AU in setting the health agenda will be discussed in more detail below.

At the national level, the political decision-making rests with the executive as represented by health ministries and legislative branches of government. Ministries of health are responsible for the organization and management of health services in Africa.[14] There are also health services managed by the private institutions and religious organizations. As stated by Chinua Akukwe,[15] effectiveness of a health system depends on an effective and functional ministry of health, including leadership and management, that can shape the national health policy and set norms, standards, and training. He goes on to say that managers of health services need to focus closely on the felt needs of clients and their families, and that health services must respond to needs and priorities.

Global governance has undoubtedly impacted the extent to which African governments can set priorities and plans because of the multiplicity of role players and the weak position they occupy during negotiations. The multiple memberships, the multiplicity of role players, and unclear roles brings into sharp focus the question of balancing global decisions and national ownership, sovereignty, and state obligations, subsidiarity of the different role players in setting the health agenda and the contradictory and conflicting health messages communicated as a result.

Partly because of the above, health policies and programmes become supply driven rather than demand driven and in my view Africa should fight against the uncritical acceptance of externally driven solutions and adopt a more pro-active role in taking its rightful place in the global governance for health. Unity of action and a common voice would help to achieve that.

Specific issues

Multi-sectoral approaches

There is also little inter-sectoral coordination and cooperation among the various social sector institutions and between them and the economic ministries. This tends to be the case at both the policy formulation and implementation stages.

According to the book on *Social Determinants Approaches to Public Health: from Concept to Practice* cited earlier, 'whilst people may have access to health care, they might not have access to clean and safe water, nutritious food and education'.[16] These fall under different sectors and therefore there is a need for synergy in integrated activities. Despite this awareness, there seems to no evidence of success in integration and multi-sectoral processes.

Health cuts across many sectors and the focus should not only be on health policy but rather health in all policies. As such non-health sectors take decisions that impact on health. Trade ministers attend meetings of WTO where pharmaceuticals are discussed. Whilst such ministers are interested in trade and investment issues, decisions such as on TRIPs have far-reaching consequences for health. Similarly, agriculture and food security and nutrition are very closely related. Education is also one sector that has an impact on health because an educated population will take better care of their health needs.

In this regard, there is a need to recognize that collaboration requires complementarity and dependence of action,[17] which should address health challenges in a holistic and integrated manner. This will require strengthening of inter-sectoral coordination and involve all stakeholders. There is a growing call for health in all policies rather than only health policies.[18]

Vertical programming and disease-specific interventions

Much of Africa's health sector programmes have for many years been focused on disease-specific interventions, despite the fact that one person could suffer from multiple diseases. This has led to vertical programming, which is also caused by demands made by partners in terms of their assistance and reporting requirements. Many ministries have raised concern about the conditions for receiving funding, as well as the many and different reporting structures they have to adhere to when funds are allocated for programmes.

No one doubts that HIV has caused havoc and devastation in Africa and has needed the type of response it received globally, both in terms of priority action and resources. For many years, Africa focused on HIV and Aids, TB and malaria, which were regarded as the major causes of the disease burden in Africa. Africa's response was timely and consistent, and many countries have seen reductions in HIV infections and increased access to treatment over the years, and many have put in place programmes dealing with malaria control and TB. However, this also had the unintended consequences of the development of a vertical programmes and structures within ministries.

Yet Africa was facing another silent epidemic arising from non-communicable diseases, which was not given priority because all efforts and resources were geared towards the three major diseases. Africa has the highest maternal and child mortality rates coupled with high teenage pregnancies, unwanted pregnancies leading to many unsafe abortions, and limited family planning, etc. Today, maternal and child health issues are on the continental health and development agenda with the adoption of the Policy Framework on Sexual and Reproductive Health and Rights (SRHR) and the Maputo Plan[19] but, most importantly, the launch of CARMMA in 2009. In 2010, the AU Assembly held in Kampala, Uganda, adopted Maternal and Child Health as the theme of the Summit and debated extensively and adopted key actions.

The need for an integrated approach to disease control is important because if we take a pregnant woman who is HIV positive, she is likely to receive ARV treatment prolonging her life chances but she is still faced with the risk of dying during child birth because of the lack of skilled birth attendants or lack of obstetric care. It is possible to find a common interest say in Maternal, Neonatal and Child Health and develop joint integrated programmes, which look at HIV, malaria, MNCH, etc., in a holistic manner. This will also be in line with the Maputo plan that seeks to link HIV and SRHR.

Recognizing that non-communicable diseases, particularly diabetes and cancer, and neglected tropical diseases are adding to the burden of disease in Africa, African ministers of health decided in May 2008, that the last Friday of February be celebrated as the Health Lifestyle Day and the first one was celebrated on 27 February 2009, raising awareness on healthy lifestyles and the prevention of diseases.

Despite an acknowledgement that there is a need for an integrated approach, these vertical structures have become entrenched and pose severe challenges not only in providing access to comprehensive quality healthcare, but also for multi-sectoral interventions.

Human resources for health

Africa is experiencing a shortage of health workers as many are lost to Europe, America, and the Middle East, and rural urban migration. Consequently, people are deprived of even the most basic healthcare services, information and education on hygiene, risk-free sexual behaviours, safe motherhood, and proper child-rearing. Even where these might be available, health personnel are so overwhelmed that they fail to provide proper and quality care. The question that should, therefore, occupy the minds of African leaders is what health workers are needed given the enormity of the disease burden and the shortage of health workers.

In order to deal with the human resources of health, governments including Namibia have started to invest in training of community health workers. Ethiopia provides a good example of such an initiative and the resultant impact on reducing maternal and child mortality. This is also in line with one of the recommendations of the Taskforce on Scaling-Up Education and Training of Health workers[20] for investments in the training and education of community health workers and middle-level health work force so as to effectively and practically increase the education and training of health workers quickly and on a national scale, by national governments as well as education and training bodies.

Access to medicines

Whilst Africa suffers the highest disease burden, it finds itself in an untenable situation arising from its dependency on imported essential medicines. As a result, the AU developed a Pharmaceutical Manufacturing Plan for Africa (PMPA) as mandated by the AU Conference of Ministers of Health and the 2005 AU Summit. PMPA was adopted 2007 and the African leaders collectively committed 'to pursue, with the support of our partners, the local production of generic medicines on the continent and to making full use of the flexibilities within the Trade and Related Aspects of Intellectual Property Rights (TRIPS) and DOHA Declaration on TRIPS and Public Health'. Subsequently a costed implementation was also developed.

This issue on TRIPS is further highlighted in the Report of the Commission on HIV and the Law,[21] which calls for the development of an effective intellectual property regime for pharmaceutical products. Such a regime must be consistent with international human rights' law and public health needs, while safeguarding the justifiable rights of inventors.

Related to building Africa's capacity in producing drugs is the issue of traditional medicine, which the majority of Africans rely on for their basic health needs. It is seen as the most effective means for enhancing people's access to health including medicine. During their 1st Conference of Ministers of Health in Tripoli Libya in 2003, the ministers resolved to celebrate 31 August each year as African Traditional Medicine Day to raise awareness of the centrality of Traditional Medicine in the lives of people.

Financing and sustainability

Africa has made significant progress on financing for health priorities and frameworks through domestic and external resources. During the High Level Panel Discussion on More Health for Money and More Money for Health[22] it was noted that only 6 countries out of 53 AU member states (Rwanda, Botswana, Niger, Malawi, Zambia, and Burkina Faso) have achieved the Abuja commitments of 15% of national budgets on health financing. This can be attributed to the support such countries also received through external funding but more importantly their ability to make a case for increased investment in health, and that health expenditure should not be seen as an investment and not as a cost.

In the section on 'Socio-economic and political context', I referred to multiple role players who set the health agenda. Donors, funding agencies, and institutions have done so through their funding of health programmes, which has resulted in diverse levels of funding for different aspects of health resulting in repetitions for some areas, underfunding for others, and overburdening of already strained systems with a myriad of reporting requirements. Such funds are also allocated to specific high-profile programmes (vertical programming has already been mentioned), which may not help to strengthen health systems.

Africa should avoid dependence on international financial institutions in its programmes as they tend to focus on high-profile programmes, which run counter to national ownership and local priorities. Similarly, it has been proven that the MDGs targets can be reached without a huge infusion of funds. According to a Millennium Villages' Project implemented in Kenya,[23] it primary objective was to prove that MDGs can be achieved at modest cost and in a relatively short period of time, and this entails advocacy for a more appropriate distribution of donor and government funds to support rural communities. It is also about the effective use of available resources, rather than receiving more resources.

Implementation challenges

It is important to state that the implementation of policies adopted at the AU is the responsibility of the member states, and the role of the AU is to monitor and evaluate the implementation because adoption of policies is one thing but keeping on-track and ensuring their implementation to have an impact is another.

In this regard, the DSA conducted a number of reviews on progress made by our member states in implementing some of these strategies, sharing best practices, identifying challenges, and producing concrete recommendations for the way forward. These included:

- A comprehensive 5-year review of the implementation of the Declarations and Plans of Action on HIV/AIDS, tuberculosis, and malaria.
- Review of the Plan of Action for the Decade on Traditional Medicine found that traditional medicine is still not receiving high priority by African governments, although many have incorporated traditional healers into the health system.
- Development of a Progress Assessment Tool (PAT) to assist member states for monitoring and evaluation of the implementation status of the Maputo PoA. The Maputo PoA contained 109 indicators, which were reduced to 37 qualitative and quantitative indicators in the PAT in order to facilitate comprehensive but concise reporting by Member States. Forty-three member states completed and returned the PAT on the basis of which the AUC prepared a progress report on the implementation of the Maputo PoA.
- A rapid assessment of CARMMA, which showed positive results in that there was high political commitment, multi-sectoral collaboration including CSOs, religious and traditional organizations, UN and private sector; taking an integrated approach towards FP, MNH, HIV, TB, and malaria (both at training and service delivery points) increases access to services with minimal resources; free access to healthcare for pregnant women and children; provision of scholarships for trainee nurses and midwives followed by their being bonded by government has increased availability of skilled attendants in the rural area facilities that did not have any professional or skilled health providers; addressing maternal health issues in an integrated manner with issues of gender-based violence (GBV) and female genital mutilation (FGM) with consideration and sensitivity to culture; removal of user fees to increase access to maternal and child health services; the integration of CARMMA interventions within the mainstream activities of the SRHR programme has enhanced funding possibility; allocation of budget for reproductive health divisions and assignment of credit lines for the acquisition

Whilst the AU has no shortage of policy instruments and decisions in setting the Africa Health agenda, there is a lack of effective mechanisms to monitor and ensure implementation of decisions taken by AU policy organs. The issue is not about a lack of a health agenda for Africa, but rather actions to ensure effective implementation.

It is important that AU member states focus on integrated and multi-dimensional health reforms aimed at improving the health of African populations, strengthen efforts for resource mobilization, and more effective control of major causes of morbidity and mortality. It is essential to be aware that sustainability of health reforms will largely depend on commitment, proper planning, and utilization of available resources.[24]

The African Union response to these issues

In the introduction, I stated that African leaders have provided leadership in setting the health agenda. The AU Constitutive Act[25] also provides the overall framework for human and social development, and the AU is also bound by international standards and norms.

The African Union Commission (AUC) adopted two strategic plans[26] with programmes focusing on social development, including health, population, and nutrition, which is implemented by the Department of Social Affairs (DSA). In implementing these programmes, the DSA prepare policy papers for consideration by member states experts and ministers.

During 2003 and 2012, the DSA convened the following meetings.

Technical consultative meetings

These meetings involved various stakeholders and experts to help draft policy papers and reports for submission to the AU policy organs. It also serves as a coordination of experts from various organizations, such as the Interagency Committee, which brings together the AU, RECs, and UN agencies to collaborate on HIV/AIDS, malaria and tuberculosis.

Special/extra-ordinary summits

The summit held in Maputo in July 2003 adopted the Maputo Declaration on HIV/AIDS, tuberculosis, and malaria, which re-affirmed the two Abuja Declarations.

The AU Special Summit on HIV/AIDS, Tuberculosis, and Malaria in Abuja, Nigeria, from 2 to 4 May 2006, adopted the Abuja Call for Accelerated Action Towards Universal Access to HIV/AIDS, Tuberculosis and Malaria Services in Africa. This was a follow-up to the 2001 Abuja Special Summit, where the African leaders declared HIV as an emergency, supported the establishment of the Global Fund, including a commitment to allocate 15% of national budgets to health and the establishment of AIDS Watch Africa (AWA).[27] Other related meetings that served as inputs to this summit was the Gaborone Ministerial Conference and its Declaration on a Roadmap towards Universal Access to Prevention, Treatment, Care, and Support of HIV; the Brazzaville Conference and its Brazzaville Commitment on Scaling-Up Towards Universal Access to HIV and AIDS prevention, treatment, care, and support in Africa by 2010. The First Ladies also contributed towards strengthening the fight against HIV through the Organization of African First Ladies Against AIDS (OAFLA).

Subsequent to the above, a plan of action on HIV/AIDS, TB, and malaria was developed to accelerate implementation in member states.

The 15th Ordinary Session of the Assembly took place on 25–27 July 2010, Kampala, Uganda, and the interactive debate[28] focused on maternal, infant, and child health and development. The key question was what heads of state and government will do as a collective voice of Africa in their respective countries to achieve maternal, newborn, and child health, particularly the health-related MDGs by 2015. What was remarkable about this summit debate was that it was interactive and as many as 30 heads of state and government took part in the debate. Because of this, the debate lasted for about 10 hours as leaders shared their experiences and highlighted challenges of providing quality maternal and child healthcare. The assembly adopted 10 key actions to accelerate the achievement of maternal, newborn and child health and development and thereby reduce mortality and ensure that our health systems are women- and child-centred with specific health outcomes, including investing in and promoting the health of women and children. These actions included, amongst others, to expand CARMMA to cover child mortality, and the establishment of a high-level taskforce to monitor implementation of the key actions agreed.

In addition to the above meetings, various side meetings were also held during ordinary sessions of the assembly, which were attended by some of the heads of state and government. These were the meeting on AWA, which decided on the revitalization of AWA and to expand it to cover ATM and include more heads of state.

Ministerial meetings

The 1st Session of the AU Conference of Ministers of Health (2003) was held in Tripoli, Libya under the theme 'Investing in Health for Africa's Socio-economic Development'.

The general achievements at continental and regional level that were discussed included:

1 Health issues have been put high on the Agenda of African Leaders, particularly HIV/AIDS, malaria, tuberculosis, and polio.

2 Collaboration with UN Agencies and other development partners has intensified but requires better coordination and harmonization.

3 More and more resources have been mobilized, particularly through the Global Fund, but have to be utilized rationally with good accountability.

4 Member states are more committed to fulfilling the pledges they make to promote the health and wellbeing of their peoples.

5 Regional Economic Communities (RECs), as pillars of the AU are doing better to integrate social issues into their mandates.

The 2nd Session of the AU Conference of Ministers of Health (2005) was held in Gaborone, Botswana under the theme 'Sustainable Access to Treatment and Care for the Achievement of the Millennium Development Goals'. Discussions were held on the Bamako Initiative on Essential Medicines, which reaffirmed the centrality of Primary Healthcare and traditional medicine in Africa, and also adopted the Gaborone Declaration on a Roadmap Towards Universal Access to Prevention, Care and Treatment of HIV, which underlines the need for the development of an integrated healthcare delivery system based on an essential health package and the preparation of a costed health development plan; the African Regional Nutrition Strategy (ARNS) (2005–15); the Policy Framework on Sexual and Reproductive Health and Rights, which addresses the reproductive health and rights challenges faced by Africa and mainstreaming gender issues into socio-economic development programmes and SRHR. Moreover, the AU ministers of health recommended that SRH should be among the highest six priorities of the health sector. In harmony with this ministerial recommendation the outcome of the World Summit held in New York in September 2005 reiterated the need to attain universal access to services, including access to reproductive healthcare services.

The Special Session of the AU Conference of Ministers of Health (2006) held in Maputo, Mozambique, adopted the Maputo Plan of Action[29] for the implementation of the Policy Framework on SRHR, which seeks to take the continent forward towards the goal of universal access to comprehensive sexual and reproductive health services in Africa by 2015. It is built on nine action areas: integration of sexual and reproductive health (SRH) services into primary health care; repositioning family planning; developing and promoting youth-friendly services; unsafe abortion; quality safe motherhood; resource mobilization; commodity security and monitoring and evaluation.

Today, Africa is the first continent with such comprehensive policy documents on SRHR and the Maputo plan is the most quoted reference document on SRHR in Africa. Many countries have developed roadmaps on SRHR in their own countries.

The 3rd Session of the AU Conference of Ministers of Health (2007) held in Johannesburg, South Africa under the theme 'Strengthening of Health Systems for Equity and Development'. This meeting adopted, amongst others, the Africa Health Strategy (2007–15), which serves as an overarching framework to enable coherence between countries, civil society, and the international community, with the objective of strengthening health systems in order to reduce ill-health and accelerate progress towards attainment of the MDGs in Africa. The Africa health strategy is based on the following principles amongst others: health is a developmental concern requiring a multi-sectoral response; health and access to quality, affordable healthcare is a human right; equity in healthcare is a foundation for all health systems

The 4th Session of the AU Conference of Ministers of Health (2009) held in Addis Ababa, Ethiopia, under the theme 'Universal Access to Quality Health Services: Improve Maternal, Neonatal and Child Health'. The AU is convinced that improving maternal and child health is fundamental to socio-economic development because of socio-economic factors such as poverty, low education level, and malnutrition.

CARMMA was launched by the late Prime Minister of Ethiopia, Meles Zenawi, during this meeting with the slogan 'Africa cares: no women should die while giving life'. The focus of CARMMA is to ensure accountability, coordination, and effective implementation of existing plans and strategies. Most importantly, it is an African-led and owned initiative. It is also a best practice of how continental policies can motivate and provide an impetus to national-level action. It has established common ground between global and continental initiatives, such as with the UNSG Global Strategy on MNCH.

Prior to the launch of CARMMA, AU continental workshop to harmonize/develop and institutionalize the maternal, neonatal, and child mortality reviews was held in Johannesburg, SA (13–16 April 2008). It was agreed that Africa must make every death of a mother or baby count by asking where, when, how, and why each death occurred. Since CARMMA's launch in 2009 at the CAMH4, 42 countries have launched it, nationally spearheaded by heads of state and government, first ladies, members of parliament, and other champions. What is remarkable about the country-level launches was the participation of varied stakeholders, including religious, traditional, and community leaders, representatives of government, parliament, UN agencies, and other international organizations, CSOs and communities.

Many countries choose to launch CARMMA outside of the capital cities (Ghana, South Africa, Botswana, Namibia,) so as to involve communities where most deaths occur as a result of lack of access to healthcare services. Some launches also coincided with other activities, such as the launch in South

Africa, where a conference was held bringing together senior health workers of all provinces to map out a plan for launching CARMMA in all provinces. Similarly, at the CARMMA launch in Tunisia in 2011 a conference was held bringing together African health experts to share best practices. This was because Tunisia has one of the lowest maternal mortality ratios in Africa and sets an example for other African countries. African states can and should learn from each other and adapt this to suit their own situations and to scale up such interventions.

The 5th Session of the AU Conference of Ministers of Health (2011) in Windhoek, Namibia was held under the theme 'The Impact of Climate Change on Health and Development in Africa'. This theme was appropriate given the challenges Africa was experiencing due to climate change, and to make the connection between climate change and health, agriculture, and food security, and nutrition. The ministers acknowledged that worsening morbidity and mortality rates, especially due to infectious diseases, which could be consequent to climate change, would make the achievement of the health-related MDGs more difficult. Furthermore, the already weakened health system in most African countries is unlikely to cope with the additional cost burden, which global warming and climate change could facilitate.

Special sessions

AU ministers of health organized special sessions mostly on the sidelines of the World Health Assembly in Geneva to deal with specific issues that required their consideration and adoption in-between their regular meetings. For example, a special session was held in 2010 to consider the Report on Maternal, Neonatal, and Child Health, which was submitted to, and adopted by, the 2010 AU Summit in Kampala.

Conclusion

It is with these in mind that I conclude by stating that Africa has set for itself a strategic direction as far as health matters are concerned. It has spoken loud and clear for all to hear. What is needed now is the support to be aligned to the implementation of these policies and frameworks at national level.

Africa aspires to move from commitment to results-oriented action and the key message for a better health for Africa is to focus on integrated, comprehensive, and cost-effective interventions. The role of primary healthcare is still as significant as it was more than 30 years ago, since the Alma Ata Declaration.

It is my strong belief that Africa and its partners in development by now know what the issues are, where the challenges lie, how to address them, why and when to intervene. However, this will require that Africa takes the lead in adopting a coordinated and informed African position in its dealings with principle financiers of global health and must be involved in decision-making relating to global health funding.

I remain confident that over the years, the AU has established itself as the organization that will continue to provide the leadership and create the policy space for the promotion of good health and well-being in Africa. It has also helped to transform the way in which the UN and other organizations see the AU's role in shaping the health agenda. Although there is recognition that the AU is the lead policy and decision-making organization in Africa, with a membership of 54 member states, this was more in theory rather than in practice. I am glad to note that this role has now been well established, based on partnership and mutual respect.

Despite the major challenges outlined above, there are tremendous opportunities both within Africa and at the international level, including the increasing commitment of African leaders to drive the health agenda forward. These include the current discussions on the post-2015 development agenda in which Africa must play a key role as the continent suffering this high burden of disease and high maternal and child mortality.

It is my contention that health policies and programmes in Africa must be driven by the African leadership with the support of partners and must be based on the principles of social and economic justice to reduce inequalities and inequities in the healthcare system

References

1 Report of the Commission on Social Determinants of Health. <http://www.who.int/social_determinants/thecommission/finalreport/en/index.html>.

2 WHO. *Social Determinants Approaches to Public Health: from Concept to Practice*, 2011.

3 The UN Economic Commission for Africa, African Union, UNAIDS, WHO (2004). *Scoring African Leadership for Better Health*.

4 I also made use of documents and reports developed by the Department of Social Affairs.

5 The Social Policy Framework for Africa was adopted by the 1st session of the African Union Conference of Ministers of Social Development in October 2008, Windhoek Namibia.

6 The African Union was established in 2002 as a successor to the Organization of African Unity (OAU).

7 **Mkandawire T.** 'Disempowering New Democracies and the Persistence of Poverty'. In: Max Spoor (ed.) *Globalisation, Poverty and Conflict*. Dordrecht: Kluwer Academic Publishers, pp. 117–53, 2004.

8   Commission on Women's Health, Report on Addressing the Challenges of Women's Health, WHO Regional Office for Africa, 2012 <http://www.afro.who.int/en/clusters-a-programmes/frh/gender-womens-health-a-ageing/highlights/3741-addressing-the-challenge-of-womens-health-in-africa.html> (accessed on 12 November 2013). The Commission was established in April 2010 by the WHO African Regional Committee and the AUC Commissioner also served as its member.

9   Based on current debates on the post-2015 development agenda and the AU reviews of the MDGs.

10 For example the CEDAW, AU Protocol on the Rights of Women and the AU Solemn Declaration on Gender Equality, etc.

11 AU Commission (AUC) organized the Pan-African Conference on Celebrating Courage and Overcoming Harmful Traditional Practices (HTP) in Addis Ababa, Ethiopia, 5–7October 2011. Harmful social and cultural practices include early child marriages, FGM, widow inheritance, etc.

12 The Lancet–University of Oslo Commission on Global Governance for Health, *The political origins of health equity: prospects for change* published 11 February 2014. Report can be accessed on www.thelancet.com/commissions/global-governance-for-health.

13 WHO AFRO has 46 African countries and EMRO has 8 African countries as members.

14 **See also F Omaswa and Jo Ivey Boufford (2009).** Report on Supporting Ministerial Health Leadership: A Strategy for Health Systems Strengthening submitted to Rockefeller Foundation.

15 **Akukwe C (ed.)** *Healthcare Services in Africa, Overcoming Challenges, Improving Outcomes.* Chapter 7. Adonis & Abbey Publishers Ltd, 2008.

16 WHO. *Social Determinants Approaches to Public Health: from Concept to Practice,* pp.101–2, 2011.

17 WHO. *Social Determinants Approaches to Public Health: from Concept to Practice,* pp.101–2, 2011.

18 **Leppo K** (ed). 2013. *Health in All Policies. Seizing the opportunities, implementing policies,* Department of Social Affairs and Health, Finland. www.euro.who.int.

19 This was also to operationalize the Cairo programme of action adopted in 1994.

20 Global Health Workforce Alliance. Report on Scaling-Up, Saving Lives by the Taskforce on Scaling-Up Education and Training of Health Workers. WHO, 2008. <http://www.who.int/workforcealliance/knowledge/toolkit/43/en/index.html>.

21 Report on HIV and the Law: Risks, Rights and Health of the Commission on HIV and the Law (2012) UNDP.

22 Convened by the AU at the 4th Joint Meetings of the AU conference of Ministers of Economy and Finance and ECA Conference of African Ministers of Finance, Planning and Economic Development, Addis Ababa, March 2011.

23 WHO. *Social Determinants Approaches to Public Health: from Concept to Practice,* Chapter 8, 2011.

24 **Roberts M, Hsiao W, Derman P, Reich MR.** *Getting Health Right. A Guide to Improving Performance and Equity.* Oxford University Press, 2008.

25 African Union Constitutive Act adopted at the African Union Summit (Lome, Togo) and entered into force in 2001.

26 Strategic Plan (2003–2007), Strategic Plan (2009–2012).

27 AWA was establishment with eight heads of state and government to lead the fight against HIV. In 2010, during the AWA meeting in Addis Ababa, it was decided to strengthen AWA and expand it to include Malaria and HIV and also to include more heads of state.

28 Panellists were President Yoweri Museveni of Uganda; President Armando Emilio Guebuza of Mozambique; Thoraya Ahmed Obaid, Executive Director of UNFPA; Yvonne Chaka Chaka, UNICEF and Malaria Goodwill Ambassador; and Bience Gawanas, Commissioner for Social Affairs at the African Union Commission.

29 The 2010 AU Assembly extended the Maputo Plan of Action on Sexual and Reproductive Health and Rights (SRHR) in Africa from 2010 to 2015.

Part 4

Making the best use of all the talents

Chapter 11

Introduction to Part 4: Making the best use of all the talents

Francis Omaswa and Nigel Crisp

This chapter deals with the greatest shortage in Africa—skilled health workers. It provides the background in terms of numbers, distribution, and migration of health workers, and goes on to describe some of the imaginative solutions that health leaders in Africa and elsewhere have developed to tackle these shortages. It sets the scene for the following chapters in which African health leaders describe how they have dealt with these issues, whilst developing services and professional education in tandem. It concludes with a short chapter on Indigenous Knowledge Systems.

Health workers: the scarcest resource

There are many shortages in Africa. Perhaps the greatest shortage as far as health is concerned is the shortage of skilled, supported, and motivated health workers. In reality their time is the scarcest resource and needs to be used to the very best effect.

The scale of the shortfall and the impact on peoples' lives are now well known, thanks in large part to the analysis provided in the World Health Report for 2006.[1] In this part of the book we look particularly at what can be done about this in both the short and the long term, and we illustrate this with two examples of inspiring leaders who have tackled these issues in different ways. Both of them have, like other leaders in the book, drawn on the resources available to them in the community (Chapters 12 and 13). Part 4 concludes with an account from Professor Gottlieb Monekosso (Chapter 14) of how professional education and services have developed alongside each other in sub-Saharan Africa and a final chapter on indigenous knowledge systems from Professor Catherine Hoppers (Chapter 15).

Both the editors have a special interest in this area. Francis Omaswa was Executive Director of the Global Health Workforce Alliance (GHWA) from its inception in 2005 to 2008; Nigel Crisp co-chaired a task force on scaling-up education and training with Commissioner Bience Gawanas of the African Union; and both editors have been involved in the development of the WHO Code of Practice on the international recruitment of health personnel and subsequently in the Health Workforce Migration Global Policy Council, which monitors its implementation. Francis Omaswa is also the current chair of the African Platform on Human Resources for Health.[2]

The report of the Joint Learning Initiative '*Human Resources for Health: overcoming the crisis*' in 2004 drew global attention to the health workforce crisis, which Africans had long complained about.[3] It was followed in 2006 by the World Health report '*Working Together for Health*', which provided the first global survey of the size and nature of the workforce problem. It identified a threshold in workforce density below which it was very unlikely that a country could carry out essential health interventions or meet the Millennium Development Goals. It found that there were 57 countries with critical shortfalls against this measure: 37 of them in sub-Saharan Africa. It estimated that globally there was a shortage of 2.4 million doctors, nurses, and midwives, which, together with shortages in other cadres, amounted to a shortfall of 4 million or more health workers in total.[4] Estimates for Africa suggested that there were about 1.3 million health workers in Africa and that a further 1.5 million were needed.[5]

The WHO analysis described, as far as was possible at the time, the nature of the workforce and the breakdown between professions, revealing wide geographical variations. Perhaps its most instructive insight was to compare countries on the basis of their share of the world's burden of disease and their share of the global workforce and global expenditure on health. The African Region of the WHO, which covers the whole of Africa together with Mauritius and the Seychelles, fared worst. It had at the time about 24% of the global burden of disease, 3% of the world's health workforce, and 1% of the expenditure. The position for sub-Saharan Africa by itself, without the more prosperous parts of the region, must have been even worse.[6]

In another study, the sub-Saharan African Medical Schools Survey (SAMSS), it was found that Africa, with a population of 1 billion people, trains only 6000 doctors per year, less than the UK with a population of 60 million. Further, the SAMSS found that these African medical schools were short of faculty and infrastructure.

The WHO Report and others studies have looked at the impact of these shortages on the health of populations and shown that there is a correlation between increased workforce density and reduced mortality.[7] In truth the numbers speak for themselves. There are millions of people without access to skilled health workers: mothers who can't have skilled attendants when they deliver;

people with disabilities whose conditions are eminently treatable; and children who die or are diseased because no one locally knows how to look after them when they fall ill.

Part of the global response to the WHO Report was the establishment of the Global Health Workforce Alliance (GHWA) in 2006 as a common international platform to address the crisis. It has worked with the WHO and partners to develop expertise and resources globally and to advocate for workforce issues to be become a priority in all health policies. In the 2008 Kampala Declaration, GHWA and WHO set out a strategy for dealing with the workforce crisis.[8] Subsequent monitoring reports have shown some progress but the crisis continues and health workforce issues remain very high on the list of the concerns of all governments and health leaders in sub-Saharan Africa.

These issues are complex and need to be seen in systems terms. There are problems with the supply of health workers, their recruitment and training, the social and economic environments they work in, the equipment and facilities they have to do their work, and their terms of services and pay. They are all inter-connected and affect each other. Improving one of these factors is not enough by itself and simply moves the problem to another bottleneck in the system. The root causes of the African health workforce crisis revolve around poverty, cultural and social and economic forces, and the quality of leadership and governance.

GHWA has produced a number of reports and tools over the years that cover most of these topics and identify appropriate methodologies and best practices. The biggest problem, however, remains how to implement them in an integrated fashion and sustain progress over a period of years. In this introductory chapter we will concentrate on three points, each of which has particular salience in Africa: labour markets and the migration of trained health workers; skill mix changes or task shifting or task sharing; and nursing.

Migration

The migration of trained health workers is a very significant problem both in terms of the *external* migration of people migrating from poorer countries to richer ones and the *internal* migration from poorer public health systems to better paid jobs in private organizations, international bodies, or NGOs. Both damage the public health system on which the majority of African populations depend.

The best estimates we have found are that about 150 000 people with some level of training as health workers have emigrated from sub-Saharan Africa in the last 35 years. This amounts to only about 10% of the additional numbers needed and clearly demonstrates that external migration is not the primary problem in the longer term and that the bigger need is to train more health workers. However, in the short term the high levels of migration from amongst the relatively few but highly qualified current health workers are a major problem in eroding leadership capacity.

Internal migration is mostly from rural to urban and from public to private and from government health services to NGOs, most of which are also urban. This poses an equity of access challenge that is global but worse in Africa as 70–80% of populations are rural. A tracking study by ACHEST in Uganda found that in a three-year cohort of graduates (2005–2007), 59% were located at or near the capital Kampala.[9] Approximately one-half of the global population lives in rural areas but these people are served by only 38% of the total nursing workforce and by less than a quarter of the total physicians' workforce.[10] The odds are skewed against the rural populations by the fact that people in rural communities experience more health-related problems, as they are on average sicker, poorer, and less well educated.[11]

There are no easy solutions to the health workforce problem. In the longer term the aim must be to train enough people locally and to make jobs so attractive that people will want to stay in them with better facilities, better pay, support and living conditions, and better prospects for the future for the health professionals, including education for children. African health workers should be able to work and live in dignity among the communities that they serve. In the short term many different approaches are being used within different local contexts.

Scaling-up the education and training of health workers is key to addressing the global shortages of health workers and is at the same time an important entry point into shaping a new generation of 'fit for purpose' professionals, and is currently undergoing significant rethinking. In a study commissioned by the GHWA, and co-chaired by Nigel Crisp and Bience Gawanas, it was pointed out that the education and training of health professionals should be needs based and intimately linked to service delivery.[12] The Lancet Commission on Health Professionals for the 21st Century elaborated further on this and advocated for *transformative* education in which the education system works closely with the health system to produce graduates who are not only experts and professionals, but also change agents in their communities, countries, and the world.[13] This report also advocates for team-based training to prepare health professionals to work in teams and reduce what they called 'tribalism' in the profession.

Another strong movement led by Charles Boelen is advocating for social accountability in health professionals' education and training, where health professionals are made fully conscious of the social mission of the profession.

The health profession is more than a job, it is a calling. During the 3rd Global Forum on HRH in Recife, Brazil, in November 2013, WHO released new guidelines on Transformative Education and Training of Doctors and Nurses.

In regards to addressing the problem of external migration, the WHO recognized in its Code on the International Recruitment of Health Personnel that both migrant health workers and destination countries have rights. There needs to be freedom to travel and to migrate for health workers—and some, of course, have emigrated to escape oppression—at the same time, source countries also need to benefit from the investments they are putting into educating health workers. The Code, which unfortunately still lacks any real sanctions, proposes that receiving countries should support the training and education of health workers in the 'source' countries. The Commonwealth and some receiving countries have their own codes and there are bilateral agreements between countries. Some like the UK, Norway, and Ireland have reduced inward migration massively in the recent past. Others, like the US, still have open doors.

African countries have adopted a mix of approaches to tackle emigration, including bonding and requiring health workers to work for a period after completing training before their qualification becomes official, offering qualifications that are not recognized elsewhere, and training larger numbers than are needed domestically, knowing that some will emigrate but can still benefit the country by sending home financial 'remittances'. African countries such as Ghana have arrested and reversed migration by increasing pay and improving working conditions. Interviews with medical students indicate that most prefer to work at home and serve their populations.[14] Migration is mostly caused by the 'push' factor of unfavourable home conditions, rather than by the 'pull' of a primary desire for better life abroad.

Skill mix change or task-shifting

Deploying a diverse range of health worker skill mix, also called task shifting or task sharing, are areas where Africa leads the world in creativity and application. Sharing and delegation of roles was initiated by the very first practitioners of Western medicine in Africa who were so few that it was essential for them to train a diverse group of local people to undertake tasks in the healthcare chain that suited different levels of training but could be carried out under supervision. Accordingly today, the backbone of African health systems is constituted by medical assistants, pharmacy technicians, laboratory assistants, etc. The following two chapters describe examples where people have been trained in new tasks and had the opportunity to develop their skills and use their talents outside the traditional professional boundaries. Teamwork and using all the talents is, as Dr Faal describes, the only way to deliver specialist services in a resource poor country—or, perhaps, in any country.

Sharing roles or task shifting is very often seen as a temporary measure put in place until, for example, more clinicians are available. It seems to us that this is undoubtedly right in some cases but not in others. Why would one interfere with an arrangement that is working well simply because more highly trained health workers are available? Why would African countries automatically follow the path trodden by Western countries of ever increasing specialization and costs? Evidence should be able to show what works. By contrast, we believe that countries should be proud of some of the things they are doing and in which they are leading the world. Why shouldn't Africa be proud of its achievements and build on them rather than copy Western models? After all, increasing demand for healthcare will mean that other countries will inevitably follow where Africa has led the way.

Indeed developed countries are already taking an interest and taking action. A recent study by the UK's All Party Parliamentary Group on Global Health, co-chaired by Nigel Crisp, showed that the success factors for implementing task shifting were very simple; although, of course, they required a rigorous approach to putting them into practice.

As Fig 11.1 shows, five groups of factors, starting with leadership and planning, can combine to produce an upward spiral of success. We need only turn the figure upside down to see why some attempts at skill mix change fail—through, not paying enough attentions to recruiting the right people, for example, or through failing to provide appropriate supervision or recognition. Either

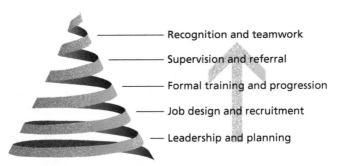

Recognition and teamwork

Supervision and referral

Formal training and progression

Job design and recruitment

Leadership and planning

Fig. 11.1 Success factors in skill mix change.[15]

Reproduced from All Party Parliamentary Group on Global Health, *All the Talents—how new roles and better teamwork can release potential and improve health services.* Copyright © 2012, with permission of the authors, available from <http://www.appg-globalhealth.org.uk/home/4556655530>.

can set off a downward spiral of failure. Dr Mocumbi's account in Chapter 12 of the training of mid-level workers to deal with obstetric emergencies reveals the rigour and attention to detail that is required for success.

Ethiopia is probably the best-known example in Africa where a government has applied the widest range of interventions to improve and strengthen the health workforce. Under the visionary leadership of Dr Tedros Adhanon Ghebreyesus, who was health minister for 7 years, it developed and largely implemented a plan to:

* Train and recruit 30 000 health extension workers, village women who had a primary role in promoting health and preventing disease but could also offer some treatments to their neighbours.
* Train and deploy large numbers of mid-level workers, skilled in particular areas of medicine or nursing such as anaesthetics or surgery.
* Increase the number of doctors trained from less than 100 a year to, initially, 1000 a year.

All of this was accompanied by appropriate policies for recruiting the right people, training them, supervising and retaining them. Ethiopia has had considerable success, although their resources are very small and their problems are immense. Minister Tedros is now Foreign Minister of his country and, whilst supportive of this book and the ideas behind it, has been unable to provide an account in his own words of his time in office. We hope that such an account will be forthcoming in due course.

Nursing

Doctors inevitably attract most of the attention in discussions about health and healthcare, although it is nurses who normally carry the greatest burden of care for patients and their families. Throughout Africa, as we have already seen and will see again in the next few chapters, nurses have taken on additional roles—sometimes with training and sometimes without—providing a very wide range of services. They are also more likely to stay in their country than the more mobile doctors and, of course, are frequently women and therefore subject themselves to the lack of power and discrimination described by Bience Gawanas in the last chapter.

We are indebted to Elisabeth Owyer, the Registrar of the Nursing Council of Kenya for setting out the position from her professional perspective in the following passages:

Nursing in Africa is largely governed by four pillars having distinct but complimentary roles. The pillars are: regulators (competent authorities/legal arm); associations/unions (welfare/political arm); educators (trainers) and departments of nursing (policy/main employers). It is important to note that many anglophone countries operate this way. However, some other countries, especially the francophone may not have the four pillars. Some may not even have a Chief Nursing Officer per se, but a coordinator of nursing activities at the Ministry of Health. Further, some may not have a Nursing Council or a Nurses Association and instead have a stand alone Midwifery association.

Nurses comprise the largest proportion of the health workforce in the region and are, therefore, the main providers of primary health care at all levels of the health system. In Kenya, nurses comprise 45% of the professional health staff and provide up to 80% of the services. Without nurses therefore, nobody can begin to talk about health systems in Africa.

The health policy and regulatory environments are changing. As a result, the consumers are concerned about rights to access and right to quality care. Indeed the Constitution of Kenya 2010 demands no less than the best level of attainable health to be provided to patients/clients.

As demand increases there is a growing shortage of nurses. According to Kerowski the demand (1.1 million) outweighs the supply (400 000). The exact demand differs from country to country with some being described by the WHO as having critical shortage. Overall, the shortage is hitting Africa hard with resultant low quality of care and a huge burden of work for the few remaining ones. Apart from that there is also faculty shortage and preparedness.

As if that is not enough, migration is still an issue in many countries. Nurses are still leaving Africa in search of green pastures elsewhere especially in the West. Currently though, in absolute terms, the numbers of nurses leaving the country have reduced from 840 per year to an average of 240 per year. The main destination is USA. This is still a worry because those who are leaving are mainly the experienced professional nurses, many of whom have an added specialization say in peri-operative nursing or critical care.

In 2011, Nelson Mandela said something I totally agree with, 'Education is the great engine for personal development'. So without the right education personal development is hindered. During my 30 years in nursing, my own dream and resolve has been to empower the Kenyan nurse. We have done this as the Council by accrediting more nursing schools to be able to cope with the growing demand for health care. In the last ten years, the numbers of schools of nursing have doubled in Kenya. However, there are still not enough opportunities for lifelong learning and workforce development. This is because, out of the 90 plus nursing schools approved, only 5 of them offer masters in nursing while none of them offers PhD in nursing. As a consequence, researchers and faculty are not being produced in sufficient numbers.

Finally, there is lack of harmonization in training and practice of nursing. As a result, there are many levels and many cadres of nurses being produced in the region. In the current situation, it is sometimes difficult to recognize training qualifications from certain jurisdictions. This complicates the spirit of reciprocal recognition and trade between the countries.

There are opportunities. Regional groupings provide platforms for knowledge sharing including the West African College of Nursing (WACN), East, Central, and Southern Africa College of Nursing (ECSACON) and South African Nurses Network (SANNAM). Opportunities for wider collaboration also exist. Recently Uganda nurses twinned with the Royal College of Nursing from the UK. Many countries and nurses associations who are members of ICN are working together in projects and programmes that strengthen the associations and nursing in the respective recipient countries.

The technological explosion means that some countries like Tanzania, Kenya, and Uganda have started eLearning to upgrade nurses from certificate to diploma level. Others like Zambia and Rwanda are considering doing the same. This helps the nurses to learn as they work so that work and families do not suffer.

I would propose that to seize these opportunities and remedy some of the challenges facing Africa we need to:

+ Establish databases on nursing to help in workforce planning and collect evidence.
+ Review and determine the ideal numbers needed and then scale up to meet these figures.
+ Sponsor masters and doctoral degrees and develop faculty and empower nurses at higher levels.
+ Ensure nurses are represented in policy making.
+ Strengthen life-long learning for nurses and provide support for nursing research.
+ Develop strong retention strategies.

Conclusion

The African health leaders writing in this book almost all mention human resources at some point. The shortage of health workers is the scarcest resource and the greatest constraint on improvement. We will return to the issue in the final chapter where we address the vision for the future.

In conclusion, the absolute key to making major changes in human resources is the existence of appropriate political will.[16] Governments and ministers of health in particular are central; whether it is Minister Motsoaledi introducing nurse-led ARV treatment in South Africa as described in Chapter 19 or Minister Mocumbi introducing *Tecnicos de Cirurgia* in Mozambique in Chapter 12. Clinical leadership is also important as shown by all the examples in this book. The people introducing changes need to have the authority and credibility to do so. Nigel Crisp has demonstrated that, even in a tightly regulated system like England's NHS, it is possible to make major changes in skill mix with determined clinical leadership and firm political will.[17]

Ominously underlying everything is the inadequate tax base in most African countries. Ministers of finance grapple with ensuring that the so-called productive sectors are funded whilst balancing this with the need to provide social services from a low GDP. There are challenges of equitable pay for the entire public service: teachers, police, and of course health workers, and there are priorities among priorities within the health sector itself. Yet all these are interconnected and interdependent and have to be supported with a focus on sustainability. Growing pressures from civil society and calls for accountability and results by development partners complicate the dilemmas faced by governments further and reinforce the need for better prepared ministries of health to play the stewardship role.

As African economies grow and the opportunity to improve health increases, it is vital that there is strong political will coupled with good leadership, governance, and stewardship of the health sector. This will be critical to identifying workable local solutions; although global solidarity and the practical support it brings will continue to be essential for some time to come.

References

1 World Health Organization: *Working Together for Health*, 2006.

2 World Health Organization: *Global Code of Practice on the International Recruitment of Health Personnel*, 2010.

3 **Chen L, et al.** *Human Resources for Health: overcoming the crisis*, 2004. <www.who.int/hrh/documents/JLi_hrh_report.pdf>.

4 World Health Organization. *Working Together for Health*; 2006, p.xviii.

5 Global Health Workforce Alliance. *Scaling up, Saving lives*. GHWA and WHO, 2008.

6 Global Health Workforce Alliance. *Scaling up, Saving lives*. GHWA and WHO, 2008, p.9.

7 Global Health Workforce Alliance. *Scaling up, Saving lives*. GHWA and WHO, 2008, p.xvi.

8 World Health Organization and Global Health Workforce Alliance. T*he Kampala Declaration*, 2008.

9 **Omaswa F, Omaswa F, Okuonzi S.** *Tracking doctors in Uganda*. 2010. <ww.achest.orgw>.

10 **Dolea C, Jean-Marc Braichet J-M, Shaw, DMP.** Health workforce retention in remote and rural areas. *Bulletin of the World Health Organization* 2009; **87**: 486.

11 **Wilson NW, et al.** A critical review of interventions to redress the inequitable distribution of healthcare professionals to rural and remote areas. *Rural and Remote Health* 2009; 9: 1060. <http://www.rrh.org.au>.

12 GHWA and WHO. *Scaling Up, Saving Lives*. 2008.

13 **Frenk J, et al.** Education of Health Professionals for a new century: transforming education to strengthen health systems in an interdependent world. *The Lancet* 2010; **376**: 1923–58.

14 **Mullan F, et al.** Medical Schools in Sub-Saharan Africa. *The Lancet* 2011; PIISP140–6736 (10): 61961–7.

15 All Party Parliamentary Group on Global Health. *All the Talents—how new roles and better teamwork can release potential and improve health services*. July 2012.

16 Global Health Workforce Alliance. *Scaling up, Saving lives*. GHWA and WHO, 2008.

17 **Crisp N.** *24 Hours to Save the NHS—the Chief Executive's account of reform 2000 to 2006*. Oxford, Oxford University Press, 2011.

Chapter 12

Tecnicos de cirurgia—assistant medical officers trained for surgery in Mozambique

Pascoal Mocumbi

Formerly Health Minister and later Prime Minister of Mozambique

Dr Pascoal Mocumbi qualified as a doctor in Europe before returning to his own country of Mozambique at independence. He became Minister of Health in 1980 at a critical time in his country's history when the health system was under great pressure because of the casualties from the civil war. It was also under attack from the rebels who were intent on destroying government infrastructure, including health facilities. He later went on to be Mozambique's Prime Minister for 10 years from 1994. This chapter describes how, faced with a severe shortage of trained workers, he initiated the training of *tecnicos de cirurgia*—assistant medical officers trained for surgery—to tackle the pressing needs of pregnant women and war casualties. This account shows that by careful recruitment, training, and consistent supervision it is possible to develop and train non-medical workers to deliver services that are only undertaken by doctors in Europe, the US, and most of the rest of the world. Almost 30 years later the programme is still in place and serving the majority of the rural populations of Mozambique. The country continues to face enormous health needs but has become, in the last few years, one of the 'frontier economies' of sub-Saharan Africa, growing fast economically and beginning to be able to offer its young population the promise of greater opportunities and better services. At the same time, other countries in Africa and beyond, faced with their own crises in how to provide healthcare for their populations, are interested in learning the lessons from Mozambique's experiences.

Exodus of the doctors

When Mozambique became independent in 1975 there was an exodus of settlers back to Portugal taking with them all their experience and skills. They left behind a very low-income country with, as a result, even fewer resources. The migration affected every sector of the economy and the country. In the health sector it took away an estimated 85% of the country's doctors and left only 80 doctors, of which I was one, to serve a nation of 14 million people. We had previously had over 500.

Mozambique is a large and very rural country; even today two-thirds of the population live in villages away from the urban areas. In United Nations terms it was classified as underdeveloped and came in the bottom 15% of the world in terms of the Human Development Index.[1] In common with other sub-Saharan African countries it suffered all the diseases of poverty (such as malaria, acute diarrhoea, acute respiratory infections, and tuberculosis), had high child and maternal mortality rates, and later the country was affected by the HIV/AIDS epidemic and all its associated diseases.

Given this background, the new government gave priority to developing human resources for the public sector and particularly for the health needs of its widely dispersed population. There was little scope to increase the numbers of doctors rapidly because at that time the faculty of medicine, and other training centres for healthcare staff, were restricted by limited pools of qualified applicants and a shortage of senior trainers. The only medical school, for example, had capacity to graduate per year about 15 doctors in the years following freedom. This scarcity of trained medical doctors and other professionals therefore motivated me, as Minister, to start the training of a new cadre of professionals, similar to the assistant medical officers in Tanzania and elsewhere in Africa, which became called 'tecnicos de medicina' or medical technicians.

This was all part of a new training policy, which set out an intensive programme to train health workers, particularly nurses, midwifes, and 'tecnicos de medicina' to take the place of doctors in many roles and tasks by delegation of responsibility. Candidates for basic health staff training were required to have attained the fourth grade in education. Starting out with this training, it was possible for an individual with determination and perseverance to proceed to middle-level training and eventually to become a doctor.

This in turn was part of a wider approach of establishing a primary healthcare system that was cited by the WHO as a model for other developing countries.[2] Over 90% of the population had been provided with a smallpox vaccine in a massive vaccination campaign, which was Mozambique's contribution to the WHO global call for smallpox eradication. However, these improvements were threatened by the civil war that followed independence.

I had worked as a doctor in the central country during this period but in 1980, four years after independence, I became the Minister of Health. By that time the Mozambican health system was being put under severe strain by having to care for the high numbers of casualties resulting from a civil war instigated by the

South African apartheid regime, which lasted until 1992. Moreover, part of the rebels' strategy was to destroy government infrastructures in an attempt to destabilise the country and the government. This, of course, included health and education systems, and much of the progress that had been made was reversed during this long period of war. The Human Development Index declined still further due to the civil war during the decade from 1980.[3]

There was a major unmet need for emergency healthcare and life-saving skills in rural areas, with the biggest problems being obstetric emergencies and war casualties. Women in particular were amongst the most affected. There was an unacceptable death toll and disability from pregnancy-related complications and injuries derived from accidents and violence—among which countless women and girls suffered the health consequences of gender-based violence, harmful traditional practices, war, and civil conflict.

As the Minister I was very concerned about the lack of health workers trained to deal with maternal and newborn health. I was also very conscious of the cost-effectiveness of training doctors and then deploying out in the rural areas the very few medical doctors who were coming out of the medical school. I knew that their skills could have a bigger impact on more people in the hospitals and the towns, rather than scattered thinly around the country.

As the Minister of Health responsible, I therefore felt obliged to create a new career for people to work in maternal and child health (*saude materna e infantile*) and, as part of this, to plan and implement the training of the *tecnicos de cirurgia* (assistant medical officers) with surgical skills. The idea of non-physician surgeons came from the observation that some of the nurses and medical assistants working in rural areas (the *tecnicos de medicina*) had begun, in the absence of surgeons, teaching themselves basic surgical techniques and practicing emergency surgery. It was clear that we could build on their experience and also learn from other countries and other professionals elsewhere about how to do this most effectively.

At the beginning, as a doctor myself, I was rather concerned about this because it was the first time that training of non-doctors for 'major surgery' was being introduced in Mozambique based on experienced nurses. On the other hand I was confident that the training of *tecnicos de cirurgia* would succeed because of the evidence coming from other African countries, such as Tanzania and Guinea Conakry. Additionally, there was already some evidence from supervision of their work in Mozambique, which indicated they performed these obstetric surgery interventions successfully.

We did not train the *tecnicos de cirurgia* as doctors because they only needed certain skills and knowledge and not the full curriculum. Other aspects, such as weaknesses in the knowledge of anatomy, physiology, and pharmacology for prescriptions, were left to be handled by the general practitioners with whom they worked as a team.

Naturally, I faced resistance to this innovation from medical doctors, particularly from surgical practitioners. It was also resisted by some members of the nursing staff who seemed to see our initiative as an adventure and that it was irresponsible to allow a non-doctor to use a scalpel. The overriding priority, however, was to save lives in more remote areas and this programme allowed us to train *tecnicos* in 3 years rather than doctors in a much longer period. The results speak for themselves. The performance of *tecnicos* and good retention in remote areas contributed widely to the reduction of maternal mortality in the country, reducing it to 408 deaths in100 000 deliveries by 2006.

Implementing the policy

The training of *tecnicos de medicina* to become *tecnicos de cirurgia* with surgical skills was started in 1983/84 by Mozambican and expatriate surgeons and obstetricians, who were concerned by the shortage of surgeons in the country. The recruitment and training of candidates were crucial in guaranteeing the quality of the scheme and ensuring that good standards would be achieved. Accordingly we recruited mainly among the best mid-level *tecnicos de medicina* and nurses who had gained substantial experience in rural areas.

The training programmes have been continuously developed over the years. Currently, the training of *tecnicos de cirurgia* consists of 2 years of clinical surgical training at the Central Hospital in Maputo, followed by an 'internship' with qualified surgeons at a provincial hospital. All candidates for the *tecnicos de cirurgia* training programme must have 2 or 3 years of basic or mid-level medical training, e.g. as nurse or *tecnico de medicina*, and several years of rural practice. Upon passing a final examination, most *tecnicos de cirurgia* are posted to district or rural hospitals where they could practice with the support and supervision of the provincial surgeon.

Supervision of their work and access, where necessary, to refreshment and re-training are vital components. There are still very few surgeons in the country and one is attached to each Province specifically to provide the necessary leadership and supervision for everyone undertaking surgery in the Province.

Medical training in Mozambique at the public university, Eduardo Mondlane, is based on a European model. The 6-year programme consists of classroom instruction in basic biomedical subjects, hospital rotations, and a final-year rural clerkship. Graduates work in rural areas for 2 years before returning for residency training. Residencies in surgery and obstetrics and gynaecology take a further 5 years. Two to three obstetricians and two to three surgeons on average graduate from the residency programme each year.

The training of the non-physician clinicians is preceded by careful selection of candidates based on the criteria already explained and a tight observation of their behavior during the initial phase of training in the hospital environment. Emphasis is placed throughout the internship on improving the quality of skills and knowledge acquired in their earlier training. It is about building on what they already know. To date 114 *tecnicos de cirurgia* have been trained and have been assigned to peripheral hospitals in the country, mainly in rural hospitals. This is slightly more than the number of surgeons who have been trained over the nearly 30 years since this programme has been in place.

It is worth noting the part that has been played by professionals from outside the country in getting this programme underway. Solidarity and assistance to Mozambique by both government and non-government partners helped us to achieve our freedom as a nation. When it was confronted with this crisis in human resources for health, our government launched calls for applicants to fill specific health needs. The urgent gaps of doctors, surgeons, obstetric-gynaecologists, pharmacists, anaesthetists, nurses, midwives, and assistant medical officers were filled for a limited time from African countries, such as Zambia, the Tanzania, and Guinea Conakry, as part of their solidarity support for the new country.

A number of individuals played very important roles. I initiated the training of *tecnicos de cirurgia* with the support of a carefully selected team of surgeons and obstetricians among national and expatriates, namely, the then Vice-Minister of Health, Professor Dr Fernando Vaz, Dr Colin Mc Cord, Dr Orlando Vieira, and Dr Antonio Bugalho. The three first *tecnicos de cirurgia* training courses were supported by three different partners. As Minister of Health I was extremely indebted to these partners and to the quality and skills of the trainers themselves.

Impact—the backbone of emergency surgical care for most of the country

Away from the three central hospitals of Maputo, Beira, and Nampula that serve 10% of the population, *tecnicos di cirurgia* now constitute the backbone of emergency surgical care in Mozambique for the vast majority of the population. *Tecnicos* perform a wide range of major surgery: 70% of which are emergency interventions. A study published in 2007 showed that 92% of all caesarean sections, obstetric hysterectomies, and laparotomies for ectopic pregnancies performed in all district hospitals in a period of a year were performed by *tecnicos de cirurgia*.[4]

There is now a series of studies published in peer-reviewed journals, which look at the work of *tecnicos de cirurgia* in terms of quality and cost-effectiveness.

One such study assessing perceptions of the standard of care provided by *tec-nicos de cirurgia* found that 90% of doctors, including surgeons, obstetricians, traumatologists, and other health workers, rated the care provided by *tecnicos* to be good.[5] A further study showed that there were no clinically significant differences in post-operative outcomes between surgical operations undertaken by *tecnicos de cirurgia* and by doctors, and that post-operative mortality rates for 10 258 patients operated on by *tecnicos* were very low at 0.4% for emergency surgeries and 0.1% for elective procedures.[6]

It is clear that *tecnicos* can deliver good quality emergency surgical care, even in remote areas where there are no doctors. The economic effectiveness of the programme has also been demonstrated through the studies referred to earlier and in other publications. They have also shown that retention is much better than for doctors. A study that looked at doctors graduating and *tecnicos* being trained in 1987, 1988, and 1996 revealed that none of the 59 doctors remained working in district hospitals 7 years after their graduation, whilst all 34 *tecnicos* were still in post 7 years after completing their training.[7] This demonstrated just how cost-effective the policy is when looking at the training and deployment costs spread over a 30-year or longer working career.

Conclusions

There are many lessons to be drawn from our experience in Mozambique. The results of this study should not be taken to imply that policy makers would or should choose one health worker cadre over another based on cost alone. Midlevel providers, such as *tecnicos de cirurgia*, are complementary to, not substitutes for, physicians. Given the magnitude of the health-worker crisis, both physicians and middle-level providers will be required in substantially larger numbers in Mozambique and eventually in other developing countries. Countries need to look at their situations to prioritize actions that relate worker needs to health policy and establish dialogue with other sectors, such as education, finance, public service, and the civil society to ensure cohesive actions.

Evidence from the Mozambique experience suggests that training more midlevel health workers in surgery is a good investment in responding to the Human Resources for Health shortage and the health and developmental challenges in sub-Saharan Africa and elsewhere in the world.

Mozambique has itself learned from its experience and has further developed its own policy, recognizing in particular the importance of teamwork in delivering quality care. From 1983/84 to date, the training of non-physician clinicians has been well-structured in a school with a syllabus, process of evaluations, and an internship programme. Subsequently, an *Institute Superior de Ciencias de*

Saude (Higher Institute of Health Sciences) was created by the cabinet decree number 47/2003 in order to strengthen the teamwork at 149 district hospitals and further respond to the human resources crisis. This ensures that all health workers are able to recognize their role in a team that provides care for patients.

In addition a new programme of training in major obstetric surgery has now been started for midwives (*Enfermeiras de Saude Materna*). The new training, based on nursing with an emphasis on diagnostic and treatment skills, practice of major emergency surgery, and the concept of teamwork, takes three and half years of theoretical and practical training plus six months of internship in a regional or district hospital.

More than 40 years on from independence there are now many Portuguese coming to Mozambique as it grows economically as one of the 'frontier economies' of Africa. At the same time it is interesting to note that, as other more developed countries experience their own crises in meeting the health needs of their populations, there is growing interest globally in our experiences of training and in deploying non-physician clinicians to meet the needs of our population.

Looking forward, there is more to do to meet the Millennium Development Goals and improve the health of our population. I believe that African leaders have to see training mid-level providers as being key to delivering quality healthcare services, improving African people's health, and developing our continent. It will also be crucial to strengthen multi-disciplinary coordination within the ministry sector—for example, in maternal and child health—assigning a lead institution to coordinate the collection and the collation of data across all sectors and units. Least but not last, the ministry might consider a disaster preparedness mechanism.

References

1 UNDP. *International Human Development Index.* http://hdr.undp.org/en/statistics/hdi.

2 **Walt G, Melamed A.** *Towards a People's Health Service.* London, Zed Books, 1983.

3 UNDP. *International Human Development Index.* http://hdr.undp.org/en/statistics/hdi.

4 **Kruk ME, Pereira C, Vaz F, Bergström S, Galea S.** Economic evaluation of surgivcally trained assistant medical officers in performing major obstetric surgery in Mozambique. *British Journal of Obstetrics and Gynecology* 2007; **114**: 1253–60.

5 **Pereira C, Bughalo A, Berstöm S, Vaz F, Cotiro MA.** A comparative study of caesarean deliveries by assistant medical officers and obstetricians in Mozambique. *British Journal of Obstetrics and Gynaecology* 1996; **103**:508–12.

6 **Vaz F, Bergström S, Vaz ML, Langa J, Bughalo A.** Training medical assistants for surgery. *Bulletin World Health Organisation* 1999; **77**:689–91.

7 **Pereira C, et al.** Meeting the need for emergency obstetric acre in Mozambique: work performance and history of medical doctors and assistant medical officers trained for surgery. *British Journal of Obstetrics and Gynaecology* 2007;**114**:1530–3.

Chapter 13

All the skills of the health team

Hannah Faal

Formerly President of the International Agency for the Prevention of Blindness

Dr Hannah Faal is a highly respected Nigerian ophthalmologist who has been a major driving force for improving eye health in sub-Saharan Africa, developing new approaches and spreading good practices. In this chapter she describes how she led the development of eye services in the Gambia by concentrating on creating a team of people of different skills who together could—and did—bring enormous improvements to the community. It was, as she says a journey in which she had to make a 'personal paradigm shift' from seeing herself as an individual clinician to someone who had to 'spearhead the effort' and make sure everyone in the wider team was able to operate optimally. The chapter shows how she systematically built up the service and team; concentrating on prevention of disease as well as treatment—all the time learning from others in her profession and from her frequent visits and observations in the villages of the Gambia. She developed a plan and a model that engaged every member of her wider team and involved patients and community members with, for example, her 'friends of vision' and 'mother hen' approaches. The chapter shows the impact this important work has had on the West Africa region and the world, as well as improving eye health in the Gambia itself. It describes how to run a specialist service in a resource-poor country and how to work across country boundaries within a region. It holds lessons in teamwork and organization for other specialties and regions of the world.

Eye health in The Gambia

In 1970, two medical graduates of the University of Ibadan in Nigeria went on a visit to The Gambia, the female for the first time and the male to introduce her to his home country. They visited the country's only two hospitals. Over the next decade they got married, completed post-graduate training in ophthalmology and obstetrics/gynaecology, respectively, and started careers in the academic milieu of universities and teaching hospitals in Nigeria. The force of the need in The Gambia was an irresistible pull, however, and in 1980 both returned to The Gambia.

The Gambia with an area of just over 11 000 km² is the smallest country in mainland Africa and lies west to east in the drought-prone Sahel belt. It is essentially made up of the River Gambia and its two banks, and stretches from an 80 km coastline of the Atlantic Ocean to about 484 km inland. Its 740km-long porous border with Senegal is artificial, a result of colonization: Senegal by the French and The Gambia by the British, with differing official languages, systems of governance, and impact on the indigenous cultures. There is high population mobility across the border because the peoples on both sides are of shared families, the same tribes, language, culture, and religion. Both countries are members of the multilingual Economic Community of West African states (ECOWAS) and its health agency, the West African Health Community and, since 2000, the West Africa Health Organization. These bi-country and regional relationships had a major impact on the eye care programme.

In 1980, the population was about 500 000. With an economy based mainly on the export of groundnuts and an estimated GDP per capita of US$250.00 in 1982/83[1], it was classified as a least developed country. The government health services were very basic with just 2 general hospitals, 15 health centres and 14 dispensaries. Unique to The Gambia was the British-funded Medical Research Council (MRC) unit located in the capital Banjul with 3 field laboratories, which later became a research partner in the trachoma control component of the eye care programme.

The health services had only in the recent past accepted the concept of specialist doctors functioning at the national referral hospital, the Royal Victoria Hospital (RVH), in Banjul. The backbone of the services was a cadre designated as 'dresser dispensers'—state registered nurses who had received extra training to function as paramedics, a task shifting. They provided services in all the other hospitals and health centres.

A recently retired ophthalmologist from the MRC provided rudimentary eye services at the RVH: general eye clinics in one consulting room, a small number of admissions (five beds) and surgeries using access to a minor surgical theatre. The support staff was one trained ophthalmic nurse and four auxiliary nurses. Patient-based medical notes were written on small sheets of paper collected from the government printing department. Prescriptions were limited to a small range of eye drugs (mainly hospital manufactured as neither the local pharmacies nor the government stocked any) and there were only three sets of surgical instruments. The Royal Commonwealth Society for the Blind (RCSB, later Sightsavers) provided diagnostic and surgical instruments, and locum cover for when the ophthalmologist went on leave.

The Swedish Government provided a Swedish optometrist, lenses, and equipment. Two Gambian school leavers, who had been trained on the job, supported the optometrist. The service functioned virtually as a stand-alone unit providing mainly aphakic glasses for the few cataract patients who had been operated on. Literacy rate was only 10% so the demand for reading glasses was very low.[2] The Swedish support ended in 1983.

I joined the staff as a second consultant ophthalmologist in 1980, from the academic environment of the department of ophthalmology of a teaching hospital.

Patients came from all over Gambia and surrounding countries, most were very poor and had travelled for three or more days to get to the hospital. They presented very late, most of them blind from preventable causes: cataract, corneal ulcers, panophthalmitis, advanced glaucoma, children with vitamin A deficiency, measles, and retinobastoma.

It dawned on me that even if I spent all hours in the hospital managing patients as they came, I would not prevent blindness and suffering. I had to ensure that what could be prevented was prevented, that what could be treated early was treated on time; and that care was provided at home or as close to home as possible. I certainly could not truly practice as an ophthalmologist providing the tertiary level care for which I had received so many years of training.

In the face of such extreme human resource constraint, the first priority was to maximize the skills and output of the few auxiliary nurses in RVH. I learned quickly to pass on knowledge and skills in the most simplified absorbable format to produce a task-oriented workforce who could function wherever the need was—in outpatients, ward, or operating theatre. I had a hard-won battle to stop the rotation of eye nurses to other clinical departments. It helped greatly throughout the years of the national eye care programme.

My personal paradigm shift

My training hitherto had prepared me to give the best possible care to each individual patient who walked into my tertiary clinic, usually following referral from elsewhere. This presumed that referral networks, all other levels of the health service, and all hospital and health systems were in place, were eye care oriented and functioning optimally. The deficiencies in my training to provide a service to a population and to enable hospital systems to meet eye care needs became frustratingly obvious.

A clinician who wants to function optimally at a tertiary level in sub-Saharan Africa, particularly from a specialist service like ophthalmology, has to spearhead the effort. He or she must ensure that all the levels and systems are in place and functioning within a comprehensive clinical and public health paradigm. Only then can mortality, disability, and morbidity be prevented and the health of the population ensured. I made a personal paradigm shift.

I decided to seek help from the legendary President of the RCSB, the late Sir John Wilson. He promptly responded and alongside the WHO Prevention of Blindness programme (started in 1978) facilitated my attendance of the 1982 General Assembly of the International Agency for the Prevention of Blindness (IAPB), which he had founded in 1975. At that assembly in Washington, USA, I was exposed for the first time to strategies for national programmes for prevention of blindness and control of the major causes of blindness.

The Assembly enabled me to network with others facing similar challenges in sub-Saharan Africa.[3] As regards human resource for eye care, I gained knowledge on primary eye care from the Kenya Rural Blindness Prevention Programme and the use of paramedics (task shifting) for eye care in Kenya, Tanzania, and Malawi.

The national eye care programme

On my return I presented a report[4] with suggestions for a national programme for the prevention of blindness to the Director of Health Services. I proposed establishing a national eye care programme, which could also be a demonstration model for sub-Saharan Africa. My recommendations were reinforced by a visiting WHO consultant and my resolve was strengthened by a country-wide tour, which exposed me to the extreme poverty of most of the population.

First, I needed to be trained in community focused eye health and was able to attend Professor Barrie Jones's innovative new course in community eye health at the International Centre for Eye Health (ICEH) in London in 1985. It covered the major causes of blindness, the factors, the solutions and eye care programming, and was a complete and holistic package. It prepared me for leadership.

An immediate outcome was the planning and implementation of the first population-based national survey of blindness and visual impairment in Africa. It was led by myself and supported by ICEH and WHO. It was also a research process to test out a new WHO record form, which would use paramedics as part of the survey team. The survey was a game changer as it provided the evidence for task shifting in the use of ophthalmic paramedics, as well as a baseline for the burden of blindness and its causes, and an estimate of the magnitude of services required. It was also used extensively by the two main sponsors of the survey (WHO and ICEH) for advocacy and for teaching and planning to the benefit of other countries.

This survey showed that the prevalence of blindness in The Gambia was 0.7% of the population with 1.4% having low vision; 80% of the blindness was preventable; 55% was cataract-related, 20% from non trachomatous corneal opacity and 17% from trachoma.[5]

A more detailed and improved national eye care plan was written as result of the survey. It set the objective to reduce the blindness prevalence rate by 50%, (to less than 0.5% and not more than 1% in any single community) and to achieve geographical coverage by integration into the primary health care system.

It was clear that the existing one or two ophthalmologists and few nurses at the RVH were grossly inadequate to the task and the programme had to make the most of what was available by drawing on the existing general human resources for health. A comprehensive situation analysis showed there was a minimal number of doctors, a small pool of general nurses, a more sizeable pool of state enrolled nurses and community health nurses trained nationally. An accepted tradition of task shifting and a total government commitment to primary health care were major strengths. The presence of institutions in Kenya and Malawi for the training of paramedics in eye health was an opportunity.

Alignment with the government commitment to primary care

The main thrust of the Gambian health service development policy, since the start of the second five-year plan period, was the establishment of a country-wide primary health care delivery system based on community operated village health services at minimal cost to government.[6] The Gambia was privileged to have a strong political commitment to primary health care, having committed to the Health for All by the year 2000, and well-designed policies, programmes, and plans. The plan was to have extensive village health services with infrastructural and administrative support, which would be clinically supported and supervised from health centres operating as the first level of referral. In addition, there would be a multi-sectoral village development committee to provide oversight of health and other activities.

The foundation of this plan was that each village of more than 400 people (PHC villages) had a village health worker (VHW), a new cadre, and a traditional birth attendant (TBA), an existing traditional group. Each group of four or five villages had a community health nurse.

The training for these workers was so busy that it could not accommodate a module on eye health. As a result it was decided to adopt Kenya's strategy of having a dedicated primary eye care trainer. An eye-trained auxiliary nurse, who was an excellent community oriented member of staff, completely familiar with the culture and languages, was sent to a similar training programme in Tanzania. On her return she was given the leeway to design the primary eye care programme herself, bringing together the community based workers in local groups.

The main emphasis was on health promotion. However, the training also covered villagers' role in early identification and providing care when patients returned after hospital visits. Practical skills were taught using patients identified during screening exercises to demonstrate eye conditions. The timing was tailored to suit the calendar of village activities. Having an open-air 'cinema' in the evenings, the slides shown using a portable battery operated projector under the tree in the village meeting point, encouraged exchanges with great fun and laughter. The village health workers were provided with torch lights, posters, vision screening charts, and other materials to use at these events, and supervision was offered by the community health nurse. Despite the appointment of the VHWs, the first port of call for care for most villagers remained the family or traditional practitioners. The survey had shown that non-trachomatous corneal opacity was the third major cause of blindness. In analysis of patients' pathology, it was noted that harmful traditional practices were a contributory factor to the visual loss observed at eye clinics due to delay in seeking treatment or in the use of harmful substances. Lessons were drawn from other countries, Malawi in particular, on collaboration with traditional healers.

A situation analysis of traditional practitioners and practice was conducted in each division covering location, range of practices, and eye practices—and noting whether these were good, harmless, or harmful. Based on the findings, a training manual, referral protocols and forms were developed and used in a collaborative way, engaging traditional practitioners as members of the health team. The numbers of patients with pathology from harmful traditional practices reduced and traditional practitioners became part of the referral network.

The programme also learned from traditional practice and culture. Health education using posters, radio jingles, and television slots worked well in the urban areas. However, these were not so successful in the countryside. The collaboration with traditional practitioners opened up the possibility of using traditional communication groups, the *Kanyelengs*, and community events and gatherings to share health messages.

Rural communities

In addition, the local health workers mainly responded to people who came with problems. They didn't go into homes to identify the visually impaired or encourage them to come for help and address their fears and concerns. In most communities, however, there was a culture of home visits by the older women and of community support. Discussions were, therefore, held with communities to see if this strategy could be used. The outcome was the 'friends of the eye' translated in Mandinka as *Nyatero*. These friends didn't deliver healthcare but addressed the period before patients and their families decided to seek help and the period after they had come back from contact with the health service. Their role was to seek out patients, address concerns, ask questions, share stories, and generally be busy-bodies. The friends worked in the homes and compounds where they were already regular visitors providing the service to about 100 people. They were typically of a non-health background—perhaps a teacher or pensioner or elderly female—were selected by the community, and had to have good enough vision themselves for the task.

Rural communities have a culture of events where clusters of communities come together for market days, funerals, and celebrations. This culture was adapted to running minicamps for cataract services and trichiasis surgery. It worked for patients and providers alike. Many more patients and their carers attended because neighbours, other members of their community, and nearby communities were attending the minicamps. The cataract surgeons or trichiasis surgeons worked together in groups of three or four providing peer support and supervision.

Blind and visually impaired people often needed persuasion and motivation to attend the camps, so the local community ophthalmic nurse (CON) would comb their communities and persuade their patients to attend. On the day prior to surgery, they would escort their cluster of patients to a convenient collection point, usually on a transport route. Transport would have been arranged and the CON would be picked up with their patients and taken to the camp. There they would 'mother hen' their patients and on discharge would take their brood back home and continue to check on them post-operatively. This was meant to address the fear of the unknown, which was a major barrier to uptake of services, ensure an accurate case selection, and high-quality post-operative care. Most of all it was responsive to the patients' needs.

The programme also made use of the local schools. Active inflammatory trachoma and epidemics of conjunctivitis were prevalent infections in children and needed treatment. In addition, school children could serve as an entry into homes, taking health education into every home, and primary school teachers were recruited to help, following the example of other community level training carried out for different purposes. A teacher training module was developed, with the participation of the teachers, and they were provided with the necessary items to work with. A partnership was established with the Ministry of

Education to mainstream the teacher training module into the teacher training college course, and later work was done with the curriculum department of the ministry of education to develop a teachers' manual and a pupils' handbook and school posters.

Health centres were the level immediately above the village health services; static facilities with general health nurses who were termed 'prescribers'. The eye health service aimed to integrate eye care into their routine work as prescribers, and training and support programmes were developed using the same principles as for the village health workers: well-trained dedicated trainers, a venue in their facilities, the extensive use of live patients, task oriented content, the provision of items required for their work. Working with the in-service training department ensured ownership and sustainability of the training.

However, periodic supervisory visits showed that this investment did not yield the expected numbers of eye patients or referrals. Most prescribers were overwhelmed by the size of their clinic attendances, the relatively small number of eye patients, the prioritization of maternal and child health services, and their own lack of confidence about seeing eye patients.

Developing human resources

The only way within a comprehensive eye service to tackle the huge backlog of surgical cases, achieve coverage, and ensure access was to adopt task shifting and rigorous supportive supervision. This involved the creation of new roles and practices.

The next level in the health service was the regional hospitals and major health centres, each serving a population of about 200 000. The sheer magnitude of the problem, the wide distribution of cataract blindness, and the precedents of nurse anaesthetists and prescribers helped make the case for the use of cataract surgeons and the task shifting of cataract surgery from ophthalmologists to cataract surgeons. This was done rigorously within a team approach with staffing norms agreed, infrastructure designed, the technology and consumables package determined, and job descriptions written. The Gambia had adopted the strategy of having a comprehensive eye service, which addressed all causes of visual loss and was part of primary health care. In order to achieve this, the cataract surgeons were termed senior ophthalmic medical assistants (SOMA) and their job description gave them responsibility for the eye health of a population. Clinical and surgical responsibilities were important but only part of their role. They needed to be leaders, managers, trainers, supervisors, advocates, communicators, and research minded. Community eye health became an essential training module or course for all members of the eye care programme and all courses it influenced in West Africa.

Success depended on the very careful selection of candidates and a multi-entry multi-exit method. This lasted a minimum of 5 years after becoming a state registered nurse and allowed candidates to add on skills gradually, undergo an internship, and expand their training to population service-related tasks. Each was given all they needed in terms of infrastructure, equipment and consumables, support staff, and a vehicle (a sturdy abuse-friendly Land Rover Defender) for work. The programme also ensured that they had staff quarters, water, and electricity back-up for work and home.

A close working relationship with the supervising ophthalmologist was critical and a quarterly visit was mandatory. The objective was fivefold (acronym SSTSS): **S**upervision of clinical and other work for quality; **S**ervice delivery for patients identified by the SOMA; **T**eaching; and **S**upport mainly for solving personal problems, such as schools for the children or housing, but could include help with advocacy locally. As with many developing countries, the availability of supplies, especially for non-mainstream services such as eye health, is a problem and part of the quarterly visit involved bringing **S**upplies to the SOMA.

The selection of candidates was gender-oriented. Males were selected to be trained as SOMAs because they were more amenable to being posted to the divisional centres, which were outside the capital. The government schemes of service were reviewed to include them and they were registered as having additional qualifications with the professional nursing council and were provided with medical indemnity by the government. They were not permitted, however, to set up private practice or to provide services to the public in cataract surgery.

The SOMAs and even the tertiary unit needed nurses trained in eye health to assist in the clinics, operating theatres, and wards. The pool of general nurses was too small, the community health nurses (CHN) and the state enrolled nurses (SEN) were locally trained and formed a bigger pool. The decision was made within the Ministry of Health to start a national training programme for SEN ophthalmic and CHN ophthalmic nurses. The SEN ophthalmic met the need in eye units at all levels and the CON formed the bridging cadre linking the community and the secondary eye unit. The CON would remain polyvalent, continuing with community duties, including maternal and child healthcare. They were to be in charge of a population of 30 000. They took over the role of the primary eye care trainer, managing the eye health training and supervision for VHWs, TBAs, the traditional practitioners, *kanyelengs*, and the friends of the eye, and school eye health programmes. They formed the backbone for trachoma screening, trichiasis case detection, and health promotion activities. They were supervised both by the SOMAs and by the general health services.

Initially, trichiasis surgery was undertaken by SOMAs in the eye units, at the community level or through the use of mini camps. This was not enough, however, to tackle the huge backlog of trichiasis. Task shifting was, therefore, adopted for lid surgery from the SOMAs to the CONs. The selection of trainees was from the CONs' pool with training and supervision by the SOMAs. Moreover, when the refractive error services were set up, the workload of the SOMAs was high and the CON pool was large enough for selection to be trained as basic refractionists.

The concept of population coverage and responsibility was adopted to combine individual care with population care in the attitude of all workers from the friends of the eye through to the SOMA and ophthalmologist. The team approach was adopted to reinforce the complimentary way of working. The vertical team was made up of the supervising staff and the supervised staff at the level below, and was aimed at population coverage. It was best exemplified by the SOMA and his group of community ophthalmic nurses in the division he covered. A horizontal team was made up of all the staff located in one facility and was reflected in the staffing norms. It needed to reflect the proper mix and match to achieve highest productivity. This was exemplified in the ratio of nurses to the surgeon in an operating theatre to achieve the highest rate of surgical output.

Expanding the programme

The size of the human resource pool was small with a high demand from all programmes, so the national eye care programme was developed in phases at a rate at which human resources were available for training and absorption by the health services. It was aligned to geographical coverage, working from the capital to the most remote region, west to east.

The first phase was the strengthening of the tertiary unit in the Royal Victoria Hospital, Banjul, to be the nerve centre offering tertiary services, coordination, planning, and training, as well as being the base for national level staff, such as primary eye care trainers. Using the division in which the tertiary centre was located, the prototype for divisional comprehensive eye services was developed: outreach services, development of static outreach points with monthly surgery, coverage with primary eye care services, and training of integrated eye care workers, was designed, tested and put in place. The process was then replicated in three phases, one division at a time and reaching the furthest division by 1996.

An evaluation of the programme in 1996/97 included a repeat national population-based survey. Though the population had increased by 51%, and life expectancy by 10 years, the blindness prevalence rate had reduced by

40% to 0.4%. A west to east gradient was found for changes in risk of blindness; this matched the west to east introductions of interventions.[7]

For each division, the first stage was to put in place primary eye care supported by monthly outreach visits to two centres from the national centre or the nearest secondary centre as these were developed. While this was happening, the SOMA and his support SEN ophthalmic nurses for the division were trained, the infrastructure was built or renovated, and the equipment ordered so that as the SOMA was ready for posting; he had all he required to perform. The population had been primed through primary eye care, he could then take over the outreach visits. What this achieved was that frustration was prevented, job satisfaction was ensured, and performance maximized.

The original human resource development plan concentrated on human resources for service delivery. However, it was quickly realized that human resources needed to be strengthened in every aspect of the system from equipment maintenance to supplies' provision. In the first decade, technicians were trained in equipment maintenance and the local production of eye drops. Later, skills such as management and teaching were taught as a module for eye health personnel; and eye health was taught to other cadres, such as medical records' clerks, where it was relevant to their work.

Equipment standing idle due to minor problems was a major constraint and lost time can be as high as 60% in some countries. A two-pronged approach was adopted to address this. The first part was to have equipment procurement, standard lists, assembly, and preventive maintenance included in the training of ophthalmologists. Each member of the staff team was trained in the care and preventive maintenance of any equipment they used. In addition, the programme invested in dedicated equipment technicians, with scheduled travel to peripheral units and a central technician workshop. Only three equipment technicians were needed, so the training was conducted in Nigeria after creating a link between the Nigerian National Eye Centre and the Aravind Eye System in Madurai.

The pharmacy unit of the tertiary hospital set up a local production of eye drops in two places in order to address the perennial shortage of drops. Initially this was done locally by the eye unit staff supervised by the pharmacist.

The results of the second population-based survey guided the next stage of the human resource development. Cataract and aphakia were still the leading causes of blindness at 58%, but trachomatous blindness had reduced from 17% to 5% and infective trachoma was increasing in the peri-urban areas. Other non-trachomatous corneal blindness, glaucoma, refractive error, and other causes accounted for 36% of all blindness. Accordingly, further human resource developments were planned to meet these new challenges.

Task shifting was adopted to train community health nurses to perform community based lid surgery. Customized courses were run to train the SOMAs and laboratory technicians in the management of corneal ulcers. Short, intensive courses were run to train the team at the tertiary level in the management of glaucoma. The training of refractionists was introduced and short courses run as a prelude to developing a recognized optometric technician course. To ensure a continuum of care for patients who ended up with low vision and blindness, short courses were run on low vision. Links were developed with an inclusive education programme for low vision and blind children and the community based rehabilitation programme for adults. The programme design evolved to a comprehensive eye service particularly focused at the community and primary level.

Once national coverage had been achieved, the country had enough staff strength in service delivery, human resources, and infrastructure and technology systems to be able to mount training programmes. It had in its own backyard, demonstrable models. This had attracted visiting trainees from medical students to ophthalmologists.

Courses were set up over a 7-year period and eventually drawn together into a single Regional Ophthalmic Training Programme (ROTP) in 2001. The fact that they were run in the country meant that The Gambia saved money on external training and generated fees from external candidates, some from as far away as Zanzibar. A small, core staff of course coordinator, administrator, and office staff managed the programme, with foreign ophthalmologists recruited for the first 3 years of the ROTP programme. Together they trained: SEN ophthalmic and community ophthalmic nurses; ophthalmic nurses/ophthalmic medical assistants: senior ophthalmic medical assistants/advanced diploma in ophthalmic nursing (cataract surgeons); optometric technicians; and provided internships for equipment technicians and enabled the local production of eye drops.

The programme needed more space and infrastructure as it matured and expanded to help neighbouring countries. Fortunately, Sightsavers and the United Arab Emirates were able to provide a purpose built prototype regional centre—the Sheikh Zayed Regional Eye Care Centre—with facilities for service delivery, training, student facilities, administration, staff quarters, and research. It became the base of the ROTP.

Influencing healthcare and human resources in West Africa

The Gambia provided a focal point and a catalyst for change in human resource development in West Africa as it provided the venue for strategic meetings and demonstrated strategies for comprehensive eye care services and new approaches to using non-medical health personnel and community level staff, as well as offering training for all cadres. Three examples show the extent of the influence of The Gambia.

First, it hosted the first prevention of blindness committee of the West African Health Community in 1989 at which the recommendation was made to train mid-level health workers and create diplomas for ophthalmology, primary eye care trainers, and optometric technicians. The diploma in ophthalmology training programme was a unique example of making the most of what was available. The curriculum was developed in The Gambia by ophthalmologists from West Africa and ICEH. The design and content was largely influenced by The Gambia experience of what expertise and skills were required of an ophthalmologist to set up a programme from scratch for a 500 000 population and to meet the comprehensive eye care needs of the population. Clinical and surgical skills, leadership, management, teaching, advocacy, communication, research, resource mobilization, and management were covered.

There was no single centre in the region that could produce the numbers required for the stated PP ratio of one ophthalmologist to 500 000 population. A modular format and multi-centre strategy was therefore adopted. The 12-week foundation module and 6-week community eye health module were run in Nigeria; the two clinical and surgical skills' modules were done at select high-volume centres across West Africa, mainly NGO supported centres, where trainees were attached at a maximum ratio of two per trainer consultant ophthalmologist. The 6-month internship done at similar accredited high-volume centres completed the 2-year training programme.

Second, The Gambia led the way in the conversion of all the SOMAs from intra-capsular cataract extraction to extra-capsular cataract extraction with intraocular lens implantation. As soon as an affordable model of an operating microscope and intraocular lens was available, an intensive conversion course was mounted, facilitated by a team of surgeon trainer and manager who not only trained the surgeons and their teams, but also instituted appropriate systems. The decision by The Gambia to make this training available not just to ophthalmologists, but to paramedics was a game changer in improving the quality and quantity of cataract surgery across the continent.

Third, The Gambia led the way in the standardization of curricula for eye health courses in West Africa, the development of manuals for community based eye health workers, and the specification of appropriate technology.[8] It also enabled agreement on staffing norms regionally. These are shown in Table 13.1.

Table 13.1 Staffing norms for West Africa[9]

Level	Cadre	Number for population of 250 000	Number for population of 100 000
	Ophthalmologist	1	1 (cataract surgeon)
	Ophthalmic nurses	4	2
	Nurse anaesthetist (access to)	1	1
	SEN ophthalmic nurse	5	3
	General nurses	5	2
	Nurse counselor	2	1
	Optometrist	1	
	Refractionist/technician	1	2
	Low vision worker/refractionist	1	1
	Equipment maintenance technician (access to)	1	1
	Nursing aide	4	2
	LPED technician	1	1
	Records clerk	1	1
	Cashier	1 (access to)	1
	Driver	1	1
	Cleaning staff	3 minimum	3

Reproduced from West Africa Health Organization (WAHO), *Recommended Eye Health Personnel Population Ratios Based on Sightsavers West Africa Staffing Norms Developed by H Faal*, Eye Care Programme Consultant West Africa, 1995–2000, by permission of the author.

The Health for Peace Initiative was set up to promote cross-border collaboration for health. The Governments of Senegal, The Gambia, Guinea Bissau, and Guinea committed to joint programming to address prioritized health problems across borders in malaria, HIV/AIDS, immunization, surveillance, and, later, the prevention of blindness. Many patients from outside The Gambia made use of the country's improving eye service and The Gambia took the lead in this area.

It faced two main challenges in doing so: first, gaining acceptance of the task shifting strategy by the professionals in the other countries and, second, dealing with the language differences (Gambia is anglophone, Senegal is francophone, and Guinea Bissau is lusophone).

The Gambia also had much wider influence in sub-Saharan Africa and globally. The programme had achieved full national coverage in 1995 and evaluation through a second national survey showed that it had achieved both a 40% reduction in the blindness prevalence rates and an economic rate of return of 19%. The experience of the programme was shared globally through lectures at the ICEH, and scientific and strategic meetings at the WHO prevention of blindness programme. It provided the evidence for the global initiative for the elimination of avoidable blindness and the development of the VISION 2020 model for a comprehensive programme for a population of a million based around the three pillars of service delivery, human resource development, and infrastructure and technology. As President of the IAPB in the first five years of Vision 2020, my main emphasis was on the roll out of the VISION 2020 one million population model and integrating community eye health modules in all eye health personnel training curricula.

The Gambia programme also learnt from other parts of the world, including East Africa, India, and the UK. Being a Sightsavers' eye care consultant from 1988, as well as an adviser within WHO Prevention of Blindness and visiting lecturer at ICEH, allowed me to influence all Sightsavers' supported programmes across sub-Saharan Africa.

Although I was an employee of an NGO, I was seconded as technical assistance to government and had the full responsibility and authority within government as a national co-coordinator. This gave me full participation in government policy and human resource development with emphasis on eye health.

My membership of the West African College of Surgeons, national professional societies, and global professional bodies allowed me further opportunities for cross-fertilization and influencing the training of ophthalmologists in Africa.

Challenges remained. An attempt was made to apply the concept of using non-para-professionals to provide refractive error services—which are normally undertaken by optometrists; however, the optometrists in West Africa were unwilling at the time to allow for, or to participate in, the training and supervision of the cadre. Eventually, however, we were able to recruit and retain an optometrist and a training course was developed for refractionists. Every professional body is responsible for defining its para-professional cadre, its training, supervision, and quality assurance. The professional turf protection can sometimes be a barrier.

Another challenge was that the number of practicing doctors was extremely small. The government policy was not to allow doctors in government service to have private practice. In practice very few doctors remained in the country and those who did moved out of the public sector. The few who stayed in public service mostly moved into public health and management.

Looking to the future there will be increased need for sub-specialty services in ophthalmology, especially as diabetic retinopathy becomes more common. The greatest challenge will be the quality assurance and maintenance of the gains made by the programme, especially as external support is reduced and the other countries, which depended on The Gambia, develop their eye care services.

Conclusions

My experiences have shown me that there are some lessons for anyone planning to develop a specialty service in a country with few resources:

1 A specialist clinician who wants to function effectively at a tertiary level must spearhead the effort to ensure that all the levels below are in place and functioning optimally. A personal paradigm shift from focusing on individual care to addressing population need is a must for any health leader in sub-Saharan Africa.

2 When there is a scarcity of human resources and a non-existent or limited service, important strategies include situational analysis of existing need and HR pools, phasing of HR and programme development, competency based training, task shifting, a team approach, norms for staffing, equipping, and supportive supervision and evidence of HR impact.

3 Where there is scarcity of human resources in the health system, and even where there is not, the community is a major resource for health—especially for taking health into homes. The community has existing practices that can be learnt from and adapted for health improvement.

4 External training institutions should be carefully selected based on their curricula and practical teaching to ensure that the products will work comfortably and efficiently in their home country environment. Backing from a trusted institution such as WHO is a critical factor for success in establishing the evidence base for a new cadre of health personnel

5 Human resources need to be developed both for service delivery and for all the support functions from equipment maintenance to procurement.

6 There is always knowledge and experience in other parts of the world. The desire and determination to seek out, learn, and network is part of making the most of what is available. Links to capacity building institutions to influence them and to be influenced is a good quality assurance and impact strategy.

7 Nationwide change needs intense advocacy at the national level. Reports of external global meetings with recommendations for local action can be a powerful advocacy tool. Most countries in the developing world respect WHO reviews and recommendations.

References

1 Health Resources Group for Primary Health Care. HRG/CRU1 Rev. 2 Country Resource Utilization Review. The Gambia. 1 December 1984.

2 Health Resources Group for Primary Health Care. HRG/CRU1 Rev. 2 Country Resource Utilization Review. The Gambia. 1 December 1984.

3 International Agency for the Prevention of Blindness Second General Assembly. Washington DC, October1982; Report.

4 Faal H. Report on Second General Assembly, IAPB to the Director of Medical Services.

5 Faal H, et al. National survey of blindness and low vision in The Gambia: results. *British Journal of Ophthalmology* 1989; **73**(2), 82–7. <http://www.ncbi.nlm.nih.gov/pmc/articles/PMC1041660/>.

6 Health Resources Group for Primary Health Care. HRG/CRU 1 Rev. 2 Country Resource Utilization Review. The Gambia, 1 December 1984.

7 Faal, H et al. Evaluation of a national eye care programme:resurvey after 10 years. *British Journal of Ophthalmology* 2000; **84** (9): 948–51.

8 Technological Guidelines for a District Eye Care Programme. Vision 2020 The right to Sight. July 2006.

9 West Africa Health Organisation; Faal H, et al. Recommended Eye Health Personnel Population Ratios Based on Sightsavers West Africa Staffing Norms Developed by H Faal, Eye Care Programme Consultant West Africa, 1995–2000.

Chapter 14

The evolution of professional education and health systems in sub-Saharan Africa

Gottlieb Monekosso

Formerly Minister of Public Health of Cameroon and Regional Director of the African Region of the World Health Organization

Professor Gottlieb Monekosso has played a leading role in the development of professional education in sub-Saharan Africa since 1969 when he became the Founding Director of the University Centre for Health Sciences in Yaoundé in his native Cameroon. He went on to become Minister for Public Health and subsequently the Regional Director of the African Region of the World Health Organization. His very long and distinguished career has given him privileged insights into the education of health professionals, as a participant as well as observer. In this chapter he charts developments from the pre-colonial period, into the colonial and through to the twenty-first century. He shows how pioneering leaders have worked creatively to overcome the shortages of people and resources, and provided trained people to meet the most pressing needs in their countries. It is a story that involves cooperation with a wide range of international partners but, as he reflects, that cooperation has sometimes been 'the best friend of health sciences' education' in providing opportunities for education but 'the worst enemy of the health system' in also providing opportunities for emigration. His own vision is of one of intellectual rigour married to a thorough understanding of local circumstances. He insisted that his students lived in the local communities as part of their education and believes it is important to 'ensure that policies are not those of the intellectual elite but that they represent the needs and wants of local populations'. Perhaps, he suggests, Africa's history of developing health sciences' education in this way may have lessons to offer the rest of the world for the future.

Professional education and health services

The evolution of professional education has gone hand in hand with the development of health services in Africa from pre-colonial times up to the present day. Sub-Saharan African peoples interacted with missionaries and traders in the pre-colonial period. There were no health systems but there were traditional healthcare practices. There were also traditional practitioners established in their villages and enjoying the confidence of their respective populations. Exceptionally, a few Africans studied medicine in Europe and returned to set up practice in major towns.

Over the centuries the peoples of Africa, south of the Sahara, like human populations elsewhere, developed concepts of health and disease onto which were grafted healing practices. In Africa, the approach was holistic. Illness affected the whole person; the physical, the mental, and the spiritual. This is why healthcare involved mystic magico-religious practices, which were passed on from generation to generation. Physical illness was treated mostly with medicinal plants, which were available in the immediate environment. There were remedies for practically all the major symptoms of illnesses, such as the relief of headache, constipation, diarrhoea, pain in the limbs, back and abdomen, fever, joint pains, even jaundice. In this regard, African traditional medicine resembled the phytotherapy of other continents. The medicine men usually established themselves in a limited geographical area where they were known and respected. They were supported by traditional midwives to assist in safe delivery for pregnant women.

The management of mental illness was also well developed by specialized traditional healers. There were also villages that were known for community mental health management. In fact until the new psychotropic drugs were discovered, there was not much to choose between traditional African and Western European practices.

The 1884 Berlin Conference, which accelerated colonialism throughout the continent, coincided with remarkable scientific discoveries. The germ theory of disease and the identification of specific illness with specific microbes laid the foundation for the discovery, a few decades later, of antibiotics and other chemotherapeutic agents, but also at the time facilitated the otherwise difficult European penetration into their new-found colonies.

Colonial governments provided healthcare services for their officials, Africans and Europeans, in the cities and towns under the supervision of a relatively small number of medical doctors. Healthcare facilities included small dispensaries and health centres of increasing size and complexity, some including beds but with few technical facilities. Hospitals were built and staffed in urban areas by government. In the rural areas, Christian missionaries filled the gap with health centres, hospitals, and maternity centres. At the end of the colonial period, there was limited population coverage of health services but there were notable efforts like medical field units, which provided mobile services and disease control, as well as flying doctor services covering vast territories.

Just before independence, local hospitals became bigger and better equipped, and some of these became central hospitals. This period saw the establishment of an administration with directors of medical services and an increasing but still small number of specialists. In some countries, there were separate African and European hospitals. In East Africa, there were separate African, Asian, and European hospitals.

There was a determined effort to identify, diagnose, treat, prevent, and control the epidemics and pandemics, mainly of malaria, yellow fever, and sleeping sickness that ravaged middle Africa at the time. The First World War did not stop disease control. In my own country of Cameroon, for example, the Germans had identified sleeping sickness as the number one priority in the zone between the great rivers of the Nyong and the Sanaga. Their energetic efforts were continued by the incoming French administration, which maintained the substantial budget the Germans had voted for the field operations against sleeping sickness. The hero was Dr Eugene Jamot who recommended the creation of a centre of medical instruction in Ayos as a backup for field work. This was really the beginning of formal training through using clinical sites and fieldwork.

The earliest health training institutions were schools for nursing aides, dressers, and midwifery assistants. To these were added assistant laboratory technicians, pharmacy assistants, dental chair assistants, and so on. In many countries one big hospital and one medical school dominated. These schools were not expected to train fully qualified doctors. Elsewhere, their graduates were licensed for practice in their home countries or region, such as the medical assistants of the Lagos Medical School and similar institutions in Francophone Africa in Dakar and Madagascar whose graduates were labelled 'médecin africain'. Some of these institutions were either upgraded or closed as the countries gained independence.

These 'African doctors' were authorized by the Royal Colleges of the UK to sit the professional examinations; and successful candidates were admitted to the UK medical register. A few made it to membership of the Royal College of Physicians. In Francophone Africa, the 'médecin africain' repeated part of the medical course after obtaining the 'Baccaleaureat'. Special arrangements were also made for the medical assistants from the Belgian Congo. At independence in 1960, there were only six medical schools in sub-Saharan Africa (excluding South Africa) that graduated fully-fledged doctors at university level.

The subsequent expansion of medical education spread healthcare coverage away from the capital cities to the chief towns of provinces or regions. There were corresponding developments in missionary hospitals with doctors being assigned as they became available to the peripheral districts. Following the Alma Ata Declaration (1978), the WHO promoted worldwide health systems based on the primary healthcare approach. It is also during the post-independence period that high-level academic clinicians were seen in the newly developed teaching hospitals and medical schools. These included Dakar, Abidjan, Ibadan, Lagos, Yaoundé, Kampala, Accra, Nairobi, Dar es Salaam, Kinshasa, and Lusaka.

After independence, there was renewed interest in traditional medical practices. 'Medicine men' sprouted up everywhere, many becoming ambulant healers. Some claimed a divine calling, combining magico-religious gestures with medicinal plant therapy. They no longer remained with the village audience. Many sold their wares in market places; others acquired a little scientific knowledge, administering not only herbs, but also antibiotics and other pharmaceutical products. A few of them sent their patients to medical laboratories, describing themselves as modern traditional doctors.

The medical establishment accused them of the illegal practice of medicine and increased regulation gradually brought their numbers down. In the 1970s some health authorities invited tradi-practitioners to see patients side by side with general medical doctors in public health centres, exchanging patients when deemed necessary. One was left with the impression that the tradi-practitioner was sometimes able to win the confidence of patients because of his holistic approach. Some countries invited practitioners to demonstrate their capacity in university public health institutes and, if successful, they were subsequently authorized to practice. In urban areas the public mixed the different approaches; they very often firstly self-medicated with modern drugs, then went for consultations in health centres, then went to tradi-practitioners if symptoms were resistant and finally resorted to expensive hi-tech medicine.

Whilst traditional practices are unlikely to be abandoned soon, their future really lies in the scientific study of medicinal plants. Some research institutes have already demonstrated the value of botanically identified medicinal plants. The challenge for African countries lies in gathering the health and economic benefits because the traditional medicine of today could be the modern medicine of tomorrow.

From health auxiliary to medical doctor in Cameroon

Cameroon is a good example of the growth and mutual interaction between the health system and health professional education. A child's education began in a village elementary primary school then moved to a middle elementary primary school in the regional capitals and finally to the only senior primary school in the capital city; a total of seven years of basic education. The last year of the programme saw the children divided into three groups: one destined for teaching in primary schools; a second destined for administrative tasks that were essential for maintaining the colonial status, such as court clerks and interpreters; and a third group destined to be health aides. The curriculum was designed to fit the task the trainees were expected to perform within the colonial system.

Many of the best students chose the health assistant category (a three-year training programme), which led them eventually, sometimes to their surprise, to increasing levels of knowledge and skills in healthcare. The trainees were then posted to health structures in different parts of the country. After varying periods of service, some of these medical assistants undertook an internship in Dakar Senegal and on successful completion earned the high status of '*médecin africain*'. By then many would have worked in general hospitals and acquired surgical, medical, paediatric, obstetrics, and gynaecology experience. In this manner, health workers were progressively provided for the nine administrative regions of French Cameroon.

Finally, the best of the graduates and the most competent had the opportunity, with independence, to become fully qualified doctors not requiring supervision. A few also went up the academic ladder and became university professors. Many contributed to the high-level management of the health services of the newly independent countries.

The development of health training institutions

Medical education developed rapidly in the first 20 years after independence. The six medical schools that existed in 1960 were linked to universities in France, the United Kingdom, and Belgium; whilst other countries devised ingenious ways of starting medical school, as shown in Box 14.1.

The following examples from some of the larger centres show how each of these institutions developed in its own way in the years before and after independence.

In Nigeria the colonial Lagos medical school was closed and the students, including myself, were transferred in January 1948 to Ade Oyo Hospital as part of University College Ibadan. These pioneer students passed the second London MB examinations after two years but couldn't continue their clinical studies in Ibadan because the University of London did not approve Ade Oyo for the London MBBS examinations. We therefore transferred to London teaching hospitals. Meanwhile, funds had been allocated by the colonial development and welfare foundation for the construction of the teaching hospital, on a substantial site, inside the city of Ibadan. The medical school remained under the

Box 14.1 Medical education developed across Africa through a variety of different routes

- Young doctors graduating in Europe were invited to return home for their internship in Lome, Togo.
- A major medical centre with experienced professional leadership became a teaching centre at Korle Bu hospital Accra, Ghana.
- A newly built city hospital was commissioned instead as a teaching hospital and college of medicine at LUTH, Lagos, Nigeria.
- A pilot teaching centre in Treichville, later University Medical Centre, Cocody, Abidjan, Ivory Coast.
- Support from an international centre in Cotonou, Benin.
- With the help of bilateral cooperation from the USSR in Guinea Bissau.
- With international and bilateral assistance from WHO and the UK in Malawi.
- With WHO support in Niamey, Niger; Brazzaville, Congo; and Libreville, Gabon.

tutelage of the University of London until 1962 when the Ibadan MBBS was first awarded. This arrangement worked very well except that public health as a discipline had been eliminated from the London MBBS finals and, paradoxically, became an optional subject for Ibadan students!

In Uganda at Makerere College in Kampala, the Mulago African Hospital, initially trained medical assistants and other health staff but subsequently graduated medical doctors. The facilities of the Mulago African Hospital were initially very poor. It was one of three hospitals in Kampala; the other two, of higher standing, were reserved for Asians and Europeans, respectively. Just before independence a new Mulago hospital was built and equipped to the standards of a university teaching hospital and Mulago became famous for its medical research. The African childhood lymphoma was described by a Mulago surgeon, Denis Burkitt. Childhood malnutrition, *kwashiorkor*, and endomyocardial fibrosis were studied by Professor JNP Davies, and the Buruli ulcer, now known to be widespread in Africa, was first identified at Buruli in Uganda. Unfortunately these achievements were obscured by political upheavals during which the medical school and the teaching hospital went through difficult periods.

In Tanzania, medical education began at the Dar es Salaam School of Medicine with a curriculum perceived initially as leaning towards the colonial medical assistant formula in spite of the excellent facilities of the newly built Muhimbili hospital. On this spacious campus, other health training schools were developed, including dental surgery, pharmacy, nursing, laboratory technology, and radiography. The medical school programme was reviewed with the aid of WHO and subsequently upgraded. It also created three field learning and practice sites: the first quite near to Dar es Salaam, the second not so near, and the third far away from it. I was privileged to become Dean and was free to implement these developments with a Tanzanian colleague as the Vice Dean, Dr Aloysius Nhonoli, who took over after my departure.

Development has continued with multi-professional education in Dar es Salaam, Tanzania, where the faculty of medicine became in 2010 a full university called Muhimbili University of Health and Allied Sciences (MUCHAS); comprising a central administration, a vice chancellor, deputy vice chancellors, schools, and institutes, as well as faculties. These include medicine, pharmacy, dentistry, nursing, radiography, and postgraduate specialities of medicine.

In Zambia, medical education was inspired by a Zambian minister of education, Professor Lameck Goma, former lecturer in Makerere, who invited me as a WHO consultant to help design the curriculum. Medical studies began with a Bachelor of Science degree in human biology to cover the first three years, followed by another three years of clinical studies. A university teaching hospital (UTH) similar to others in the Commonwealth was built with state of the art technology as the apex of the national health system pyramid.

In Cameroon, the University Centre for Health Sciences, Yaoundé, stood out as an institution established with international cooperation, bilingual teaching (in English and French), and multi-professional education in an integrated curriculum. This was done in a purpose-built infrastructure in a public health building, a biomedical science building, and a community hospital building, as well as field training areas. The Yaoundé centre, like others in sub-Saharan Africa, was a crucible for experimentation in health professions' education. It was the theatre for the implementation of the global agenda of educational concepts like community orientation, problem-based learning, and competency-driven education. I was the foundation Dean from 1969 to 1978.

Despite the differences in their history, the new medical schools followed a similar pattern in the development of their activities. Each new medical school was partnered with its own teaching hospital. The partnership was maintained even when the two entities were supervised by the ministries of higher education and public health. The advantage was that the top management of both institutions was in the hands of the same group of senior professors. They ran the medical advisory committee of the hospital management board, as well as the academic committee of the medical school that had responsibility for the curriculum.

The second-generation medical schools created after 1960 started as small enterprises of less than 20 teaching staff under the direction of the Dean, who had exclusive responsibility for the affairs of the new school. The major disciplines were represented by a senior lecturer or professor with a few lecturers. There were no departments as such. The number of students admitted was generally between 20 and 50, graduating about half or three-quarters after 5 or 6 years training.

The next stage was that of a dean supervising departments, each with a small number of teachers. For example, the department of medicine in Makerere in 1960 was run by a professor, two senior government medical specialists, and three lecturers in medicine, including myself. The total medical school staff generally did not exceed 50, although additional staff were recruited by the teaching hospitals (senior registrars, registrars, and house physicians).

The curriculum generally followed the Flexner pattern—pre-clinical, para-clinical, and clinical sequence. However, some new institutions attempting an integrated curriculum divided the staff and departments into three academic divisions, such as: biomedical sciences, clinical practice, and public health. Sometimes stakeholders delayed creation of discipline-based departments by postponing the establishment of such departments until an integrated curriculum had been achieved. This was the case with Dar es Salaam in 1968/70. As academic and professional staff increased in numbers, pre-clinical, para-clinical, and clinical departments were established, usually when integrated teaching and other innovative approaches were reasonably well-established.

As the new medical schools grew to maturity, there would be as many as 20 to 30 staff in each department, with a total of 200 or more staff in the medical school. They would admit as many as 100 students each year and graduating almost as many.

The tendency was then to create sub-departments (for example, a department of surgery or of medicine) would have 5 to 10 sub-departments for each sub-specialty like cardiology and neurology, and these medical and surgical specialized departments (for example neurology and neurosurgery) would collaborate at the summit. There might be as many as 20 to 30 surgeons in the department of surgery and just as many in medicine, not to mention other major areas like paediatrics, obstetrics, gynaecology, medical imaging, etc. Such large faculties of medicine have developed into autonomous colleges within the university hierarchy. Inevitably, the growth of the teaching hospital and its technology followed the trend in the medical school and vice versa.

The major difficulty has been, and continues to be, the very high cost and the focus on tertiary care at the expense of primary and secondary care. It then becomes imperative for undergraduate medical education to be carried out in regional and district hospitals with a view to maintaining the balance in the curriculum.

Working together across Africa

There were some aspects of our work that were distinctly African. Probably the most important was the new approach to teaching health professionals, which we developed using the concepts of field learning and practice sites. The idea was that students who studied medicine in urban modern cities should gain experience about the health situation of rural populations who formed the majority of people in African countries. Some of these sites were specially designed for the teaching of public health in rural settings. Others were designed with the same objective but with student and staff accommodation that replicated life on the campus, to some extent defeating the original purpose.

In Yaoundé, on the other hand, I insisted that students rented accommodation in the houses of villagers and lived with the same population that they met in the health centres. These sites excited international interest and quite a few medical schools in Europe and North America visited the centres and some sent their students for tropical field assignments. Initially established for public health or community health, the teaching and work of these sites were later integrated into the social and economic development of these zones. I am a biomedical researcher and believe that a physician must care with his or her head *and* heart.

This was in many ways a very exciting time, which produced some extraordinary research results as higher educational institutions and medical schools explored their environments. There were diseases and disease patterns waiting to be 'discovered', such as endomyocardial fibrosis, idiopathic cardiomegaly, tropical neuropathies related to chronic cyanide intoxication, iron deficiency anaemia due to hookworm disease in adult male farmers, susceptibility to meningitis and malaria in pregnant women, the complex immunological effects of malaria (on the kidney, liver, spleen, and brain), the phenomenon of sickle cell disease, childhood malnutrition (*kwashiokor*), Kaposi sarcomas, African childhood lymphoma, histoplasmosis, tuberculosis (pulmonary and generalized), buruli ulcer, chemotherapy of leprosy, and control of river blindness; the evolution of cancer in Africans compared to African Americans, the latter being closer to the North American and European patterns.

This formidable list of pathologies provided major challenges to physicians and other health practitioners. Fortunately the challenges came with some solutions—antibiotic and chemotherapeutic agents. This proved to be an exciting period for the care of patients, for teaching of students, and research. I myself undertook clinical, laboratory, and field epidemiological studies and demonstrated the relationship of chronic cyanide poisoning from cassava diets with endemic neuropathies in Southern Nigeria.

These developments were supported by the way that the Medical Schools worked together wherever we could. The deans had been meeting together since 1960 thanks to a grant from the Rockefeller Foundation. These meetings allowed us to share experiences and led to a consensus as to how the teachers felt that medicine should be taught in sub-Saharan Africa. Encouraged by the Association of American Medical Colleges, whose executive secretary accompanied us, we created an Association of Medicals Schools in Africa (AMSA) and I was elected foundation president. Over time, AMSA became influential and its members created professional associations, which were able to establish medical education programmes that cut across post-colonial influences. AMSA participated in the Constituent Assembly of the World Federation for Medical Education (WFME) in Mainz, Germany, and I was signatory to the WFME constitution on behalf of Africa.

Professional education in medicine and other health professions received strong support from WHO AFRO. The first conference on medical education in Africa was held in Yaoundé, Cameroon, in 1966 and attempted harmonization of the Anglophone and Francophone traditions. The WHO regional director, Dr Comlan Quenum, brought together deans of the first- and second-generation medical schools in Brazzaville in the 1970s, as well as teachers of public health, and we agreed that there should be a public health orientation in the curriculum of the respective schools.

This period also saw the development of professional associations. An Association of Physicians of East Africa already existed in 1959/60, as well as an association of surgeons, both created by expatriates. I was able to bring the idea to Ibadan after a two-year assignment in Kampala, and associations of physicians and of surgeons were created there in 1962. Members were specialist physicians and surgeons from practically all West African countries. Both associations grew to become Colleges of Physicians and of Surgeons, with sufficient authority to develop, teach, and organise professional examinations, awarding specialists certificates that were recognized by countries.

Health systems were developing in parallel over this period. In most African countries, health systems were established in a top-down manner, beginning with structures in the capital cities. They generally followed the culture of the ex-colonial powers. In some cases, like in Cameroon, bilateral agreements provided for different patterns in the regions. German, French, American, UNICEF, and Belgian experts were assigned to different regions of the country. The national authorities 'learnt' from these different influences and developed a system based essentially on the African health development framework—the three-tier community focused national health system supervised by a minister of health.

WHO AFRO organized inter-country cooperation for health systems development during the decade of 1985–94.

Looking to the future with international cooperation

A new phenomenon of the proliferation of medical schools occurred at the turn of the new millennium. People and governments raised their voices in support of a movement to increase the doctor-to-population ratio in the belief that the falling quality of care was related to the low doctor-to-population ratio. Government-owned medical schools were forced to increase their student intake, sometimes by a factor of five, and the private sector was encouraged to join in the fray. The consequence was that instead of six in 1960, by 2010 there were over 120 medical schools in sub-Saharan African countries. The increase in numbers was not matched by increases in facilities, equipment, or finances. In some countries, the medical schools seemed to have been hastily created with only a handful of teachers and limited opportunities for practical clinical teaching.

This was the difficult situation observed by the sub-Saharan African Medical School Study (SAMSS) financed by the Bill and Melinda Gates Foundation.[1] I took part in this exercise: we visited a sample of medical schools and the rest were surveyed. It was clear that many of these countries and their medical schools needed help and some help came quickly through a collaborative effort between sub-Saharan countries and the USA, including twining US medical colleges with African institutions.[2]

Looking to the history of the last few decades, we can see that international cooperation was essential for the development of health systems and in the growth of medical education. Paradoxically, international health cooperation was the best friend of health sciences' education but at the same time perhaps the worst enemy of the health system. On the educational level, young Africans won scholarships to study medicine (and other professions) abroad but many did not return home. Some had acquired skills in the use of technology that could not be practised in their home countries at that particular time.

International agencies would observe a weak health system and yet seduce some of its best elements for expatriation. Often technical advice is excellent but cannot be implemented because of cultural barriers. Not infrequently, the visiting expert assumes he/she understands a culture and provides advice that only weakens the health system. Quite often contributions come as gifts that aggravate the dependency syndrome and divert young governments away from their own priorities.

What is needed ideally is for external cooperation to clearly assist in the implementation of indigenous policies, taking care to ensure that the policies are not those of the intellectual elite but that they represent the needs and wants of local populations. The Millennium Development Goals were a great step in this direction, making humankind work together, looking in the same direction and targeting goals in which they can recognize themselves. The new post-2015 development agenda should ensure that the outcomes of our common endeavours can be seen and felt by local populations everywhere.

Conclusion

Teachers in the new African medical schools created before independence faced the challenge on the one hand of the unusual methods of the colonial administration, whilst on the other hand we realized that the teaching of medicine in Europe and America was not entirely appropriate. We witnessed the phenomenal growth in knowledge, including of science and technology, economics and management, which virtually transformed doctors, previously humanists and philosophers, into technologists and entrepreneurs. This called for a renaissance of humanism in medicine.

Practising medicine in the African setting also called for a return to the basics. The doctor–patient relationship defines the profile both of a doctor and the healthcare seeker in behavioural terms: the health professional will be caring, competent, and supportive; sick persons expect relief of suffering, if not cure of disease, and, eventually, better health. When a doctor attends to a patient, his/her caring humanitarian attitude and analytical scientific thinking engage him/her to apply his/her knowledge and skills to the benefit of the patient. The doctor–patient relationship should, to a large extent, determine the configuration of health systems and consequently the agenda of medical education, medical care, and medical research. The medical school is a repository of professional skills and knowledge, and the staff are role models of desirable professional attitudes and critical scientific thinking.

These ideas are the basis for proposals for reinventing health professions' education in African countries. This should be done in multi-professional university centres of health sciences where, trained together, health professionals will work in health teams to deliver quality healthcare. Each training institution would have responsibility for the care of target populations in health districts or regions. This was the mission assigned to the University Centre for Health Sciences created in Yaoundé, Cameroon, in 1969.

The Independent Commission on Health Professions' Education at the turn of a new century has clarified many concepts and ideas, such as community oriented, problem-based, and competency driven curricula; the identification of core themes, instructional strategies—informative, formative, or transformative learning; instructional methods in relation to institutional missions and systems of governance adapted to new situations.[3] Some African medical schools have been able in the last 50 years to implement many of these innovations, operating in virgin territory relatively free of vested interests. A century ago the crisis in American medical education led to the Flexner Report that revolutionized the teaching of medicine worldwide.[4] The current health crisis in Africa could be the opportunity for creative innovations for Africa to contribute significantly to global health.

Whilst we can learn from others, we have our own distinctively African approach, which has much to teach the rest of the world.

References

1 Sub-Saharan African Medical Schools Study. <www.samss.org>.
2 Through the Medical Educational Partnership Initiative (MEPI), www.fic.nih.gov, and other routes.
3 Frenk J, et al. Education of health professionals for a new century: transforming education to strengthen health systems in an interdependent world. *The Lancet* 2010; **376**: 1923–58.
4 Flexner A. *Medical education in the United States and Canada*. Carnegie Foundation, 1910.

Chapter 15

Indigenous knowledge systems

Catherine A. Odora-Hoppers

Research Chair in Development Education at the University
of South Africa

Professor Hoppers holds a South African Research Chair in Development Education at the University of South Africa. Prior to that, she was a technical adviser
on Indigenous Knowledge Systems to the Parliamentary Portfolio Committee
on Arts, Culture, Science, and Technology. In this chapter she describes the tensions that exist between Western scientific approaches and Indigenous Knowledge Systems. She illustrates the way in which traditional knowledge of, for
example, herbal medicines, has a potentially very high economic value and
describes how this can be developed in partnership between local and global
interests. She goes on to describe her role as Professor of Development Education in creating a new interdisciplinary field of study, which strengthens the role
of Indigenous Knowledge Systems in the social and economic development of
Africa and opens out new ways of seeing the world and acting to improve it.

Knowledge systems around the world

Many societies in the developing world have nurtured and refined systems of
knowledge of their own, relating to such diverse domains as geology, ecology,
botany, agriculture, physiology, and health. Within this, the emergence of
terms such as 'parallel', 'indigenous', and 'civilizational' knowledge systems
are also expressions of other approaches to the acquisition and production of
knowledge.

I would argue that Indigenous Knowledge Systems (IKS) need to be strengthened—particularly with regard to their links with education, rural development, improvement of existing skills and grassroots' innovations, job creation,
primary health care, and human resource development. In doing so, I would
suggest that the IKS process is seen as helping to facilitate and engender mindset change in all public institutions with regards to IKS in particular and towards
knowledge and people-centred development in general.

IKS, therefore, reminds us that it is a fitting time to reaffirm the commitments made 50 years ago to strive for even more effective, rigorous, and balanced implementation of human rights for all. Within this, the relationship between intellectual property and human rights lies in the confluence between traditional knowledge, the right to health, the obligations of democracy and transparency demanded of science in its links with society, in cultural heritage, and in the principle of non-discrimination.

In 1999, the World Conference on Science for the 21st Century took place in Budapest. In its Declaration published in 2000, it states that full and free exercise of science, with its own values, should not be seen to conflict with the recognition of spiritual, cultural, philosophical, and religious values of traditional knowledge. An open dialogue needs to be maintained with these value systems to facilitate mutual understanding. It states that for the development of an all-encompassing debate on ethics in science, and a possibly ensuing code of universal values, it is necessary to recognize the many ethical frameworks in the civilizations around the world.

> . . . traditional societies, many of them with strong cultural roots, have nurtured and refined systems of knowledge of their own, relating to such diverse domains as astronomy, meteorology, geology, botany, agriculture, physiology, psychology and health. Such knowledge systems represent an enormous wealth [both material and non-material]. Not only do they harbour information as yet unknown to modern science, but they are also expressions of other ways of living in the world, other relationships between society and nature, and other approaches to the acquisition and construction of knowledge. Special action must be taken to conserve and cultivate this fragile and diverse world heritage in the face of globalization and the growing dominance of a single view of the natural world as espoused by science. A closer linkage between science and other knowledge systems is expected to bring about important advantages to both sides.[1]

Modern scientific knowledge and traditional knowledge systems, the Declaration elaborates, should be brought closer together in interdisciplinary projects dealing with the links between culture, environment, and development in such areas as conservation of biological diversity, management of natural resources, understanding of natural hazards, and mitigating their impact.

According to the World Intellectual Property Organization (WIPO) worldwide Fact Finding Missions report (1999),[2] it is noted that TK practitioners in the area of health were now increasingly collaborating with modern practitioners with whom they exchange information and cooperate to find treatments in the most difficult cases. However, lack of government support or systematic recognition of their contribution to health still persists. This has led communities to emphasize *getting recognition* as being a higher priority over and above financial reward.

Quite often, African *izangoma*/traditional healers and *amakhosi*/traditional leaders are major custodians of IKS. Indigenous religious leaders, *Shembe, Lekganyane, Nehanda, Modjadji*, to name a few, are both seen as, and practise as, healers and spiritual heads whose intervention in social issues are critical to the social health of the community. In Nguni culture, for instance, *Inkosi yohlanga* (hereditary) king/queen mother symbolize the health of the nation (we here distinguish between hereditary *amakhosi*/traditional leaders from the missionary and apartheid imposed ones). These people are part of the culture developed over many years and are socially acceptable, charge affordable fees, and take a holistic view of the circumstances of the patient

The World Health Organization (WHO) defines traditional medicine as:

> the sum total of all the knowledge and practices, whether explicable or not, used in diagnosis, prevention and elimination of physical, mental or social imbalance and relying exclusively on practical experience and observations handed down from generation to generation, whether verbally or in writing.[3]

The issue of access to and use of indigenous knowledge in medicine in particular is becoming increasingly important globally, not least because of the huge economic implications of the use of traditional knowledge. A good example is the 60 billion dollars world market of herbal products, which is expected to grow to 5 trillion dollars by the year 2020. Healthcare providers worldwide, including major pharmaceutical giants, are starting to incorporate many of these herbal products into their mainstream activities without the actual knowledge holders being aware of this.

As traditional medicines are largely based on medicinal plants indigenous to developing countries, where the indigenous system has been in vogue for several centuries, there is great interest in accessing them either directly or through the use of modern tools of breeding and cultivation, including tissue culture, cell culture, and transgenic technology.

Knowledge and technology sharing

Nigeria offers a good example of how to resolve the tensions involved in this relationship between Western manufacturers and local people. Here patent protection has been identified as a key prerequisite for generating benefits to local practitioners based on their knowledge. The Nigerian Institute for Pharmaceutical Research and Development (NIPRD) entered into an agreement with the herbalists whose knowledge they used to develop drugs. The agreement provides a very comprehensive framework for obtaining the informed consent of the local herbalists for using his or her knowledge to develop commercial products.

The Institute is obliged to furnish to the herbalists in writing, the results of every scientific test or analysis carried out on material derived from the herbalists.

The benefit-sharing arrangement includes a detailed documentation of the philosophical and empirical context of the investigations. The problems of translation across different worldviews were also factored into the process rather than ignored, as is the norm with modern scientific research. They applied the principle 'when in doubt, record and report rather than ignore and omit'. The Nigerian case also illustrates that there are some commonalities between the medical thinking of ancient Western philosophers and the Igbo worldview.

For instance, there is a similarity in the scepticism about the corpuscular theory (i.e. relying too much on empirical understanding of the way parts of the body work), and the Igbo's rejection of the explanation of diseases or health based on some microscopic constituents of material objects.

It is also felt that Western definitions of certain diseases and their treatment are focused on the major outstanding symptoms while ignoring the 'subtle-but-chronic' and debilitating symptoms of the disease. Traditional medicine emphasizes not only the physical properties of the herb, but also the natural life force within the plant and the spiritual role of the ancestors and the gods in the healing process. A herbalist is thus not just a herbalist, but also the custodian of the religious life of the community.

In the context of this agreement, a herbalist was given the post of lecturer in traditional medicine at the University of Jos. A clinic was also set up, which is run and managed by the healers themselves. Healers and modern doctors sometimes jointly diagnose the patients.

It was with this sensitivity and openness that the concept, well known in African societies as ethical conduct and generosity even in poverty, was beginning to be understood and even valued again. The sacred institutions for conserving trees, rivers, and plants were all recognized as part of the institutional context for promoting the conservation and sustainable use of biodiversity.[4]

Bodeker and Knoneberg have written about how traditional medicine, a term used here to denote the indigenous health traditions of the world—and complementary and alternative medicine—have, in the past 20 years, claimed an increasing share of the public's awareness and the agenda of medical researchers.[5] Studies have documented that about half the population of many industrialized countries now use traditional and complementary medicines, and the proportion is as high as 80% in many developing countries.

Most research has focused on clinical and experimental medicine (safety, efficacy, and mechanism of action) and regulatory issues, to the general neglect of public health dimensions. Public health research must consider social, cultural, political, and economic contexts to maximize the contribution of T/CAM to healthcare systems globally.[5]

The integration of the traditional and other knowledges, including technology, requires developing awareness and creating policies and strategies that aim at the recognition, development, promotion, and protection of the traditional or indigenous knowledges. The need for this recognition, promotion, and protection arises from several factors. Indigenous people around the world are the caretakers of the land on which they live. Their care of the land contributes to the sustained biodiversity in those areas and has allowed people to live in one place, often for thousands of years. Their ecological knowledge is massive, and may surpass that of modern science.[6]

These people have been forced aside by outsiders and often taken from the land they sustained for so long. This marginalization has distorted the possibility of evolving an understanding of the lifestyle, the knowledge systems, and living cultures that govern the lives of indigenous or rural communities.

Because these rural communities often live without modern amenities, do not have access to other infrastructure benefits that are available to a sizeable proportion of a national or regional population, and are economically deprived, the intellectual property rights of these communities have been susceptible to theft. They have also often been targets of badly conceived interventions that have been detrimental to the sustenance of their lifestyle and their knowledge systems.

McNeely states that indigenous peoples do not use the concept 'technology' in their vocabulary, and development groups seldom mention the social and cultural experiences of their interaction with indigenous and/or rural populations, a permanent grey area has sedimented, which has the effect of blocking new or potentially constructive interventions, especially in the area of technology transfer.[7]

The future—creating new structures and new disciplines

South Africa is the African country that is leading the way, and where innovative steps have been taken in policy, legislative, and practice. The indigenous knowledge policy was passed by parliament in 2004. New and reformed intellectual property laws are just being passed and there 10 ministries that work together to incorporate IKS into their policies, strategies, and practices. The Medical Research Council (MRC) set up the National Reference Centre for African Traditional Medicine (NRCATM) in the Western Cape. A similar centre has been set up in Pretoria.

Current estimates suggest that more than 60% of the world's population rely on traditional medicines, and in South Africa, this figure is over 80%. Traditional healers in South Africa are the first healthcare providers to be consulted in up to 80% of cases, especially in rural areas. The new National Centre will also provide potential for trade, job creation, and poverty alleviation. It will establish an information system on African traditional medicines; research medicinal plants; identify education and training on traditional medicines; protect indigenous knowledge through patents and intellectual property rights; promote research into diseases; and establish a processing business.

The centre is led by the Department of Health, the Medical Research Council, and the Council for Scientific and Industrial Research, and will be used by traditional healers, the government, regulatory authorities, scientists, medical professionals, conservation authorities, communities, and businesses.

Botswana is also creating a policy to protect, preserve, and promote its indigenous knowledge and mainstream it into the country's macro-economic framework. Development of the policy will involve identifying, documenting, and gathering local traditional knowledge practices from areas including agriculture, health, culture, and religious beliefs, and then feeding them into a legislative framework. It has isolated policies on natural resources, such as the National Policy on Natural Resource Conservation and Development and the National Policy on Culture, which fit within international frameworks including the Nagoya Protocol, an international agreement to combat bio-piracy and share benefits from national resources research fairly.

The African Regional Intellectual Property Organization is also developing a protocol to protect holders of traditional knowledge from any infringement of their rights and the misappropriation, misuse or exploitation of their knowledge. In other words, indigenous knowledge debates have become more complex and academic, particularly when viewed in the context of intellectual property and the expectation that regional collaborations should be encouraged and developed.

The question for the future, epitomized by these approaches, is about how Africa will reconcile and integrate the disciplines coming from a Western epistemology with the very different traditions and patterns of indigenous knowledge systems?

As part of its wider approach to development, the South African Government decided to create 200 research chairs under the Ministry of Science and Technology with the core mandate to advance the frontiers of knowledge through focused research in identified fields or problem areas, and create new research career pathways for highly skilled, high-quality young and mid-career researchers, as well as stimulate strategic research across the knowledge spectrum.

Most of them are in the natural sciences, but I have been privileged to be appointed to the Chair in Development Education, which combines the social and the natural sciences and bypasses the usual split between basic and applied research.

Established in January 2008, the DST/NRF (Department of Science and Technology/National Research Foundation) South African Research Chair in Development Education is hosted by the University of South Africa (UNISA), which has positioned itself as 'the African University in the service of humanity'.

The Chair introduces a new pedagogy in academic research and citizenship education, which takes development and the acute lessons drawn from it as *a pedagogic field* and has human development as the goal. Its exploration through research, post-graduate teaching, and community engagement seeks answers to some of the most taxing and exciting questions about development, knowledge production, and science. It asks the questions:

- What kind of transformative actions must be brought to bear to enable both restorative action and sustainable human development to occur in Africa and elsewhere?

- How can key areas of disciplinary knowledge production (such as science, economics, education, and law) be reconstituted in order to bring about a just and human-centred development on the continent?

Development Education reframes human development within a paradigm of restorative action and cognitive justice. It is premised on an epistemology of hope, and from there it articulates transformation from the standpoint of second-level indigenization. Putting hope at the centre of our epistemology prevents 'the limits of reality to reign supreme'. Hope probes the future and thereby illuminates the possibilities of the present. Hope tells us that our present existence is not ultimate and that there is an alternative. It is a vision of a possibility that might be realized.

This DST/NRF Chair in Development Education straddles a number of strategic policy areas in South Africa: science, technology, and innovation policy; higher education policy and the indigenous knowledge systems' policy. In addition, it draws on the University of South Africa's 2015 *Strategic Plan: An Agenda for Transformation*.

The Department of Education White Paper 3 on Higher Education Transformation states that the democratic transition requires that 'all existing practices, institutions, and values are viewed anew and re-thought in terms of their fitness for the new era'.[8] Therefore, the goals and orientation of higher education, and science and technology systems and policies need to change in order to support the new political project of a democratic society based on social justice. This has implied a concerted search for the best possible conceptualizations and institutional forms to discharge this task.

The White Paper of Science and Technology has the National System of Innovation as a key architecture to achieve its policy objectives. It calls for a greater understanding of social processes and social problems as a source of social innovation, and urges for the production of new knowledge and an informed critique of the transformation of South African society and its economy. The human and social sciences, in particular, are expected to design interventions to help the inclusion of previously disadvantaged people into the National System of Innovations, function as change agents, and as educators—responsible for a range of capacity development interventions geared to enhance the transformation agenda at systems level.

The problem of the limited paradigms guiding knowledge production, the poor partnership between the social and natural sciences, and their overall effect in limiting the understanding of society's problems had already been noted in the review of the science and technology institutions.[9] In that review, and later the DST Research and Development strategy, the role of the social sciences in developing more holistic understandings of societal problems, helping to delineate the contours of problems facing society, and, in particular, of probing the possibilities for using local knowledge as the platform for implementation of innovation-based strategies, had also been outlined. One of the three areas of multi-disciplinary research mentioned explicitly was indigenous knowledge systems.

The IKS Policy registers a commitment to the recognition, promotion, development, protection, and affirmation of IKS in South Africa. It provides an enabling framework to stimulate and strengthen the contribution of indigenous knowledge to social and economic development in the country. The main drivers of the policy include:

- Affirmation of African cultural values in the face of globalization.
- Practical measures for the development of services provided by IK holders and practitioners.
- Contribution of indigenous knowledge to the economy.
- Interfaces with other knowledge systems.

Universities were originally established as transmitters of culture, learning, and independent thought. However, over time the business of the academy has become that of transacting mainly in data and information, but not knowledge, insights, or wisdom. Increasingly its traditional role of fostering scholarship, original research, and critical thinking is losing ground.[10] This poses a number of ethical issues that need to be discussed, if not resolved.

In addition, a tension exists between the role of the university as on the one hand providing a platform for engaging and critiquing elite global economic interests; but on the other hand, it is steeped in the elite culture, and is a product of elite interests rather than community ones. It is also a major 'credentialing' institution for a certain social class rather than an intellectual community bound by 'social contract' to less formally recognized intellectual ones.

Furthermore, in spite of many well-intentioned community outreach projects, in reality, university communities are more 'closed loops' of discourse than they imagine. As they go forward in finding a place in the 'international knowledge economy', what then, are the conditions for a new social contract between universities and society?[11]

Conclusion

Indigenous knowledge is seen as part of the subaltern and heterogeneous forms of knowledge that had no place in the fields of knowledge that grew in compact with colonialism and science. By linking the memory of its survival from the 'epistemological death row' and casting this emerging drama within the task of renegotiation of human agency, indigenous knowledge and their carriers and holders in communities around the African continent and the global South at last have a place.

And by their stirring presence, they become revolutionary heuristics in a post-colonial transformation agenda. In my role as Chair I affirm that local knowledges, tribal knowledges, civilizational knowledges, dying knowledges, all need a site, a theatre of encounter, which is not patronizing, not preservationist, not fundamentalist, but open and playful (Visvanathan 2000). The moral and pragmatic task is to develop new cognitive tools and propositions capable of deciphering the erasure cryptogram that hierarchized and excised the majority of African people from the global collective memory as a positive and substantive contributor to world civilization—hence denying them active citizenship in key areas of contemporary global currency including knowledge and science.

What this means in practice is that there will be an underlying process of continuously and critically examining through research, the legacy of Africa's relation with international systems, while engaging in building new scenarios for action and policy formulation looking at the future. The way to do this in a teaching and learning context is to introduce trans-disciplinary focal areas for theoretical, applied, and strategic research explorations, e.g. science, culture, and society; peace and human development; indigenous knowledge systems and innovation; university and society in Africa—all of which contain powerful heuristics in terms of theory building, methodological perspectives, and practical interventions in a new ethical dispensation.

References

1 UNESCO. World Conference on Science for the 21st Century, 2000. <http://unesdoc.unesco.org/images/0012/001207/120706e.pdf>.

2 WIPO. Fact Finding Missions, 1999.

3 WHO. Traditional and complementary medicine. <www.who.int/medicines/areas/traditional/en/>.

4 **Berlin OB and Berlin EA.** Improving health care by coupling indigenous and modern medical knowledge: the scientific bases of Highland Maya Herbal Medicine in Chiapas, Mexico. In: *Science for the Twenty First Century. A New Commitment.* UNESCO, 2000, pp. 438–9.

5 **Bodeker G and Kroneberg F.** A public health agenda for traditional, complementary, and alternative medicine. *Am J Public Health* 2002; **92**(10):1582–91.

6 **Durning AT.** Supporting indigenous peoples. In: LR Brown, C Flavin, S Postel, and L Stark (eds). *State of the World.* WW Norton & Company Inc., 1993, pp. 80–100.

7 **McNeely.** *Successful Technology Transfer to Indigenous Peoples*; National Renewable Energy Laboratory. James Madison University 2000.

8 Government of South Africa. Department of Education White Paper 3 on Higher Education Transformation, 1997.

9 Government of South Africa: The SETI Report. 1998.

10 **Peat D.** *The Role and Future of the Universities.* Pari Centre. Italy, 2000.

11 **Odora Hoppers CA.** 'Re-assessing Community Engagement on the African Continent'. Address to the board of the South African Higher Education Community Engagement Forum (SAHECEF), Pretoria, 18 March 2011.

Part 5

Health for the whole population—leaving no-one behind

Chapter 16

Introduction to Part 5: Health for the whole population— leaving no-one behind

Francis Omaswa and Nigel Crisp

This chapter addresses the way in which universal health coverage has become one of the most important concepts in global health. It sets the scene for the following chapters in which leaders discuss the implementation of universal health coverage in Rwanda, South Africa, and Ghana.

Leaving no one behind

This part of the book is concerned with strengthening health systems, including their financing, so that they can provide healthcare for the whole population.

It contains three remarkable stories from three of the African countries leading the way—Rwanda (Chapter 17), South Africa (Chapter 18), and Ghana (Chapter 19). Each faces very different challenges. Rwanda is re-building its country after the genocide and has espoused a community based system that draws everyone together. In South Africa the Government has to confront the massive HIV/AIDS epidemic and its legacy, as well as establish a national system in a context where there is already a large and strong private health sector serving a small proportion of the population. Ghana, which is growing fast overall, has the problem of delivering healthcare coverage to the poorest parts of its population and ensuring that nobody is left behind.

The countries are taking different approaches, appropriate to their very different contexts; but they are similarly focused on serving their whole populations and on seeing health and healthcare as being absolutely central to the future wellbeing and prosperity of their countries. All of them are also taking a measured phase by phase approach to the enormous task of introducing universal healthcare, with pilots and evaluations at every stage. Both Rwanda and Ghana have already been developing their systems for more than a decade, whilst South Africa, currently piloting its approach, is planning for implementation over the next decade and more.

The last chapter 'Health for the whole population' in this part of the book takes an overall view of the challenges facing African countries in planning and achieving universal coverage. It is written by an economist and a medical doctor and is based on their experience across Africa. Taken together, we believe Chapters 17–20 can offer very relevant insights to other countries in Africa and beyond.

The global context

These national developments take place in a wider global context where the attainment of universal health coverage is becoming a new global goal with strong support from leaders both in the WHO and the World Bank. Dr Margaret Chan, Director General of WHO, has written: 'Universal Health Coverage is the single most powerful concept that public health has to offer'.[1]

Meanwhile at a World Bank and WHO conference in Tokyo in December 2013, World Bank Group President Jim Yong Kim was unequivocal—'achieving universal health coverage and equity in health are central to reaching the [World Bank] global goals to end extreme poverty by 2030 and boost shared prosperity'.[2] The most significant outcome of the conference was the release of a joint World Bank and World Health Organization proposed framework for monitoring progress towards UHC. The framework sets out clear commitments to reduce out-of-pocket payments and improve access to healthcare for the poor with two new targets:

◆ Halve the number of people impoverished by healthcare payments from 100 million to 50 million by 2020, and eliminate the problem altogether by 2030.

◆ Double the number of poor people (the poorest 40%) with access to healthcare services by 2020—from 40% to 80%.[3]

The importance of these approaches was reinforced by a recent review of financing that argued that most low- and middle-income countries will be able to see major improvements in health in the next 20 years, bringing both health and economic benefits to their people.[4] It seems clear from these and many other statements and developments in recent months that universal health coverage will be a core part of global health policy in the post-MDG years after 2015.

At the same time European countries, which have had universal coverage for years, are finding difficulties in maintaining it. Their immediate problem is financial, caused by the global crisis and the rapidly growing costs of ageing populations and expanding technologies. However, the deeper problem is that they have health systems designed for the problems of the last century—when they operated very successfully—but which are ill-suited to the needs of the twenty-first century with its explosion of non-communicable diseases. It is becoming increasingly clear that they are outdated and need radical change.

The conjunction of the ambitious expansion of health systems in Africa and other countries around the world with the crisis in health systems in Europe and North America provides some interesting dynamics and tensions. The developing systems can gain insights from the more developed ones but need to be careful not to adopt their models and practices wholesale. The developed systems can similarly learn from the developing ones which, without the same legacy of structures and behaviours, can and are innovating and developing new approaches.

Much of the global debate on universal health coverage revolves around economics with discussion of 'fiscal space', what can be afforded, and who needs to pay what. Even the language of 'coverage' implies the use of an insurance-based system of some sort. It may also imply the introduction of top-down national systems. The examples here, particularly that of Rwanda, challenge this economic and top-down dominance with their alternative emphasis on health, communities, and local ownership. It is the editors' view that we need to understand much better the role of individuals and communities—and their non-financial contributions to healthcare—if we are to achieve universal coverage. This debate, however, is for another time.

In Chapters 21–23, regardless of these sometimes very theoretical global discussions, we can see health leaders getting on with the task in hand and, in the words of our title, *making change and claiming the future*.

References

1 The Lancet. *Universal Health Coverage*; themed issue. 7 Sept 2012 <http://www.thelancet.com/themed-universal-health-coverage>.

2 The World Bank. *Speech by World Bank Group President Jim Yong Kim at the Government of Japan-World Bank Conference on Universal Health Coverage.* http://www.worldbank.org/en/news/speech/2013/12/06/speech-world-bank-group-president-jim-yong-kim-government-japan-conference-universal-health-coverage.

3 UHC FORWARD. *New World Bank and WHO Targets Announced on Health Coverage for the Poorest 40%*, available from <http://uhcforward.org/headline/new-world-bank-and-who-targets-announced-health-coverage-poorest-40> accessed 22 Dec 2013.

4 Jamison DT, et al. Global Health 2035: a world converging within a generation. *The Lancet*, 10.106/SO140-6736(13)62105–4, 3 Dec 2013.

Chapter 17

Twenty years of improving access to healthcare in Rwanda

Agnes Binagwaho

Minister of Health of Rwanda; Senior Lecturer at Harvard Medical School; and Clinical Professor of Paediatrics at the Geisel School of Medicine at Dartmouth College

Dr Agnes Binagwaho is a Rwandan paediatrician who was trained in Europe before returning to her own country after the genocide. She was Permanent Secretary of the Ministry of Health from 2008 until she became the Minister of Health in 2011. In this chapter she describes the establishment and development of a patient-centred healthcare delivery platform, breaking geographic barriers by ensuring equitable distribution of health facilities aligned to the administrative structure of the country, and also by mitigating financial barriers with a community based insurance system that has provided coverage for more than 90% of the population by 2011. She emphasizes the importance of a holistic approach to providing care that is community based, driven by Rwandan leaders with international support, and being part of the wider development of her country. She describes many important principles that were applied in developing the system: from conceiving of 'our mission as fulfilling the right to health of each person over the entire course of their life' and recognizing that 'when you focus on the poorest first, you take the rest with you. When you focus on where the greatest gaps are, you make the biggest gains.'

Healthcare as part of the wider recovery and development of the country

This chapter is based on my experience as, first, Executive Secretary of the National AIDS Control Commission followed by Permanent Secretary, and now Minister of Health. It is important to emphasize that accomplishing all that we have has been a team effort, involving many people who are engaged daily with improving the lives of others. Also, the consistent gains we have made for our people would not have been possible without their own contribution, political will, and the support of our development partners.

It is 20 years ago that the country was destroyed during the genocide against the Tutsi. Extreme violence, including sexual violence used as a weapon of war, caused unbelievable suffering.

At the time, I was a paediatrician in France, and I observed with extreme despair the horrors occurring in my birthplace. Two years later, I joined with many others in the diaspora in returning to Rwanda because we believed in the promise for a better future, and that this was worth fighting for. We will never forget this part of our history, and we will continue to fight through all segments of society so that this never happens again. Today the shared notion of '*ndi Umunyarwanda*' meaning 'I am Rwandan' defines our vision, our unity, our achievements, and our future. It strengthens our nation's character.

I mention this background because it underpins and explains why we have taken the approach that we have to creating a patient-centred health system in the country; one that is based on social solidarity and the importance of making sure that every citizen gets access to the quality care available, regardless of who they are, where they live, and how much they can pay. We view it as part of the wider recovery and development of the country.

In this chapter, I will focus on three of the major barriers that were preventing our people from accessing the care that they needed: geographic, financial, and informational. The following pages describe how we started to overcome these three barriers. Our approach gives insight into how we understand the wider determinants of health and the way that improving health is intimately linked with improving education, transportation, and economic opportunity.

Geographic equity

When I first returned to Rwanda in the summer of 1994, the health system was non-functional. The infrastructure was destroyed. The majority of health professionals and their families had been killed or fled the country.

When I came back, I began to understand the organization of my country, which is now organized into four provinces and Kigali city. In these provinces, we have a total of 30 districts. Districts are divided by 416 sectors and each sector has approximately 10 cells, each of which is comprised of an average of 10 villages.

To improve access, the leadership wanted to mitigate the distance from healthcare services, and thus built our primary healthcare system in a way that is sensitive to where care is needed. Meaning today, the time to reach a health facility in Rwanda, it is 60-minute walk, on average.

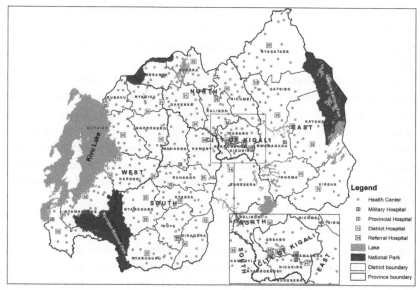

Fig. 17.1 Map of health facilities in Rwanda, December 2012.

Reproduced with permission from the Rwanda Ministry of Health/Health Management Information System, June 2013.

Each district now has one or two district hospitals, totalling to 42 district hospitals. We also have 502 health centres spread throughout the sectors; only 10 of the 416 sectors do not have one. Additionally, at the cell level, we currently have over 200 health posts run by nurses and are actively preparing to build 1000 more over the next 24 months (Fig. 17.1).

But health facilities were not enough—we needed people who are trusted and respected at the local level to also promote health. As such, we developed a community health worker network of over 45 000 people. In each of our 15 000 villages, we have three community health workers (CHWs), consisting of two women—with one woman trained and devoted to antenatal care, post-delivery, and care for children under 1 year of age—and one man. He and the second female CHW are trained by the Ministry of Health to identify, treat, and provide general care to their neighbours.

The CHWs are elected by their village to serve in this role. They are from the communities in which they serve, and must be able to read, write, and transmit monthly reports. Each CHW has a cell phone that they use for their reporting via SMS/text, which they also use for calling ambulances, seeking advice, and alerting officials of possible outbreak of disease. They are able—among other health services—to treat gastroenteritis and respiratory diseases, diagnose and treat malaria, mobilize for prevention and rapid treatment of TB and HIV, and malnutrition. They are key to all prevention programmes, and they have performed very well with providing antibiotics, antimalarial treatment, and family planning.

A key reason to maintain such a robust network of well-trained CHWs is to address 80% of the burden of disease in the country at the village level. Also, by having the CHWs—who are neighbours, friends, and fellow villagers—in such close proximity to our people, this can accelerate the transfer of those with health problems beyond the scope of the CHWs to health professionals. With this approach, we have broken geographic barriers, drastically reduced the rate of premature mortality, and improved timely access to care and treatment for our people.

Financial equity

After 1994, we were determined to create a system that removed the financial barriers to healthcare. This led to the development of a community based health insurance system called *Mutuelles de Santé*. The basis of the fee-based scheme is very simple, and it covers 90% of healthcare costs for enrolees, with patients paying only 10% of the costs out of pocket at the point of care.

The *Mutuelles* is a community owned system, which provides access to treatment and care in the health centres, and in both state owned and non-state hospitals that have an agreement with the government and the *Mutuelles*. It has been developed over the years to provide a greater range of services and to ensure that it reaches everyone in the country. We learned from and adapted our approach as we went—and we continue to do so. We have taken many steps to achieve higher levels of population coverage, including the creation of a strict referral system for health service delivery from the community to hospitals.

The first step towards the creation of a community owned health insurance system started with a pilot in three districts in 1999. The immense success of this pilot encouraged the government to develop a mechanism for making the community based health insurance (CBHI) system available to the entire population. The scaling up occurred when the First Lady of Rwanda submitted a project jointly with the Ministry of Health to the Global Fund. The successful submission led to a project granted with funding to strengthen the health system by paying the premium for around the 800 000 poorest Rwandans. Universal access to health insurance in Rwanda would not have been made possible without this project.

Given that the government of Rwanda pays the premium and the co-payment at the point of care for the poor, this initiative became very popular to the less poor who were starting to recognize that the poor had better access to health insurance than they did. As a result, they rushed to pay the fee to be covered, which was $2 dollar per household at the time. While the financial contribution was not that large, the enthusiasm to purchase insurance represented a shift in mind-set of the people of Rwanda. It was the first time that our population would pay to have access to healthcare services without actually being sick. This has allowed us to educate the population about the value of health insurance and reducing catastrophic expenditures.

As recognition of the value of being enrolled in *Mutuelles* began to spread, we were able to start our journey for financial sustainability of the *Mutuelles* by increasing the contribution paid by households to $2 per member per household. Uptake did not suffer even with this increase in premium paid by families.

Even through the subsequent financing shifts related to the *Mutuelles*, the poorest members of the community never paid anything for their membership fees or co-payments.

This is due to our collaboration with development partners, increased domestic funds invested in the health sector by the Rwandan government, as well as reinvigorating the *ubudehe*. The ubedehe is the traditional pro-poor community solidarity system that was adapted to become a community driven socio-economic classification system, which is based on the assets of each household as evaluated by their surrounding village.

As the population has understood the value of the benefit of the package of services covered by the *Mutuelles*, the family take-up of insurance remains very high.

In the current system, which has been in effect since July 2011, we have stratified the affiliation of the *Mutuelles de Santé* according to the socio-economic classification of *ubudehe*. Today's system is fee stratified, with the wealthiest members of the population paying the most (about $12 a year per member of the household), the middle class paying less ($6 per capita), and the poorest in our county paying nothing. And uptake continues to be very high, with over 90% of Rwandans having health insurance (Table 17.1).

Table 17.1 Coverage and utilization (percentage of population) of the *Mutuelles* insurance system, 2003–10

	2003	2004	2005	2006	2007	2008	2009	2010
Enrolment in CBHI	7	27	44	73	75	85	86	91
Utilization rate	31	39	47	61	72	83	86	95

We have coupled the new stratification with a roaming system that allows patients to receive care from any health facility across the country, no matter their contribution level to the *Mutuelles*. In Rwanda today, enrolment to health insurance really is a universal benefit, and the *Mutuelles* itself is more sustainable.

Underlying the success in both the financing and uptake of *Mutuelles,* has been our focus on making it a community owned system. Members pay their fees near their health centre at *'Sections of Mutuelles'*, which are managed by professionals who report to a Board elected by the community. From this local pool of funding (from about 10 villages at each section), 40.5% is forwarded to the corresponding district to cover the costs of care provided at the district hospital should a patient transfer be made from a health centre. Another 4.5% of the collected funds is sent to the Ministry of Health to pay for services delivered in another district or in referral hospitals (the tertiary level). Over time, we are developing local bodies to assume management of the funds so that the central government can step back to take on a more strategic role. After all, this system will always be community owned.

Now that the system has been well incubated, the Ministry of Health is handing over the financial management of the *Mutuelles de Santé* to the Ministry of Finance and related institutions because it is the governmental body with jurisdiction to monitor health insurance and financing.

Establishing this type of community based health insurance system has not been a simple process. Its achievement is a testimony of the entire government working as one for the welfare of our population. The effort has been led by the Ministry of Health and has enjoyed the great support of other ministries, including the Ministry of Local Government and the Ministry of Finance. Once again, it has been a team effort.

Right to information

As we aimed to overcome both geographic and financial barriers to care, we used a participatory approach because the people at the community level are directly part of the governance system. We also recognized the importance of equitably delivering health information to our people. As such, we have prioritized this 'right to information' because if the people do not know about these services that we have created for them, they will not seek them. In other words, we needed to create a type of demand for high-quality healthcare that did not exist when I returned to Rwanda after the 1994 genocide against the Tutsi.

To do this, we have provided the population with information on the major killers, how they can be infected, how they can protect themselves against infection, how and when they can be treated, and what they should expect from a system that is focused on improving customer care. We still have a long way to go but we are progressing (as evidenced by the annual Citizen Card, which is an annual survey on client satisfaction reported to Parliament).

Of course, due to the high rate of illiteracy in the past, this took time—and we still have a long way to go for our people to understand what health risks exist, as well as what it means to have a right to quality care. Since health is a participatory process, we aim to do all that we can to improve the options available to people to live a healthier life. Day after day we are working to improve this.

Holistic approach to health services

Over the last decade, there has been an unprecedented global solidarity to fight HIV, TB, and malaria. Without this movement, funds mobilized at the global level would not exist to mount such a strong fight against these diseases in the developing world. In Rwanda, however, we rejected the idea that a vertical approach could achieve the health gains that we desired for all of our people.

Our holistic approach has required us to leverage vertical funding sources to not only fund our response to HIV/AIDS, TB, malaria—which includes universal access to treatment for the three diseases and declines in mortality by more than 80%—but also to build a better health system. In other words—we 'horizontalized' this vertical funding in order to strengthen and expand our health response for our entire population.

Our experience in Rwanda provides evidence that there is a false dichotomy present within the evolving debate in the global health arena regarding the merits of so-called 'vertical' or disease-specific initiatives versus those of 'horizontal' or health systems-oriented efforts. It does not have to be a choice.

This holistic approach to providing care to our people is not simply an effort to integrate funding sources in order to strengthen our entire health sector. From the earliest days of the HIV/AIDS response in Rwanda, we have also learned that urgency can be the enemy of the future. To explain, we do not have to choose *either* to provide access to urgent treatment to save a life *or* invest in prevention *or* develop sustainable primary care infrastructure. Rather, by outlining a clear vision and coordinating the activities of all groups and stakeholders working in the health sector, we can accomplish *all three*: simultaneously, addressing the immediate or urgent crisis at hand while also investing in the future by improving prevention and creating a sustainable primary care infrastructure.[1]

This was important because the same HIV-positive parents want the pregnant mother to prevent mother-to-child transmission of HIV to her unborn baby and avoid the child from being a future orphan by being themselves provided with ARV treatment, and to ensure that the child is delivered in a safe environment.

This child—when born HIV-free—will also need access to a full course of all vaccinations—and, in Rwanda, 90% of our children are vaccinated against 11 vaccines—but also access to prevention and rapid treatment of malaria and other major killers such as pneumonia and gastrointestinal diseases. To accomplish this, we also need to assure that high-quality drugs are available (with no stock outs), provided in a timely manner, and delivered at the right location by qualified personnel. To achieve this, we have used vertical funding to build a safe and efficient procurement chain to appropriately manage the treatment of these three specific diseases—HIV, TB, and malaria. This procurement chain, however, also helps us to provide care for all diseases that burden our people.

As our response to these three major communicable diseases has improved, we are seeing a shift in the disease burden within Rwanda. People living with HIV/AIDS are also more vulnerable to many kinds of cancers, for which they require diagnosis, treatment, and palliative care. In order to meet these growing needs of the Rwandan people now living with HIV, whom we have kept alive with ARVs and proper follow-up, we need to provide the country with the capacity to control this new frontier of diseases that our population now faces. Now that our country's life-expectancy has doubled, these non-communicable diseases are of greater concern. This is our duty given our mission to fulfil the right to health of each person over the entire course of their life.

We did not reach this in one day. In practice, when the Ministry of Health has built capacity for HIV testing, we did so in such a way that the laboratory could be used for many other diseases and the technicians were trained in all the current procedures according to our norms and guidelines. And today, we go a step further by training them in more advanced techniques that broaden our capacity to treat our people. We have also built antenatal clinics, delivery wards, and drug supply chains. Using vertical funding, we installed high-speed internet connections in our facilities across the country. We have created a more sophisticated health sector, using e-management to better serve our population. Though we still have strong limitations, we strive to ensure that whatever we do for a single disease serves the entire population for the entire scope of diseases that burden our people.

It was not easy in the beginning because some of our partners did not understand our vision, despite the Rome Declaration, the Paris Declaration, the Accra call for action and Busan meeting, the commitment to channel aid through country systems and to strengthen national plans and accountability towards results was not there. This was a challenge for us as we aimed to pursue this holistic approach to care for our people, because when our partners were talking HIV, we were responding with information and communications technology

(ICT). And at many points in time over the years, they did not understand our vision and how we could get there.

Now that our system has been independently evaluated by the United Nations and others,[2] our approach has gained credibility and those who did not think that it would work in the past are starting to look at our vision in another way.

But I need to acknowledge that globally, there is still resistance on the part of some donor countries to channel their aid through national systems, even if we have proven that it works: with this approach, the same dollar produces more health.

The channel of funding is important to address because impact is diluted and aid is ineffective when we have multiple and parallel funding mechanisms. But it is true that donors are not the only ones to blame for bypassing national systems. Some are weak, non-functioning, or simply led by corrupt governments that should not receive direct funding without first changing. But why not use aid to build up and strengthen these systems?

It is the responsibility of states to govern and secure benefits for their whole populations. Donors on their side are responsible for fulfilling their commitments and they are to blame when they fund corrupt systems. The world has reacted extremely softly and slowly in addressing the vanishing funds sent to corrupt governments, institutions, and civil society organizations. In reality, we have to operationalize the principle of mutual accountability. Partners should be made accountable when they—for no justifiable reason—fail to fulfil their signed commitment to support development, as we often face in Rwanda.

Unfortunately, mutual accountability so far is only one way. There are high demands made on the backs of developing countries but there is often acceptance of non-fulfilment on the donor side. For example, we spend too much time and energy on procedures, accounting and reporting on hundreds of indicators to donors because each intermediary in the channel of funding asks for its own report. For example, for an HIV-positive woman of 35 years, we are asked for her fertility rate, the number of children she plans to have, the children she does have, the ones she probably will have during her life time, the projected rate of child death (not to be confused by the real rate of child death), the comparison of her use of family planning with all women ages 15 to 45, and also the comparison of the uptake of family planning of all HIV-positive women, her nutritional status during pregnancy compared to all pregnant woman, and so on. I have more than 15 other indicators for this very same HIV-positive woman of 35, and even with all this we still don't know if she eats well, if she receives her treatments correctly, or has access to family planning and safe delivery.

It is imperative to decrease the number of indicators and promote national implementation, monitoring, and evaluation systems.

Results

Like many countries, we have made major advances in reducing premature mortality, over the last two decades (Fig. 17.2). Our commitment to community participation, horizontalizing vertical funds, equity, and universal coverage has put Rwanda on track to achieve the health-related Millennium Development Goals (MDGs).

If we look more closely at this decline in child mortality figures, we can see that the poorest benefited the most (Fig. 17.3). This is a very important point: when you focus on the poorest first, you take the rest with you. When you focus on where the greatest gaps are, you make the biggest gains.

Achieving MDGs 4, 5, and 6—which target, among others, the reduction of child and maternal mortality, as well as access to HIV and essential medicine— have been of particular concern to me as a paediatrician. As such, it is rewarding to see the results that we have made as a country, as shown in Table 17.2. These are not just numbers, but real people in Rwanda who are no longer dying unnecessarily from disease that we know we can overcome with this holistic approach.

Specifically, 20 years after we had the highest child mortality rate in the world, we are now in reach of achieving MDG 4 for child survival. This is not by chance, but due to hard work, a strategy focused on equity, participation, and strong national ownership. As you can see, it works. The work is not finished, however, but the achievement to date is reason for great hope. As my President,

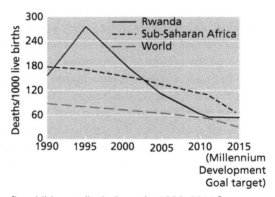

Fig. 17.2 Under-five child mortality in Rwanda, 1990–2011.[3]

Reproduced from *British Medical Journal*, Farmer PE et al. Reduced premature mortality in Rwanda: lessons from success, Volume 346. Copyright © 2013 British Medical Journal Publishing Group, with permission from the BMJ Publishing Group Ltd, available from <http://www.bmj. com/content/346/bmj.f65#ref-36>. Includes data from Levels and Trends in Child Mortality, Report 2012, Estimates Developed by the UN Inter-agency Group for Child Mortality Estimation. Copyright © 2012 by the United Nations Children's Fund, available from <www.unicef.org/media/ files/UNICEF_2012_IGME_child_mortality_report.pdf>.

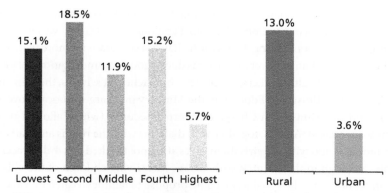

Fig. 17.3 Annual rate of decline in child mortality by wealth quintile and residence, DHS 2008–10.

Data from National Institute of Statistics of Rwanda (NISR), Ministry of Health (MOH) and ICF International, 2012, *Rwanda Demographic and Health Survey 2010*, Calverton, Maryland, USA: NISR, MOH, and ICF International, available from <http://dhsprogram.com/pubs/pdf/FR259/FR259.pdf>; and Ministry of Health (MOH) [Rwanda], National Institute of Statistics of Rwanda (NISR), and ICF Macro, 2009, *Rwanda Interim Demographic and Health Survey 2007–08*, Calverton, Maryland, USA: MOH, NISR, available from <http://dhsprogram.com/pubs/pdf/fr215/fr215.pdf>.

Table 17.2 Reduction in mortality in Rwanda related to HIV, TB, and malaria

Indicator	Source	Timeframe	Total reduction (%)
AIDS-related mortality rate (deaths per 100 000 population)	WHO 2012	2000–09	78.4%
Tuberculosis mortality rate among HIV-negative people (deaths per 100 000 population)	WHO 2012	2000–11	77.1%
Malaria deaths (total reported by Rwanda to WHO)	WHO 2012	2005–11	85.3%

AIDS-related mortality rate data from World Health Organization (WHO), *World Health Statistics 2012*, Copyright © WHO 2012, available from <www.who.int/gho/publications/world_health_statistics/2012/en/>; tuberculosis mortality rate data from World Health Organization (WHO), *Global tuberculosis report 2012*, Copyright © WHO 2012, available from <http://apps.who.int/iris/bitstream/10665/75938/1/9789241564502_eng.pdf>; and reported malaria deaths data from World Health Organization (WHO), *World malaria report 2012*, Copyright © WHO 2012, available from <http://www.who.int/malaria/publications/world_malaria_report_2012/en/index.html>.

His Excellency Paul Kagame, has said, 'the MDGs are a floor, not a ceiling.'[4] We will not be satisfied until these lines on the graph drop to the very bottom. No mother or child should die from preventable or curable diseases.

We have learned to think out of the box, and to develop home-grown solutions, all while maintaining the integrity of our nation's vision that has been built upon wide participatory consultation. Let me give an example: in 2011 we were able to launch a national Human Papillomavirus (HPV) vaccine programme in the school setting. It was immediately a success, with more than 93% of the target population covered. This was due to good communication between the community health workers, the nurses, the teachers at schools, the Ministry of Health, the Ministry of Education, the Ministry in Charge of Local Government, and the Ministry in Charge of Internal Security (which allowed us to borrow their cars). All this, together with dialogue with the mums and dads, in communities and with the girls themselves at school resulted in a 4-day vaccination campaign in the country, with CHWs identifying children of the village not in school those days so that we could propose to families a catch up vaccination for them.

This approach is based on a vision anchored in a human right to health and also the right to information. On top of improving access to health, we are tackling the social determinants of health, because this would not have been possible without improving our electricity distribution, our primary, secondary, and tertiary education, or without developing our drug procurement, cold chain supply, and transport capacity.

It has taught me that we need to have the same dialogue at the global level so that we create effective systems with effective use of aid based on these principles. We need to advance this discussion in the global arena by disseminating this debate through open-access journals, the internet, and conference meetings and exchanges so that we truly advance access to both information and to health for people miles away. But for this to happen, people everywhere need to be able to access information, to be active actors in the global dialogue around aid; this starts with having the basic right to participate in decisions concerning their own lives.

The future

Despite the tragedies of 20 years ago, we can take a positive view of the future in Rwanda.

Because deaths from infectious diseases and during childbirth have continued to decline, Rwanda has turned its attention to the unmet challenges of premature mortality caused by chronic and non-communicable diseases, which grow as a percentage of our disease burden each year. This does not mean that we will lose for one second our focus on conditions like HIV/AIDS or obstructed labour or neonatal sepsis. It means that we have our eyes open to track the next burden. We need to keep thinking outside of the box to develop our health system and the platform of patient-centred service delivery.

For example, cervical cancer is the leading cancer among women in Rwanda, and many women die from this disease around the world. This may be well known but we do not have any global goals dedicated to reducing the impact of cervical cancer or breast cancer, or the respiratory diseases caused by unsafe global pollution or our indoor cooking smoke (that disproportionately affects women and children). We need to prepare our health sector to respond to these new situations that threaten the health and wellbeing of our people.

Fair aid should never oblige us to fall into the trap of not being able to respond to new challenges that may arise. As I told you, the current situation gives us hope. The results we have witnessed have opened the minds of our partners to a new way of development, and we hope it will continue. We have accomplished these great gains because of dedicated health professionals, community health workers and community leaders that are all expert in their field. They are the true experts. Without them, Rwanda's health sector would not be what it is today.

References

1 For further reading on integration of HIV clinical services in Rwanda, please see: Price J, Leslie JA, Welsh M, Binagwaho A. Integrating HIV clinical services into primary health care in Rwanda: a measure of quantitative effects. *AIDS Care* 2009; 21(5):608–14.

2 For reviews of Rwanda's health system, please see: Farmer PE, et al. Reduced premature mortality in Rwanda: lessons from success. *BMJ* 2013;346:f65. doi: 10.1136/bmj.f65.

3 **Farmer PE, et al.** Reduced premature mortality in Rwanda: lessons from success. *BMJ* 2013;346:f65. doi: 10.1136/bmj.f65.

4 President Kagame's address to the 68th UN General Assembly. New York, September 25, 2013. Available at: <http://www.newtimes.co.rw/news/index.php?a=70765&i=15492>.

Chapter 18

HIV/AIDS and National Health Insurance in South Africa

Nigel Crisp

This chapter has been written by Lord Crisp following conversations with South African health leaders including the Honourable Dr Aaron Motsoaledi, the Minister of Health for South Africa

When he became the South African Health Minister in May 2009, Dr Motsoaledi was faced with two of the world's biggest health challenges. First, how to lead the fight on HIV/AIDS in South Africa, at the epicentre of the global epidemic. This task was made much more difficult because of controversy over the link between HIV and AIDS before he was appointed as Minister, the sheer scale of the problem, and because there was no consensus on the way forward. His predecessor had started to make the necessary changes, but there was still a great deal to do. Second, how could he introduce a national health insurance scheme in order to offer healthcare to every person in the country? Here, too, there was a major complication: South Africa has a large and expensive private sector serving about a fifth of the population and a poorly resourced public sector catering for the majority. How could he reconcile the two and build a national system on these disparate foundations?

This chapter describes how Dr Motsoaledi set about tackling these issues by building on the work that was already underway. It is a complex story, with many confusing cross-currents and elements of conflict and intrigue. In reality, a large part of the Minister's role has been to try to cut through the confusion, offer a clear pathway for the future, and communicate, communicate, communicate.

Tackling HIV/AIDS

South Africa is at very different stages with the two challenges. Enormous progress has been made on HIV/AIDS and the country was praised in 2013 by both President Obama as 'leading the way'[1] and by Michel Sidibé, Executive Director of UNAIDS saying, 'South Africa will lead the way to the end of the AIDS epidemic'.[2]

Meanwhile, the introduction of the national health insurance scheme is a far larger task, and far more complex, and offers many more opportunities for confusion and conflict. There was a broad international consensus about what needed to be done on HIV/AIDS. There is no such international agreement on national health insurance and no road map to follow: each step needs to be determined and lessons learned as they are taken. Here the South Africans are building the road as they walk on it.

Interestingly, as we shall see, Dr Motsoaledi has started by concentrating on improving services in the public sector, rather than focusing at the outset on how to fund an insurance scheme. It provides a sharp contrast with most other countries where much of the early policy making inside government about universal health coverage concerns finances rather than quality and services.

Does HIV cause AIDS?

Journalists besieged Dr Motsoaledi from the moment he was appointed Minister. They had a simple question to ask him: 'Did he believe that HIV caused AIDS?'.

Dr Motsoaledi was both prepared and unprepared for the question from the media and for the task ahead. He was delighted to be summoned to the Presidential Palace after the 2009 election but was surprised to be appointed Minister of Health. He had been a provincial minister in his home province in Limpopo over many years, but he was never appointed in health. He thought it would be the same this time around. As a doctor he knew about health but he didn't know the Health Ministry nor did he know the policies, programmes, and controversies surrounding it in any detail. At that first press conference five days after his appointment, he laughed off the question. Did he believe HIV caused AIDS? He was a doctor, what did they think he believed? It bought him just enough time to prepare himself to deal with the underlying issue and change the government's policy on HIV/AIDS.

He was, however, in other ways very prepared for the task. He was not only a doctor but was a member of the African National Council's (ANC's) Sub-committee on Education and Health that had for 2 years been developing policy. As elsewhere in Africa, the post-independence—or here, post-apartheid—euphoria and optimism about the future had been replaced by a hard realism about the difficulties of making improvements. The ANC knew that there had been progress made on health since they took power in 1994, particularly in the first 5 years, but a lot of gaps still existed and people demanded action. There had been increasing levels of public protests about the poor quality of services in the last 2 years.

In 2007 at its Polokwane Congress, famous as the venue for the election contest for leadership of the party between Thabo Mbeki and Jacob Zuma, the ANC made health and education its priorities for the next 5 years and set up a subcommittee under the chairmanship of Dr Zweli Mkhize to address them. Dr Motsoaledi was a member and over the next 2 years participated in the discussions that involved about 100 of the ANC's activists on health and attempted to understand the mistakes and failings of the past. It culminated in a 10-point plan for the future.

This plan, as described in Box 18.1, was included in the government's Programme of Action published in July 2009 and later became the foundation for the health Negotiated Service Delivery Agreement signed by the Health Minister and the President of the Republic of South Africa.[3]

This broad and far-reaching plan contains within it both the commitments to tackling HIV/AIDS and the establishment of National Health Insurance (NHI). The most urgent issue, however, was HIV/AIDS because of the devastation it was causing in the country—which was well reflected in public and media concern.

Box 18.1 The 10-point plan for the improvement of the health sector

1 Provision of strategic leadership and creation of a social compact for better health outcomes.

2 Implementation of National Health Insurance (NHI).

3 Improving the quality of health services.

4 Overhauling the healthcare system and improving its management.

5 Improving human resources management, planning, and development.

6 Revitalization of health infrastructure.

7 Accelerated implementation of the National HIV and AIDS and STI National Strategic Plan (2007–11) and increased focus on TB and other communicable diseases.

8 Mass mobilization for better health for the population.

9 Review of the drug policy.

10 Strengthening research and development.

Dr Motsoaledi may have known what he believed as a doctor but he also understood that his first task would be to convince the government of the need for radically new policies to tackle the pandemic. He found in the Ministry what he described as 'a well' of information, and collected more from colleagues and associates outside. There were analyses, figures, and graphs from South African bodies such as the Medical Research Council; African bodies like the African Union; and international ones such as the World Health Organization and UNAIDS. Put together, he knew that all this information could be made to tell a powerful story. Previously, when seen as purely separate bits of data, they had simply been ignored. He set about creating the narrative he needed in those first few days in office.

The first item on the 10-point plan, as Dr Motsoaledi points out, is strategic leadership. He needed to provide it but he also needed support from the President, the Deputy President, the Cabinet, and the whole Government on new radical plans to turn the tide of the pandemic. At the same time, however, he needed new implementation plans and new resources.

Thanks to the actions of a number of determined South African health leaders who understood the nature and scale of the problem, and had worked on it though the dark years of denial, the South African National Aids Council (SANAC) chaired by the Deputy President of the country, already had a strategy. Moreover, the Treatment Action Campaign (TAC) had, virtually from the outset of the epidemic, set out both to challenge drug companies on pricing and the government on the need for treatment and, more recently, access to ARVs. Barbara Hogan, Dr Motsoaledi's predecessor as Minister, had employed one of its leading figures as an adviser and begun both to change policies and, crucially, to build bridges between the TAC and the government. This foundation, as Dr Motsoaledi, says, has been absolutely crucial to the later success of the campaign against the disease.

The existing strategy was referred to in the 10-point plan and formed a good basis for action. There was, however, a significant gap between it and what was needed in order to support the new government approach. The SANAC needed to develop additional policies and an 'accelerated' plan needed to be created.

The central issues were that there were severe limitations on the availability of ARVs and more funding was needed. At the time ARVs could only be prescribed to patients with very weakened immune systems by doctors in accredited hospitals that had a full complement of therapists. This restricted access to relatively few people in urban areas. Dr Motsoaledi wanted access to everyone that needed it and took the bold decision to develop a nurse and primary care based service operating from clinics throughout the country. There had been a few pilots in South Africa and elsewhere but this was essentially a new policy that had not been tested at this scale.

Officials who worked with him at the time give him great credit both for his ability to create a consensus on the way forward and for his vision in establishing this new policy and making sure it was implemented across the country. The new policy—the extension to the old strategy—was approved by the National Health Council.[4] The President himself lent his authority to the new treatment guidelines when he announced them on World AIDS Day in 2009. They were essentially the same as those promoted by the WHO in 2009 and offered treatment to all pregnant women, children under 5, people with a diagnosis of TB as a well as HIV and with a CD4 cell count of 350 (it had previously been 200).

The new consensus and policies helped with the need for more funding. International agencies and partners had been working on HIV/AIDS in South Africa for years, often at cross-purposes with the government and in covert opposition to their policies. They welcomed the changes and Dr Motsoaledi was able to negotiate new arrangements and funding from major donors such as the UK's Department for International Development (DFID) and the United States' President's Emergency Plan for Aids Relief (PEPFAR).

He had also worked hard with his own government, and hence the President instructed the Treasury to provide additional funding to support the new strategy. He argued cogently that the scale of the crisis was such that 'You soon won't have enough people to build the roads or other investments unless you tackle HIV/AIDS'.

All these developments came together on World AIDS Day, 1 December 2009, when the President announced the new policy and an additional 3 billion Rand to tackle HIV/AIDS. He was accompanied by the Deputy President and Michel Sidibé, the Executive Director of UNAIDS, as well as his Minister of Health Dr Motsoaledi—thereby demonstrating the national and international strategic leadership that had been missing for so long and that set South Africa at last on a new course.

It was a great triumph for Dr Motsoaledi. He had brought together political will, a new implementation plan and increased resources. The first part of the task had been accomplished but the rigours and difficulties of implementation were ahead.

Implementation began in April 2010 and, whilst there have been continuing challenges and difficulties, the results are showing through thanks to the efforts of many different people and organizations across the country. The new approach allowed the Ministry of Health to bring together the many disparate groups involved in tackling different aspects of the epidemic, to share learning, and build on good practice.[5]

Progress has been good. In February 2010, at the start of the period, 2 million people a year were being tested for HIV and AIDS, 18 million were tested in the 18 months from April that year. In February 2010, 923 000 people were on treatment, but by March 2013, 2.1 million were on treatment. In February 2010 there were 490 facilities able to provide anti-retroviral therapy (ARVs) and 250 nurses able to initiate ARVs without a doctor; by March 2013 there were 3540 such facilities and 23 000 nurses trained.[6] All of this was accompanied by public campaigns and education throughout the country.

As we noted at the beginning of the chapter, this increased activity has resulted in South Africa being praised for the drop in transmission rates from mothers to their children, the reduction in deaths, and the sharp decline in new cases. In 2002, nearly 600 000 people were infected with HIV during the previous year and virtually no-one was on treatment. A decade later in 2012, there had been 367 000 new infections in the previous year and 449 000 were added to treatment for the first time and 80% of those eligible for treatment were receiving it.

As Dr Motsoaledi says, the battle isn't won; but the improving trend is now well established. Looking forward, the biggest issues are about quality of care and about integrating the HIV/AIDS programme more fully into the wider health system—and ultimately into the national health insurance programme.

NHI—a national triumph or a disaster?

In many ways NHI got off to the worst possible start. The first that most of the public heard of it was from leaks from some of the people who were consulted by the ANC's Special Committee on Education and Health. Some of them, it appears, didn't like the way NHI was developing and felt their advice was not being followed. Others who hadn't been part of the process but opposed the whole idea of NHI for personal, ideological, and commercial reasons added their criticisms. Together they set off a media storm.

NHI, it was said, would wreck the existing health systems, benefit nobody, and leave the country with a disaster to deal with. There were three main lines of attack, each from different groups and each rather different from the others. The first was that the successful private sector with its high standards would be destroyed as the government would compel it to take thousands more patients without adequate reimbursement. The opposite view came from those who thought it would force everyone to 'go private' and join high cost medical aid schemes to fund their use of services. The third line of attack was that it would lead to vastly increased taxes; these opponents of the scheme argued that the country simply couldn't afford it.

The government had a crisis on its hands. Doctors were saying they would leave the country if NHI was implemented, the media stirred the arguments for all they were worth, and the public became ever more concerned. It was said that there was a small group that was meeting in private to construct a secret plan to be imposed on the country. The failure to communicate early and seize the initiative placed the government as a whole, and Dr Motsoaledi in particular, on the defensive.

These arguments took place in a context where South Africa was spending 8.5% of its GDP on health; very similar to the UK and European average and very different from the rest of sub-Saharan Africa. This figure by itself was misleading, however, because it concealed the fact that 16% of the population, the middle classes, made use of a well-resourced private sector, which accounted for 4.1% of GDP, whilst 84% of the population only had access to the government system and consumed the other 4.2% of GDP.[7]

It is easy to see why private providers of healthcare, the hospitals and clinics, and their patients might be fearful of how a national health insurance scheme might affect them. There were also about 90 Medical Aid Societies (not-for-profit health insurance organizations) whose existence might be threatened by a national health insurance scheme. There is no other country that aspires to introduce a national health insurance system that has anything like such a large and well-established private sector to work with and around. The other African Governments that have introduced new national systems, such as Ghana and Rwanda, did so in countries with healthcare provided overwhelmingly by government and charities. In South Africa, by contrast, there was a strong private sector, which could offer opposition to the government's plans or might, just conceivably, present an opportunity.

Dr Motsoaledi, characteristically, reacted to the initial opposition by going out and meeting the critics in the media and holding many meetings with GPs and others who might be affected. He described it as fighting a battle for alternative views to be heard and felt himself subject to interrogation from a hostile media. It was a very difficult period.

The analysis he presented was very straightforward. South Africa had two problems. One was a very under-resourced and poorly performing government-run health sector. The other was a very well-resourced but extraordinarily expensive private sector. (In parenthesis one might note that the costs of the sector are such that if 16% of the population were consuming 4.1% of GDP in healthcare, then extending this to the whole country would cost about 25% of GDP—a level far exceeding American let alone European expenditures). The problems of the public sector were well known but the profligacy of the private sector was not at all understood by the public at large. Both sectors, he argued, needed reform.

It was very important, as he knew, to show what a national health insurance scheme could deliver if he were to convince a sceptical public of its value. He set out the ambitious aspiration that 'every citizen has the right to good quality affordable health care and access to it should not be determined by the socio-economic status of the individual'. He recognized that it would take years to fulfil; nevertheless, it was an ambition worth working towards. He did not start out, however, as others have done, by concentrating on the insurance and financial aspects, but, rather, recognized that the first step was to improve the public service.

He explains that this was due to a number of insights he had gained both from others and from his own observation. Dr Luis Sambo, Executive Director of the WHO in Africa and author of Chapter 6 of this book, said in a speech to the African Union in Tunis in 2011 that African countries that wanted to introduce universal health coverage for their populations needed to have a strong infrastructure in place, in terms of facilities, human resources, technologies, and information systems.

This point was reinforced for him by the fact that some other countries that had introduced free healthcare without the adequate infrastructure of staffing and facilities in place had led to little if any improvements for their population. Even in South Africa, the free care for mothers and children introduced in 1996 had released pent-up demand but was seen as being of such poor quality that very few people appreciated it. He was also influenced by learning that the British NHS provided services to everyone in the country. The highest quality hospitals in the UK are in the public sector and everybody uses the NHS in emergencies, and almost everyone uses it for primary care and the most specialized services.

All of this led him to the view that the first thing he needed to do was to improve the public service. Quality of service was the key. Improving the public sector would enable him to introduce a national health insurance system that offered real improvement for patients in ways that they would recognize. The NHI Implementation Plan as outlined in the Government's Green Paper of 2011 accordingly says that the first 5 years will be devoted to strengthening the public sector.[8] As part of this, 10 pilot districts across the country have been chosen to demonstrate what can be achieved. He has also recognized the long-term nature of this endeavour with the full NHI not in place till 2026.

It is worth noting that Dr Motsoaledi is in the relatively fortunate position, compared to most African health leaders, that he has strong government support for his policy—it is one of the two main ANC priorities—and he is working in a relatively affluent country, which is able to make a growing investment in public healthcare. Despite all the uproar at the time of launching the policy, authoritative external sources have calculated that South Africa can afford to develop a universal health system provided it is done in a reasonable and measured fashion.[9]

Against this background, the pilot districts were chosen carefully to be broadly representative of the country with some rural ones and others urban, some with the highest burden of disease and others with more healthy populations. The Tshwane District around the capital Pretoria was included, with its mixed rural and urban population, but the other main metropolitan areas were excluded. In addition, the Province of KwaZulu Natal decided to add a district and to fund and support it alongside the pilots supported by the National Government.

The pilots are based around five key elements. First, there is a large and very broadly based investment in infrastructure underway. Existing hospitals and other facilities are being renovated, new ones constructed, and improvements made in electricity and water supplies. Second, there is a parallel investment in human resources with a number of initiatives to improve staffing, leadership, and management. These include the creation of a Leadership and Management Academy for Health: with an initial focus on training Chief Executives who will be delegated greater local autonomy to manage their organisations. They also include the training of more specialists and the introduction of new systems to manage staff and relate staffing levels to workloads.

At the heart of the pilots is the third element, quality. Here, the government has established an Office for Quality Standards, which is based broadly on the British NHS's Care Quality Commission and other examples from around the world. It has carried out a survey of facilities and is setting six core standards, which will be used for monitoring quality. These cover topics that are directly aimed at patients' experiences: from safety and infection control to cleanliness, waiting times, and drug shortages or 'stock outs'. The standards apply across the whole country and inspections will be carried out in all health facilities—starting with public hospitals but progressing over time to include clinics and the private sector. Facility improvement teams have been appointed in the pilot Districts in order to help organizations improve performance.

The final two elements are re-engineering primary care and contracting private sector GPs to provide services in government facilities. There is already a great deal of activity underway here. There is a new school health system, which was started with help from the European Union, and picks up problems with eyesight, nutrition, HIV/AIDS, drugs, and alcohol. There are now also 10 000 primary healthcare workers operating in 4200 local government municipal wards and providing local surveillance, health advice, and some treatment in a model based on practice in Brazil. These and other primary care workers are supported by teams of specialists being recruited in each district, which will include a principal obstetrician and gynaecologist; a principal paediatrician; a principal family physician; a principal anaesthetist; a principal midwife and a principal primary healthcare professional nurse, with others added over time as the need arises. This whole system will also be supported by building improved links to the hospital sector.

In one of its more radical initiatives, the government is also contracting 600 GPs to provide 4-hour sessions in public clinics. Dr Motsoaledi emphasizes that this is being managed slowly and carefully to ensure that the GPs add new services to the clinics and don't simply fill existing gaps. He doesn't want them to be forced to cover existing services because of shortages of nursing staff or to become frustrated at lack of equipment or facilities. He is very keen to make the scheme a success and demonstrate two absolutely key points for the future: that public services can be improved and can deliver for *everyone*—not just the poorest—and that private sector health workers can work effectively alongside the public sector.

Dr Motsoaledi argues that the 'present system doesn't want GPs'. He points to the evidence that private sector expenditure is becoming ever more hospital focused. Of the 84.7 billion Rand spent by the Medical Aid Societies in 2010, 30.7 billion went to private hospitals, 19 billion in specialist fees, 14 billion on pharmaceuticals, 11 billion on administration, and only 6 billion on GP's services. There is a continuing downward trend and the expenditure on GPs in 2011 was lower still.

GPs are aware of this trend and there is evidence that some are leaving the country as they are squeezed in the private sector. Dr Motsoaledi sees this as an opportunity to bring them into partnership with the public sector. This is all part of the far bigger issue of how the public and private sectors could work together to make National Health Insurance a reality for South Africa. There is still a long way to go and this remains perhaps the most difficult challenge facing Dr Motsoaledi. No other country has this particular combination of a weak public sector and a very strong private one. No other country, as Dr Motsoaledi says, has such an expensive private sector. It is, as he points out, dominated by three large for-profit companies, which have roughly equal shares of the market. A Competition Commission Inquiry is being set up to investigate the private health market.

This is not the only remaining challenge, of course. He also has to work with the Treasury to design all the financial aspects of the scheme from questions about whether there is to be a single payer or several to ones about what exactly is covered and whether there will be co-payments as well as tax contributions to the scheme. These will be answered in a forthcoming White Paper.

Human resources and leadership

One theme that stands out from these conversations with health leaders is the emphasis on human resources and the need not only for more health workers, but also for appropriate training and skill mix, good human resource management, and good leadership. As has been described elsewhere in this book, these are also the major concerns of health ministers and service providers throughout Africa and, indeed, globally.

Dr Motsoaledi is concerned about migration of health workers from South Africa but is also very concerned about the so-called 'internal migration' of health workers away from the public health services to NGOs and, most significantly of all, to the private sector where their skills are not available to the majority of the population.

He also recognizes that South Africa is both a sender and a recipient of migration: it has also benefitted enormously from migrants from elsewhere in Africa who have been attracted by the wealth of the country and the greater opportunities it can offer them. As such the South African Government, like the UK, has come under criticism from other African countries and feels a responsibility to support other African nations where it can. Dr Motsoaledi points out that South Africa provides education and training, particularly in medical specialities, for citizens from many of its neighbours.

Throughout these conversations Dr Motsoaledi and other South African leaders have continually stressed the importance of being part of the wider health community globally and of learning good practice from other countries. He and his staff have visited the UK, Brazil, and other countries in pursuit of what will work best in South Africa. He is particularly interested in issues of leadership and management.

Leadership and management are crucial to success in South Africa. As Dr Motsoaledi has pointed out, whilst there are many good Chief Executives, there were, until he intervened, many others who had been appointed through wrong policies and didn't have the skills for the job. This is why he has insisted on a new process for appointing Chief Executives and set up the Leadership and Management Academy to define standards and ensure they have the necessary competences.

Dr Motsoaledi's own role as a leader is made more difficult because responsibility for health and healthcare is split between Provinces and the Federal

Government. He has the power that stems from the ability to provide some funding and the setting of standards nationally. He has, characteristically, used this combination in a very creative way by insisting that there are 'non-negotiable' elements in the Provinces' budgets, which require them to spend a proportion of their finances on particular activities such as infection control—and has then made sure that they are held to account for this in the annual budget processes and reviews. In reality, of course, he must also rely on his considerable powers of persuasion to make sure there is consistent progress across the country. Here, as with the relationships with the private sector, the Minister must play a very strong but subtle leadership role in negotiating, guiding—and sometimes goading—partners into making changes.

Lord Crisp writes

I have known Dr Motsoaledi since shortly after he took up post as Health Minister in 2009 and had the chance to discuss many issues with him and other leaders over the years, culminating in the conversations that are the basis for this chapter. I knew something of his personal background in the struggle against apartheid and a little of how much this and other factors have helped him in his role as Minister of Health.

As this account shows he has personal credibility, great determination and energy, is a skilled politician and leader, and communicates very effectively. He is well equipped to take on these great challenges in South Africa. All of us can learn from what is happening there.

References

1 UNAIDS press release. *President Obama says South Africa is leading the way to an AIDS-free generation*; 8 July 2013.

2 UNAIDS press release. *President Obama says South Africa is leading the way to an AIDS-free generation*; 8 July 2013.

3 Department of Health of South Africa. *National Department of Health Strategic Plan 2010/11–1012/13*; 2010, p.20.

4 The National Health Council brings together representatives of National and Provincial Governments to advise the Minister on national policies and plans.

5 **Mate Kedar S, Ngubane G, Barker P.** A quality improvement model for the rapid scale up of a program to prevent mother to child HIV transmission in South Africa; *International Journal of Quality in Health Care Advanced Access*, 24 May 2013.

6 Information provided by South African Ministry of Health in December 2013.

7 Republic of South Africa. *National Treasury Intergovernmental Fiscal Review* 2011.

8 Department of Health of South Africa. *National Health Insurance in South Africa: Policy Paper*; Government Gazette No 34523, 12 August 2011. <http://www.samedical.org>.

9 KPMG. *A spoon full of sugar*. 2012.

Chapter 19

Coverage of the poor— innovative health financing in Ghana

Frank Nyonator

Dean of the School of Public Health, University of Health
and Allied Sciences, Ghana and formerly Acting Director General
of the Ghana Health Service

Dr Frank Nyonator is a Ghanaian public health physician who has had a long and distinguished career in his country's Ministry of Health, culminating in the role of Acting Director General of the Ghana Health Service from 2011 to 2012. He has played a leading role in the development of the country's national health insurance scheme, which seeks to make healthcare affordable for the poorest people in the country. In this chapter he describes the journey that Ghana has been on since 2003 as it sought to bring together existing community based health insurance schemes of many sorts within a single national framework, which offered a package of care to all its citizens—however poor and from whatever background. It has been a journey of 'learning by doing'. There have been challenges in integrating the existing schemes, in applying different aspects of the policy, in funding, and in reaching the poorest. The government has changed and with it some aspects of policy. Nevertheless, after 10 years about a third of the population are active members of the National Health Insurance Scheme and there is a foundation in place for continuing the journey to ensure that health services are available to everyone as the country continues to grow and prosper.

National health insurance in Ghana

We set out to create a national health insurance scheme in Ghana in 2003 with an ambitious plan to roll this out to cover the entire population within 10 years as part of the Ghana Poverty Reduction Strategy. Legislation was passed and significant revenues were earmarked for the plan. The scheme, scaled-up from smaller community based health insurance schemes, attempted to include poor and vulnerable population groups in the first stages of implementation by exempting these groups from contributions and providing financing for their coverage.

In this chapter I describe the country's vision for the scheme, before going on to discuss the practical details of implementation and the extent to which the scheme has managed to provide coverage for the poorest people in the country.

Ghana's vision for universal health coverage was set out in the Ministry of Health's (MOH) Medium-term Strategic Plan (1997–2001) and recognized that the government has the prime responsibility for ensuring good health and economic success for its citizens. There had been considerable progress in improving health status and longevity of Ghanaians in recent years—more and more children were surviving and total fertility rate (4.0) is one of the lowest in the sub-Saharan African region and the adult population is living longer.[1] However, whilst Ghana has also made efforts to increase its health workforce during the mid-2000s, the population's access to, and utilization of, primary healthcare services were relatively low and funding for primary healthcare was inadequate.

Like other low-income countries worldwide, Ghana was faced in the 1970s through to the 1990s with the dual challenge of achieving accessible and equitable coverage of health services while providing healthcare more efficiently within a constricted budget. Financing healthcare in Ghana had evolved from the post-independence policy of free medical care through to the token fee system in the 1970s, to the establishment of user fees (with some exemptions) in 1985 with full cost recovery for drugs (the 'cash and carry' system).

This evolution—with its increasing user fees—was partially responsible for the low access to, and declining use of, health facilities throughout the country. These growing costs and the fact that the exemptions were largely non-functional have exacerbated inequities in access to health services. A study in the Volta Region of Ghana showed that while user fees clearly contribute to financial sustainability in most health facilities, this was at the expense of equity, as reflected in the largely non-functional exemption mechanisms.[2]

Ghana, like many other developing countries, saw its vulnerable populations excluded from any social security coverage. This, coupled with the constant reformation of the role of the extended family (driven largely by globalization and urbanization) that had previously played a significant part in risk-pooling and social protection, meant that many were now left exposed to the harsh dynamics of national and global social and economic risks.[3]

The government in power in the year 2000 understood very well the problems associated with the out-of-pocket health financing 'cash and carry' system. Consequently, it decided to abolish this financing mechanism and replace it with a health insurance scheme, which it envisioned would be national and cover all vulnerable groups. The objective was to pool the risks, reduce the individual financial burden, and achieve better utilization rates, primarily so that patients did not have to pay out-of-pocket at the point of delivery. The declared objective was that at least 50–60% of resident Ghanaians would belong to a health insurance scheme within the next 5 to 10 years. Subsequently, the then President of Ghana categorically promulgated that the 'cash and carry' system of healthcare in Ghana had to be abolished by the end of 2004.[4]

In principle, all the political parties in Ghana accepted that rolling out health insurance was indeed a step in the right direction in the face of the worsening inequities that the user fees had introduced. However, the opposition parties and some social organizations, including the labour unions, worried about the undefined nature of the scheme and the hasty pace at which the government was moving to implement it.[5]

Nonetheless, equity concerns were paramount and the government persisted in moving away from the user-fee system to a mandatory social insurance system and passed the 'National Health Insurance Act' (Act 650) in August 2003 to make this operational.[6] This decision, according to its analysts, was to enable the government to achieve its health goal in the Ghana Poverty Reduction Strategy (GPRS) and the Health Sector five-year Programme of Work (2002–2006). The government had made it clear that the decision was not necessarily to use health insurance to increase funding for the health sector as an 'additional' source, but was focused on removing financial barriers to accessing healthcare (which the 'cash and carry' had in large part contributed to) and promote end user or purchaser participation in decision-making in health.

The suggested organizational structure was innovative. It was a fusion of a Social Health Insurance (SHI) concept and the Mutual Health Organization (MHO) concept into one National Health Insurance System (NHIS) concept that had never been tried before. The organizational structure though not fully determined was to evolve as implementation continued. The policy makers in government recognized it would be difficult to implement the final organization *en bloc*, but expected that the ultimate system would emerge over an unspecified time.[7]

The decision to adopt this concept was influenced in large part by Ghana's experience in social financing schemes or the *'susu'* organizations. Indeed, Ghana had a range of existing voluntary health insurance schemes, including a wide range of community based Mutual Health Organizations (MHOs), and a small, but growing private commercial health insurance sector, which covered a limited number of formal sector workers in the capital and other large urban areas. The MHOs were autonomous, not-for-profit organizations based on solidarity between members and were democratically accountable to them. Their objective was to improve members' access to good quality healthcare through risk sharing based on their own financial contributions. The MHOs also aimed to improve the lives of members and all citizens and to promote democratic decision-making.[8]

These schemes had a range of different benefit packages and contribution levels. In late 2002, it was estimated that there were over 159 MHOs in Ghana, covering over 220 000 people[9] Some of these schemes were essentially prepayment schemes linked to a specific health facility, while others were more 'traditional' insurance schemes that reimbursed the costs of a range of services for their members. Most were relatively small scale with substantial community involvement in their management. Despite the existence of this growing number of voluntary health insurance schemes, user fees paid on an out-of-pocket basis were still important sources of revenue for health services in Ghana.

The new policy sought to replace these existing community financing schemes with a National Health Insurance System (NHIS) that aimed for universal coverage of the population. This would be achieved by bringing together the various schemes so that there was basic health insurance available to everyone, but the schemes would still have scope to develop differently. The scheme would be based on the District-wide Mutual Health Insurance Schemes (DMHIS) present in each district in Ghana. These mutuals are governed by Community Health Insurance Committees, which serve as premium collection points and elect representatives to the District General Assembly, the ultimate decision-making body for the scheme. The day to day management of the individual DMHIS is left to the Board of Directors/Trustees, elected from the General Assembly, and to the salaried Scheme Management Team.

Implementation, financing, and sustainability

As we have seen, the Ghana NHIS is a combination of the Social Health Insurance and the Mutual Health Organization concepts. It is social because it is compulsory for every person living in Ghana to belong to a health insurance scheme in the light of the spirit of national solidarity and social responsibility. The law permits two types of schemes to operate at the district level: the District Mutual Health Insurance schemes I have described, and Private Health Insurance Schemes, which can either be commercial or mutual schemes.

Both the district-wide and the private mutual schemes operate along the principles of MHOs, the distinction being that the District MHIS receive a government subsidy, whilst the Private MHIS do not. The Private Commercial Health Insurance Scheme is primarily a business venture. This arrangement therefore means that, at the district level there is only one DMHIS belonging to government. All other schemes (existing or new) either had to merge with the DMHIS (to benefit from National Health Insurance Fund) or become a private scheme, whether commercial or mutual.

This policy decision and directive by law had implications for the survival of existing small schemes. In the majority of places as the policy was being developed, the existing schemes were on the verge of collapse or simply stalled because of the fear that they would not be subsidized. Whilst government encouraged the integration of existing schemes to form part of the district-wide schemes, the majority of the existing schemes felt that the government was simply pulling the 'rug' under their feet and forcing them into the integration. The district-wide concept was ambitious, given the fact that communities in nearly all districts in Ghana are not homogenous and there was scepticism about solidarity beyond the traditional communities. This difficult and uncertain situation was further complicated by the fact that initially the majority of districts thought that government subsidies would pay everybody's premium.

Financing the district schemes was also complex. It involved pooling resources from social insurance contributions from the formal sector; government and donor budget support for health; the National Health Insurance Levy (NHIL); premium contributions by the informal sector; and Internally Generated Funds (IGF) from the uninsured (in both public and private sectors). A National Health Insurance Fund (NHIF) was created from a NHI levy of 2.5% sales tax on almost all goods and services, 2.5% payroll deductions for formal sector employees as part of their contribution to the Social Security and Pensions' Scheme Fund and government revenue allocations authorized by parliament. The NHIF allocates subsidies to each district MHIS, which transfer the contributions of formal sector workers secured from the payroll contributions, and serve a risk equalization and reinsurance function. Those outside the formal sector make their contributions directly to their district MHIS. There are provisions for contribution exemptions for indigent members.

The long-term objective of this mandatory health insurance was to have every resident of Ghana belong to a health insurance scheme that adequately covers them against the need to make out-of-pocket payments at the point of service. They would obtain access to a defined package of acceptable quality and necessary health services. This was initially a relatively comprehensive entitlement package that included general and specialist consultations and a range of inpatient services, as well as certain oral health, eye care, and maternity services. In the medium-term the aim was to achieve enrolment levels of about 60% of residents in Ghana within 10 years of starting mandatory health insurance schemes.[10]

Financial sustainability was obviously important. In this context it refers to the ability of the NHIF to mobilize and efficiently use domestic resources on a reliable basis to achieve current and future target levels of utilization of health services within the health sector. The financing model used by the NHIC makes some basic and simple assumptions that:

◆ In the long run, the scheme will cover 100% of the formal and informal sector.

◆ The uninsured informal sector will access services at the same rate as the formal sector employees.

◆ The present fees will represent the price of healthcare.

◆ Government budget support (including donor support) to hospitals and health centres will directly support service delivery.

Sustainability will, crucially, depend on the level of usage. Various scenarios for increases in utilization have been used to compute the income and expenditure projections of the NHIS. Whilst International Labour Organization projections suggest that the scheme will not be sustainable in the long run, the National Health Insurance Council projection shows that the scheme is sustainable. This is not the only factor affecting sustainability. The premium contribution of between GH¢7.20 and GH¢48.00 per contribution is not sufficient to make the scheme sustainable by itself so, as described earlier, other sources of funds (NHIL, SSNIT, and Budget Support) were expected to fill the funding gap. Any shortfalls in any of these will affect the sustainability of the scheme. An assessment of the sustainability of each of the funding sources is critical to the sustainability of the scheme.

A further consideration is the rate at which the scheme increases its coverage of the population. The government policy framework proposed that the scheme was expected to cover at least 30–40% nationwide coverage in the short term (within five years from the start in 2003). The medium-term objective (for the next 5 to 10 years) was to cover at least 50–60% of the entire population. This is shown in Fig. 19.1. Thus, by the year 2008 it was expected that about 35% of the population will be covered, whilst by the year 2013 coverage would reach 54%.

Against this background, analysis showed that the share of direct government funding on health as a percentage of total government expenditure would remain stable throughout the period. This demonstrated that the introduction of the NHIS would probably allow the health sector to grow in financial terms.

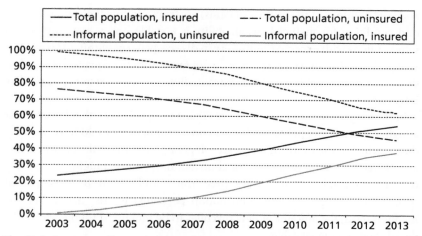

Fig. 19.1 Coverage of insured and non-insured, total and informal populations 2003–2013, base scenario.

The real challenge for managers in the sector is to make sure that the increase of resources is commensurate with the increase in access and quality of care.

This, however, also depended on the rate of utilization of services by people covered by the insurance scheme. Here, the underlying assumptions were that public healthcare expenditure would grow rapidly over the 10-year period succeeding NHIS implementation. Whilst revenues to the public healthcare delivery system were also expected to increase, the expectation was that the National Health Insurance Act would mobilize new resources into the health sector. However, the increase in health service utilization by insured persons has led to a subsequent increase in overall expenditure that has outpaced the growth of resources, hence creating a financing gap. The faster the extension of actual insurance coverage the earlier that imbalance could emerge. However, there is a period of 4 to 5 years during which the overall system should remain in surplus. This provides some breathing space to fine-tune the financing system and install effective cost-containment mechanisms.

A critical condition for financial equilibrium during the coming years is that the government will not reduce its financial commitment to the health sector and hence all new sources of revenues (contributions for SSNIT, levy on VAT, and contributions of the insured persons) are truly additional resources. A second condition for financial sustainability is a stable policy environment on interventions with expected continuity in disease patterns within the basic service package. The above projections do not factor into the equation changes in disease patterns, epidemics, and introduction of new and more expensive interventions.

In the long term, the Government of Ghana will probably either have to bear a higher share of the public health expenditure bill, or it would have to introduce—which is the more unlikely case—higher premiums to the district insurance schemes, higher formal sector contributions, and/or a higher health levy or a suitable combination of these three. This would need to be accompanied with a fair exemption from contribution payments for the needy. For the medium term, the amount of new revenues to be mobilized till the end of the decade appears manageable.

Measures to provide cover for the poor

The DHMIS is designed to cover both the formal and non-formal sectors (i.e. those in and out of formal employment). The DHMIS is mandatory for all formal sector employees, as we have seen, whilst community level and non-formal groups will pay premiums to the district MHOs. As stated above, tax revenues will continue to form part of the overall health financing strategy for a long time to come and the Ministry of Health will continue to finance the major part of the public sector health service delivery system. Therefore, at the national level, funds for exemption of certain diseases and categories of the population will continue to be provided by the government.

In addition, the National Health Insurance Fund aims at providing funds for exemptions and to pay premiums outright for the core poor and indigent. Communities are therefore mandated to adapt means' tests to identify the poor and indigent persons for registration by the district schemes. Each district is then required to keep and publish a list of indigents in its area and submit the list to the governing body of the NHIS—the National Health Insurance Council.

Whilst these were laudable plans to ensure that the poor and vulnerable are not excluded, there are fears that these are not far-reaching enough and might lead to stigmatization within the society and unwillingness to enlist by those who actually are in need. Currently, efforts are being made to categorize the contribution levels based on socio-economic stratification. The policy proposes six main types of categorization: core poor, very poor, poor, middle income, rich, and very rich. However, the schemes are faced with the huge challenge of operationalizing the policy. There is no clear-cut definition either of the various social groups or of the premium levels to be paid by the different groups as an alternative to the flat GH¢7.20 per capita premium based on equity.

Clearly there is a problem in really defining the poor and core poor in Ghana, and there is a caution not to trivialize the issue. Already social groupings are calling for a clearer definition of 'indigent' in the Act and making sure that social differentials in the payment of premium are captured in the act. Meanwhile the schemes were being encouraged to be innovative in the definition of the social grouping.

Since the inception of the scheme in 2003, there have been a lot of controversies surrounding its operation and purpose. The first one was to do with members of the opposition National Democratic Congress (NDC), whose members claimed that the scheme was one made for members of the then ruling New Patriotic Party (NPP). As such many members of NDC did not want to register with the scheme. On the other hand it was reported that members of the NPP did not encourage members of NDC to join since it was a policy that had come during the time when the NPP was in power. All the propaganda that surrounded the scheme at its inception was revisited in 2009—with the different parties on the opposite sides—when the NDC took over government and with it control of health policy.

Currently, there is controversy over the proposal, included in the ruling party's election manifesto, that members should a pay a one-time premium only. This has not yet been implemented. Many critics of the proposal claim that it is just not possible to support the scheme with a one-time premium, since the sustainability of the scheme would not be possible if premiums were not paid yearly.

The current status of NHIS

Controversy has also surrounded the governance and administrative procedure for the provision of health insurance set out in the founding Act of Parliament.

To overcome this, the old Act (Act 650) has been repealed and replaced by a new one—the National Health Insurance Act 2012 (Act 852)—which provides a new governance, institutional, operational, administrative, and financial framework to address the many challenges that impede the effective implementation of the National Health Insurance Scheme.

It abolishes the district schemes and sets up a unitary National Health Insurance Scheme to be operated by a National Health Insurance Authority, answerable to the governing board of the Authority. The Authority is required to set up regional offices in each administrative region and the district offices considered necessary. The Act provides for the Private Commercial Health Insurance

Schemes and Private Mutual Health Insurance Schemes to be regulated by the National Insurance Authority.

The new Act also broadens the category of exempt persons to include pregnant women, children under five, and those over 70, as well as other vulnerable groups such as persons suffering from chronic psychiatric disorder. However, all categories of exempt persons, with the exception of children and women receiving antenatal and post-natal care, must pass a means test.

Against this background of uncertainty with the scheme, active membership has not grown as expected. A Parliamentary memo from the National Health Insurance Authority dated 30 September 2012 showed that 18.5 million of Ghana's population of 25.03 million had been registered. However, of this number, active membership was 8.64 meaning that about 34.5% of the total population were active members of the NHIS.

The Authority plans to intensify efforts through massive membership campaigns and policy reforms to encourage enrolment and renewal of membership. It is therefore estimated that 38% of the population or 9.93 million will be active members of the NHIS in 2013. This is about 14.9% increase over the active membership base in 2012.

The average premium rate per member in the informal sector in 2012 was GH¢10.81. In 2013, it was planned to strengthen controls over the registration system in order to improve premium collections and accountability, and also reduce leakages. It is expected that the average premium per member would increase to GH¢13.56. The average claim bill per active member in 2011 was GH¢66.82. In 2012 the cost rose by 10.9% to GH¢74.12 per active member.

The average use of the scheme per member, however, declined from 3.27 in 2011 to 3.1 in 2012. At the same time, the average cost per encounter rose from GH¢20.43 in 2011 to GH¢23.91 in 2012. In 2013, it is anticipated that there will be a 25% increase in claims' cost per use of the scheme on account of the following factors:

- Expected inclusion of the following in the benefit package: family planning, mental health, prostate cancer, childhood cancer, physiotherapy, and the physically challenged.
- The effect of the recent increase in tariffs by 20.5%.
- Expected increase in medicine prices by 22.5%.

Conclusions: the way forward

The National Health Insurance Scheme (NHIS) in Ghana was established with the view to improving financial access for Ghanaians, especially for the poor and the vulnerable, to quality basic healthcare services and to limit out-of-pocket payments at the point of service delivery. It is clear that the challenges of establishing an innovative National Health Insurance Scheme for Ghana are many.

In implementing the NHIS the Ghanaian authorities are 'learning by doing'. This was reflected in the progress of the rolling out of the district schemes. A recent study to evaluate the impact of NHIS on health service utilization and out-of-pocket payments in Ghana points to a critical lesson that instituting insurance is by itself not adequate to completely remove the financial access barriers to healthcare.[11] This is particularly because insured clients still incur out-of pocket charges for items that should be covered by insurance and for informal care.

Looking back, Ghana has come a long way in its efforts to use innovative financial schemes to provide healthcare services for poor people. It has been a long and often quite difficult journey. Lessons have been learned at every stage about how to achieve this in practical terms. Looking forward, therefore, we have a foundation on which to build—and to truly ensure that no-one is left behind as health services and health continue to improve in Ghana.

Ghana has, thus, embarked on innovative ways of financing its health delivery organizations. This has drawn local and international attention, with experts wondering whether this is a hazardous experiment or a way forward or lessons for African countries.

Acknowledgement

This manuscript was edited and revised by Ms Mabel Y Segbafah of the PPMED, GHS.

References

1 Ghana Statistical Service (GSS), Ghana Health Service (GHS), and ICF Macro (2009). Ghana Demographic and Health Survey 2008. Accra, Ghana.

2 **Nyonator F and Kutzin J.** Health for some? The effects of user fees in the Volta Region of Ghana. *Health Policy and Planning* 1999;**14** (4): 329–41.

3 **Asomadu-Kyereme R.** Doctoral Seminar Paper: Extending Pro-poor Social Security in Ghana. 2006. Retrieved August 2013 at: <http://www.uni-bielefeld.de/soz/igss/pdf/proposals/proposal_asomadu_r.pdf.>.

4 International Labour Organization. Ghana Social Trust Pilot Project: Financial Analysis of the National Public Health Budget and of the National Health Insurance Scheme. Discussion Paper No. 4, 2004.

5 **Agyepong IA and Adjei S.** *Public Social Policy Development and Implementation: A Case Study of the Ghana National Health Insurance Scheme.* 2007. Accessed August 2013 at: <http://heapol.oxfordjournals.org/content/23/2/150.full.pdf+html>.

6   Government of Ghana. National Health Insurance Act (Act 650), August 2003.

7   International Labour Organization (2003). Ghana Social Trust Pilot Project: comments on the planned national Health Insurance System in Ghana. March 2003.

8   **Atim C (ed.).** *Training of Trainers Manual for Mutual Health Organisations in Ghana.* Partnerships for Health Reforms (PHR) ABT Associates Inc. September 2000.

9   **Atim C, Grey S, and Apoya P.** *A Survey of Mutual Health Organizations in Ghana.* PHRplus, Bethesda, 2002.

10 Ministry of Health. National Health Insurance Policy Framework for Ghana. Revised Version. August 2004.

11 **Nguyen HT, Rajkotia Y and Wang H.** The financial protection effect of Ghana National Health Insurance Scheme: evidence from a study in two rural districts. *International Journal for Equity in Health 2011;10:4. Retrieved at:* <http://www.equityhealthj.com/content/10/1/4>.

Chapter 20

Health for the whole population

Patrick Kadama and Peter Eriki

Dr Kadama is Director for Health Policy and Strategy and Dr Eriki
is Director of Health Systems at ACHEST, both having previously
worked for WHO and the Ugandan Ministry of Health

This chapter, written by two medical doctors, Dr Patrick Kadama and Dr Peter
Eriki, draws on their extensive experience of health, both in Africa and in international organizations.

They describe the way in which the support system provided by the traditional African extended family has given way in recent years to a new dependency by individuals on state organized health systems, charities, and private
concerns. The result has been increasing health costs and growing inequalities.
It is now the poorest people who pay proportionately the highest amount for
their healthcare out of their own pockets. The chapter sets out in broad terms
the challenges faced by countries seeking to offer universal access to health and
healthcare for their citizens. These are challenges that, as we have seen in earlier chapters, require countries to find a way to meet these challenges that is
based both on their culture and history, and on their financial capabilities and
circumstances.

Family, customs, and history

The extended family is an almost universal feature of traditional societies in
Africa. There are widespread variations in tribal customs or culture, socio-
economic structures, geography, politics, and history; many are related to the
external influence of colonialism. However, these extended families have many
shared attributes of collective, kinship-oriented systems of production and
consumption of goods and services.

The extended families in effect represent the building blocks of the traditional
African society, their perception of health, and their influence on health-
seeking behaviour. It is in this context that the extended family has traditionally
provided a form of social safety net for households in African societies, ensuring traditional healthcare that leaves no-one behind.

Effect of new world economic pressures on African social values and health systems—and public policy responses

New health systems were 'technocratically' introduced in the last century, with little participation from the demand side of healthcare in society. This approach has in many countries inadvertently transferred much of the extended family social responsibilities to governments, with healthcare provided through networks of public sector service outlets, largely funded through tax revenue. It has contributed to the breakdown of collective, kinship-oriented social values and systems in many African family settings, at a time when many families are living below the poverty line. It has created a situation in which collective interests are at odds with private interests and has created a social dilemma.[1]

It is in this context, that the financial burden of healthcare has significantly grown at a time of rapid population growth, when there has also been a series of economic crises and political upheavals that have greatly disrupted the operation of free tax revenue funded public sector health services. Many families are now faced with having to seek care from full fee-for-service networks of formal and informal private healthcare providers, where services are accessed on the basis of out-of pocket payments at the time of accessing care.

The subsidized health services provided by faith-based non-state organizations and a full fee-for-service network of formal and informal private health providers have at all times complemented the free tax revenue funded services, but their prominence has lately risen as the latter got disrupted through under-resourcing by the public sector.

Shortly after the Alma Ata pronouncements on primary healthcare as a philosophy to guide the attainment of health for all by the year 2000, macro-economic pressures begun to emerge across Africa, as elsewhere. These were followed by government austerity measures that sought to introduce fee-for-service systems in the hitherto free tax revenue funded services in many parts of Africa as a means of sharing the burden of their financing. This cost-sharing effort was in effect a 'cost-shifting' initiative from the public sector to private households, most of which were known to be living in poverty and had to meet the cost of care through out-of-pocket payments. In light of this, the social response was quick to build the evidence to illustrate the negative impact of out-of-pocket payments for health services. The widespread practice of out-of-pocket payments for health services in the African low-resource setting still underlies the slow pace of progress towards universal health coverage in the region.

Recent analysis by the African Regional Office of WHO (2013)[2] has reviewed the status of health financing in Africa, including the status of out-of-pocket payments for healthcare as a share of total health expenditures (THE). First, in 45% of countries assessed, the out-of-pocket payments account for more than 40% of the total health expenditure in Africa. There is evidence that catastrophic health expenditure and impoverishment remain low in countries where out-of-pocket expenditure is less than 15–20% of the total health expenditure, few households are impoverished and catastrophic health expenditure drops to negligible levels.[3] The analysis, however, shows that there has been little progress towards improving on the out-of-pocket expenditure situation in Africa over the last 10-year period studied between 2001 and 2010.

Second, there is a more complex relationship between out-of-pocket payments as a share of total health expenditure and GDP per capita. While there is an overall trend of decrease in out-of-pocket expenditure with the rise in economic development, total health expenditure is in some situations significantly different between countries at the same level of economic development. On the other hand, some countries have similar low shares of out-of-pocket spending but very different income levels. This suggests that there are other constraints besides economic factors that are bringing down the share of out-of-pocket payments. It may well be a result of health financing policies that can drive down out-of-pocket payments even in poor settings while, on the other hand, in some rich countries out-of-pocket payments can be high.

The WHO analysis generally indicated that countries implementing health financing reforms that increase government health expenditure through various strategies and mechanisms will witness a decreasing share of out-of-pocket spending. The findings demonstrated that, as you might expect, low levels of public health expenditure (measured as a share of GDP) have high levels of out-of-pocket spending (as a share of total health expenditure), and vice versa. In other words, lowering financial barriers to access health services, and increasing government health expenditure, provide mutually positive benefits. Finally, efficiency savings as a means of increasing government health expenditure should be kept in mind as a necessary complementary measure.

Emerging concerns with inequality in health outcomes

Significant misdistribution of household incomes (wealth) is not restricted to low resource settings but is, in practice, just more often found in such settings. Apart from Equatorial Guinea with a GNI per capita higher than US$12 275 in 2010, which was classified as a high-income country by the World Bank, all other African countries have low- to middle-income status. About 60% of countries (26 of the 45 countries in the WHO/Afro region) with a GNI per capita below US $1005 in 2010 (in current prices), are classified by the World Bank as low-income countries. This shows the broad disparity in wealth distribution of the African region in a global context.

Recent demographic health surveys in the region show a widening gap in health outcomes between the lowest and highest quintiles.[4] The global, regional, and country level disparities in wealth are related to disparities in health outcomes; health outcomes that are a matter of human rights. Access to healthcare according to need and not just according to means, has come to be firmly perceived as a right. Access to needed healthcare is a critical factor in sustaining good health outcomes in society at all stages of the human life-cycle.

'Health from the womb to the tomb'

When Alan Johnson[5] addressed health professionals in September 2007 he echoed the sentiments of the 1940s, when the British National Health Service (NHS) was created in 1948 by Clement Attlee's Government under the direction of Health Minister Aneurin Bevan. The service was set up with a promise to provide people with healthcare from the 'cradle to the grave'. Setting out plans to reduce health inequalities, Mr. Johnson said that many factors determine health and may be established before babies are even born. He pointed to the body of research on how a baby's weight at birth determined their health in the future. It is known that in the short term, lower birth weight can lead to increased risk of cerebral palsy, visual impairment, and deafness. In the medium term, it can slow down cognitive and physical development. In the long term, it can lead to chronic diseases such as diabetes and cardiovascular disease. If their mantra in the 1940s was 'from the cradle to the grave', then their vision for the twenty-first century should perhaps be 'health from the womb to the tomb', Johnson concluded.

Life should be celebrated by discovering the wonders of human development in the 'womb to tomb'. This exposes the topics relating to the beginning of life, physical development, stages of life, geriatrics, as well as death and dying. Effectively, humans firmly adhere to the fact that without a beginning to life at conception, people could never exist at all. However, we should aim to acknowledge every aspect of human life, dignifying its worth, celebrating its presence, and appreciating its miracle. In the USA, a bill to provide a womb to tomb medical care to the nation runs into serious criticism. Similarly, larger changes are needed in Japan where the 'womb to tomb' employment system had collapsed. In sub-Saharan Africa, there are tendencies to compartmentalize the various segments of the life-cycle of health from the 'womb to tomb', leading to the loss of focus and recognition of the intertwined relationships of these segments. Instead of segregating into 'pregnant women, newborns, infants, children, adolescents, youth, married couples, and the elderly', it may be more prudent to look at these as a continuum.

The health systems developed should be robust and sensitive to the needs of the entire life-cycle stages of the population's life-cycle. These systems should be accessible and affordable to all those who may need them. This leads to a daunting question: at what cost and who pays?

There are significant challenges in designing pro-poor risk-sharing schemes for health financing of universal health coverage and themes for the future.[6] Strong health systems are the common objective for populations, while health financing mechanisms are the universal means to ensure their operation to produce critical goods and services required for households in society to perpetually generate and sustain (good) health. Countries are working to improve spending on health in order to strengthen health systems for universal access. Generally, in the African Region as elsewhere, funding for health is from multiple sources but with the prominent peculiarity that the bulk of funding for health originates from direct household out-of-pocket sources. The other usual source of funding for health includes flows from government, donors, employers, and non-governmental organizations.

The World Health Report 2010 indicates that estimates by the High Level Task Force (HLTF) on Innovative International Financing for Health Systems expect a low-income country to spend on average US$44 per capita in year 2009 to provide an essential package of health services.[7] Analysis by WHO Afro shows impressive progress by African countries in moving to this level of financing. It is noted, for example, that Rwanda more than doubled its per capita expenditure on health over a period of 10 years, with a large part of this increase attributed to external funds. The number of countries in the WHO/Afro region with total health expenditure above the minimum level of US$44 per capita recommended for 2009, more than doubled in the 10-year period between 2001 and 2010, rising from 24% (11 out of 45 in 2001) to 51% (23 out of 45 in 2010), respectively. Unfortunately, however, this leaves almost half (49%) of the countries in the region with a level of funding for health lagging below the minimum level of US$44 per capita recommended for 2009.

Fig. 20.1 illustrates that the number of countries spending less that $29 per capita annually on health has fallen dramatically in 10 years, whilst those spending more than $44 has grown equally rapidly.

Globalization is taking place against a background of complex population dynamics, which are compounded by political upheavals, as well as the recent world economic downturn. All this together has changed spending priorities

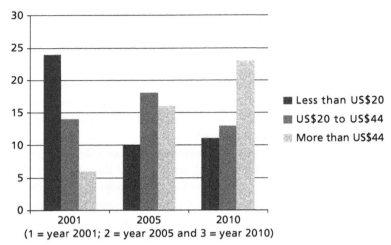

(1 = year 2001; 2 = year 2005 and 3 = year 2010)

Fig. 20.1 Trends in total expenditure on health by African countries over 10 years.[8]

Data from WHO Regional Office for Africa, *State of Health Financing in the African Region*, Copyright © WHO Regional Office for Africa, 2013.

for health and healthcare the world over. As set out above, the vast majority of African countries are ranked in the low- and middle-income category of countries. This is where scarcity of funds for health presents the most acute financial barrier to the provision of health services. WHO Afro estimates that the average total health expenditure in African countries stood at US$135 per capita in 2010. This is just about 4% of what is spent on health in an average high-income country. Despite the progress in Africa that was reviewed, there is an absolute lack of finances for health in the African region and this is a fundamental barrier that must be tackled. This scarcity of funding is set in the face of an adverse situation of environmental challenges, as well as adverse trends in other social determinants of health, including the disproportionate double burden of diseases in Africa. All these constitute barrier to progress towards universal health coverage.

In this setting of severe scarcity of financing for health, the predominant mechanisms in use in the African region to support operations of the health systems constitute additional barriers. They are highly inefficient in the public system and significantly pervasive, as well as ineffective, in the largely informal, and barely regulated, traditional private sector, which has the highest number of financial transactions (flows). In about half of African countries, 40% or more of the total health expenditure is constituted of household out-of-pocket payments, which is the most regressive way of funding healthcare. The reliance on this payment mechanism creates financial barriers to access health services and puts people at the risk of impoverishment.[9] Furthermore, the current financial flows within the health systems, especially the public sub-sector, are exacerbating inefficiencies and inequities; for example, through skewed allocation of funds to urban areas and specialized care for the elite.

While this set of barriers represent a complex platform for action in Africa, this is at a time when 'The science of complex adaptive systems provides important concepts and tools for responding to the challenges of healthcare in the 21st century'.[10] Traditionally, action for progress on the road towards universal health coverage has often been positioned on modifications of a three-pronged policy framework of health system financing functions[11, 12] aiming at:

- Developing fair and efficient mechanisms for collecting funds for health not just collecting more.
- Articulating modalities for sharing risk through pooling of funds for solidarity between and across strata of household income quintiles.
- Agreeing modalities for purchasing and/or provision of care from suppliers for an appropriate life-cycle based on an effective set of health interventions in the most efficient and equitable way while containing costs.

An increasing number of African countries are making progress with traditional approaches for risk sharing to finance universal health coverage. As earlier chapters show, Ghana has in over 10 years achieved about 30% coverage with a national health insurance scheme. A largely external funded effort in Rwanda, but with very high political commitment, has attained significant coverage. Traditional health insurance schemes are covering employed persons, especially in the public service employment; while private schemes are found predominantly in urban areas.

Conclusions

Innovations for health financing in Africa are required during the transition towards social transformation. The predominantly rural setting of African households today, as well as the large number of households living in the low-income strata of society, need to be consciously factored into programme designs to attract sufficient participation, even in those African countries that have launched traditional risk-sharing schemes. Many of these schemes cover those in formal employment and those able to meet the premiums. This excludes the bulk of households, usually in the rural areas, and those working in the informal sectors. Community based models, with the notable exception of Rwanda as described in Chapter 18 where the poorest quarter of the population pay no fees, have had limited impact to date.

Schemes need to be designed with rural-based poor households and informally employed persons in mind to take account of a transitional period of heavy public sector subsidies during a process of social transformation of the African communities to be covered. The design needs to consider options comprising a dynamic mix of 'fund-collection modalities' and 'fund-pooling' arrangements over the transition period, because the health financing system is a complex adaptive system interacting with a constantly changing socio-economic situation of households, quite often in a very unpredictable manner.

The heavy burden on public spending implied by the situation in Africa will require governments to evoke non-traditional sources of tax revenue to finance healthcare. Countries such as Mali have introduced earmarked taxes for health on high-value/high-turnover consumer products as, for example, cigarettes and alcohol and mobile phone usage, with some promise of success. There is increasing confidence that these non-traditional sources of health financing support will be critical in managing the financing burden for the transitional period in Africa, while prudently managed growth drives progress to higher proportions of people/households to participate in risk-sharing schemes.

Transitions may take quite some time in many countries and will require a sustained effort supported by sustained political commitment to the attainment of universal coverage in all African countries.

References

1 Kerr NL. Motivation losses in small groups: a social dilemma analysis. *Journal of Personality and Social Psychology* 1983;**45**: 819–28.

2 WHO Regional Office for Africa, 2013. State of health financing in the African Region.

3 Taskforce on Innovative International Financing for Health Systems. Constraints to scaling up the health Millennium Development Goals: costing and financial gap analysis. Working Group 1 Report, 2010, Geneva.

4 Uganda Bureau of Statistics and ICF International. Uganda Demographic Health Survey, 2011—Final Report (English). 2012.

5 Johnson A. Womb to tomb replaces cradle to grave as focus for health service. *The Guardian*, 12 September 2007. <http://www.theguardian.com/uk/2007/sep/12/politics.health>.

6 WHO Regional Office for Africa, 2013. State of health financing in the African Region.

7 World Health Report, 2010. Health Systems Financing: key to Universal Coverage. Geneva. World Health Organization.

8 Data from: WHO Regional Office for Africa, 2013. State of health financing in the African Region.

9 Borghi J, Ensor T, Somanathan A, Lissner C, and Mills A. Mobilising financial resources for maternal health. *Lancet*. 2006;**368**: 1457–65.

10 **Plsek PE, and Greenhalgh T.** Complexity science—the challenge of complexity in health care. *BMJ* 2001 ; **323**(7313): 625–8.

11 **Kutzin J.** A descriptive framework for country-level analysis of health care financing arrangements. *Health Polic* 2001; **56**: 171–204.

12 **Carrin G. and James C.** Key performance indicators for the implementation of social health insurance. *Appl Health Econ Health Policy* 2005; 4: 15–22.

Part 6

The future

Chapter 21

Introduction to Part 6: The future

Francis Omaswa and Nigel Crisp

This chapter turns to the future. It describes the different challenges that three generations of leaders have had to face in Africa—from colonial times, via the HIV/AIDS epidemic, and on to a time when Africa takes its place fully on the world stage. Lessons are being learned from each stage for the future.

Turning to the future

Chapters 22 and 23 are written by younger and future leaders, and describe their experiences as well as their hopes and fears. The first of these is by Miatta Kargbo who became Minister of Health and Sanitation in Sierra Leone in 2013 and discusses the issues she faces as she helps to lead her country towards a brighter future in the wake of the civil war, which only finished 10 years earlier.

Chapter 23 draws on contributions from three women and three men, from different backgrounds and different countries. They are all already playing leadership roles in health. In it they describe how they see the current state of health and health services in Africa and what they see as the encouraging trends and potential threats for the future.

The authors of the earlier chapters all have many years of experience and have great achievements to their names. It is possible to see three generations of African leaders here, starting with those who, like Francis Omaswa, lived through independence and the great hopes it brought in its train. They also had to cope with the distorting legacy of colonialism, which meant, amongst other things, that access to any form of organized or scientific health care was severely limited among African populations. Miriam Were in Kenya, Gottlieb Monekosso in Cameroon, and Pascoal Mocumbi in Mozambique were all engaged in setting up new systems and services to reach the wider populations when the British, French, and Portuguese, respectively, left their countries.

The next generation, who took up leadership roles some time after independence, have found their working lives dominated by other concerns such as the scourge of HIV/AIDS and the extraordinary explosion in aid and development of the last 15 years. They, too, have had to struggle with their own particular colonial and national legacies to build new systems and services, as we have seen with Agnes Binagwaho following the genocide in Rwanda and Aaron Motsoaledi after apartheid in South Africa.

The younger and future leaders, as Chapters 22 and 23 show, are world citizens, educated abroad like many of their elders, but enabled by technology and changing global politics to participate in global debates and thinking. They have the rich legacy of the earlier generations to build on—the many remarkable achievements described in this book—as they take up their struggle to improve health and health services in Africa. Hopefully they will be working with access to more resources and to a world that looks at Africa in a different way.

The final chapter of the book (Chapter 24), written by the editors, brings together many of the main themes that have emerged from the earlier chapters, gathering together insights from the leaders of the present and the past. It goes on to set out a vision for the future, which demands action from Africans themselves and from the rest of the world, and shows how the African experience and perspective can help shape improvements in health globally.

Chapter 22

The future: view from a Minister

Miatta Kargbo

Minister of Health for Sierra Leone

The Honourable Miatta Kargbo MBA became Minister of Health and Sanitation in Sierra Leone in February 2013. She had previously served as Presidential Adviser, a post she came to with several years of experience in management, strategy development, global implementations, and strategic process improvement. The editors were keen to get the views of one of the newest and youngest health ministers in Africa about the future of health and healthcare in Africa, as well as for her own country. In this chapter she sets out an optimistic vision whilst at the same time describing very clearly the many challenges that will have to be met. She also describes the practical steps that can and are being taken to improve health and ensure access to healthcare, even for the poorest.

The state of health and healthcare in Africa today

Healthcare in Africa is in a state of recovery and revival. If you look back over the history of health services in sub-Saharan Africa, the colonial period saw the construction of great hospitals and systems. The post-colonial period was marked with challenges to meaningful socio-economic development, personal ambitions, and political unrest that prompted wars and conflicts. This has led to damage across the continent, having an effect like a stroke or a heart attack on health services, which includes massive destruction of infrastructure and loss of health workers.

We are now transitioning across Africa into a period of revival. There is an increased consciousness about the central importance of a healthy nation. The Millennium Development Goals (MDGs) have focused minds on tackling poverty and ill health. There is widespread recognition and awareness about the threat of non-communicable diseases (NCDs), especially in countries like Sierra Leone that are facing a double disease burden of communicable and non-communicable diseases.

This is a good time for health in Africa with blossoming awareness. The change is being driven in part from the recognition at the highest political levels of the link between health and wealth. Health has started to make a much better business case within government that it is an integral component of growth and poverty reduction.

A great example of this is family planning. If you are a mother in a rural village with nine children, there is limited chance you are going to be able to send them all to school. They are going to grow up with limited prospects and little to contribute to the economy or country as a whole. They are also going to struggle to get good nutrition or to access health services, which will drive up the risk of stunting and of high infant mortality. So family planning in this context becomes a fantastically high-value intervention by empowering women and parents to have families that are healthier and better educated, improving not only their own prospects, but that of the nation as a whole.

The role of women is central to the improvement of health across Africa. Women act almost as health advisors at the local level, having responsibility for everything from their children, family nutrition, hygiene, and the household. As women become better educated and better informed about health, they become a key local driver for improved health at the family and village level.

The encouraging trends for the future . . . and the worrying ones

The improving state of health in Africa rests on a number of encouraging trends. There is much greater consciousness of health issues and the importance of health—both by government and the public. There is increased investment in health by governments and development partners. There is growing awareness and understanding of women, even at the village level, about maternal and child health, and even non-communicable diseases.

There are also some worrying trends, however, that need to be recognized and addressed, as they threaten to undermine this health revival in its early stages. Adolescents lie at the centre of this. What we are seeing with adolescents is a whole series of interrelated health problems, such as teenage pregnancy, sexually transmitted infections, drug abuse, mental illness, trauma from war, and non-communicable diseases.

If we fail to take fast action on these, we will be overwhelmed. The rapid rise in cancer across Africa is a good example. We need to prioritize early cancer diagnosis and treatment if we are to keep this threat under control.

These growing health problems largely rest on the inevitable trend of the growing Westernization of lifestyles in Africa, such as increasing smoking and consumption of pre-packaged foods. Many African communities have been protected from non-communicable diseases by a healthy culture that includes natural foods and athleticism. This traditional culture is fast disappearing and at risk however, and governments have got to increase awareness and sensitize the public to create more value on healthy lifestyles.

Much of the debate around health in Africa over the last two decades has centred around HIV/AIDS and there are grounds for cautious optimism here. In Sierra Leone, older generations are well informed about HIV/AIDS and they are being more responsible and taking steps to protect themselves. As a country, we have been able to stabilize the HIV/AIDS prevalence rate at 1.5%, but we should not let this achievement reduce our efforts to control the epidemic. It is critical that we increase awareness among the younger generations as part of a constant process of education and learning. We must also focus on specific high-risk groups, such as sex workers, men who have sex with men, and drug users, who are mostly left out of most programmes The stigma associated with these groups can foster an attitude in government or amongst the public that their risks are their problem, but we instead need to adopt an approach that this is all of our business.

These patterns in health problems are complemented by a set of positive trends across Africa in health systems.

The rise in community health programmes stand out as an exciting development that are allowing us to reach people even in the most remote areas. Community health workers are rapidly extending access to critical health services, covering issues such as nutrition, malaria, and reproductive health. Community health workers are able to reach out into villages and people's homes, allowing us to address problems early, improve the local environment to prevent disease, and not overwhelm the system with issues that could have been address at the community/household level.

These programmes are complemented by the widespread adoption of a task-shifting approach, where the traditional roles of health workers, such as of doctors and nurses, are redistributed to make the best use of the limited staff available and rapidly increase the availability of critical health services at low cost. In Sierra Leone, we are taking this to the next level with the introduction of clinical officers, who will be able to undertake a whole range of basic medical and surgical procedures. Within the next three or four years we hope to see 50–70% of emergency obstetric surgeries carried out by clinical officers. Task-shifting will particularly benefit patients outside of the big cities, as clinical officers are willing to work and live in remote rural areas where doctors have been unwilling to go.

There continues to be great hope across the continent that we will see a much greater number of people from the African diaspora returning to their home countries, after years or decades of training and experience in the West, to offer their skills to the badly understaffed public sectors. This trend has been much slower than expected. Low-income countries are unable to compete with the salaries and lifestyles of health workers in the West and until the playing field is evened out, we are unlikely to see much change here. High-income countries need to reconsider recruiting staff from Africa to help build capacity in Africa, and low-income countries need to significantly strengthen their recruitment and retention strategies.

One way of responding to the on-going haemorrhage of health workers out of Africa is to significantly scale up health worker training, and this is exactly what we are starting to see. In particular we need to increase the number of doctors working in maternal, newborn, and child health. In Sierra Leone we have prioritized the establishment of post-graduate training programmes for doctors and nurses, so that health workers no longer have to go overseas for post-graduate training to specialize, and therefore avoid the temptation of not coming back home. This also increases the number of senior trainees, who provide needed services within the health system and the tertiary hospitals.

For many countries in Africa, to strengthen post-graduate training they will need the help of their stronger neighbours, which for Sierra Leone would include Ghana and Nigeria, who can lend their specialist expertise where there is none locally. We are definitely seeing an increase in regional collaboration within Africa that is a very encouraging trend for the future.

This regional collaboration is complemented by the strengthening of South–South collaboration, such as with Cuba and China. Sierra Leone and other African countries are definitely benefiting from this, but some of the programmes are quite young and face teething problems. The challenges are in the details, including issues such as language barriers, appropriate qualifications, and professional registration.

A damaging legacy from the past has been the system of patient fees and health financing that has reduced access to health services for the poorest and most vulnerable, and sometimes starved critical parts of the health system of funding. In Sierra Leone, which has a population of six million, more than 60% of the population live under the poverty line. These people either cannot afford life-saving health services or have to make catastrophic health expenditure, which pushes families that had been just coping financially into bankruptcy, and therefore into a downward spiral of unemployment and poverty that can continue for generations. There is no way for these people to pay for health services on their own, making risk pooling and social solidarity essential. Ghana and Rwanda are two countries that have led the way in expanding coverage to health services and many other countries are following their example.

Sierra Leone introduced its Free Health Care Initiative for pregnant women, lactating mothers, and children under-five in April 2010. This initiative has led to an enormous increase in access to health services for these groups but it cannot continue to rely on donor funding. Sierra Leone and other countries therefore have to find a way to transition these schemes into initiatives that can be sustained into the future. The Free Health Care Initiative is Sierra Leone's first step in a journey towards universal health coverage that covers all groups.

The final and most fundamental trend has been the strengthening of leadership in Africa and a reclaiming of the health agenda. In our lifetimes we have not seen enough leaders stand up and talk about health, but we are now seeing Presidents and Ministers setting the health agenda for their countries. Respect for leaders in Africa used to be based on their revolutionary stances, but now we are seeing leaders on the covers of magazines for being catalysts for change in healthcare. We are seeing this trend for strong leadership in health from across the continent, from President Ernest Bai Koroma in Sierra Leone to President Goodluck Jonathan in Nigeria, President Kikwete of Tanzania, and President Macky Sall of Senegal. This has restored a much more appropriate and effective balance in agenda setting for health in Africa, with the agenda coming from African leaders.

My greatest hopes and fears for the future

My greatest hope is that we will continue to see the current upward trajectory and not lose focus on the ultimate goal of quality and timely healthcare for everyone. This can be achieved if we are able to revolutionize the way people think and feel about their health.

I am worried that we are starting to lose the adolescent population in healthcare, which would have terrible consequences. Other groups, such as children under five, pregnant and lactating women, and to some extent, older people seem to have health-related programmes that cater for their healthcare. Adolescents are getting lost in the system, however, and this is due to a whole array of factors relating to how we run our health services. We are failing to train health workers to understand or communicate with adolescent patients, who do not access services and do not get the treatment they need as a result. Even the way our facilities are designed and managed can be hostile to this group. Improved family planning amongst adolescents will be critical to the health of the whole nation; we cannot achieve good health for all, if we do not address this problem. We are at risk of seeing a next generation of smokers and diabetics or of women with six children who we lose from the system, first professionally and then socially.

My vision for health in Sierra Leone

My vision for healthcare in Sierra Leone is for people to get the quality and affordable services that they require and deserve. To achieve this, we will need to build infrastructure, capacitate hospitals, and strengthen our human resources. Developing community health programmes and expanding the Free Health Care Initiative to include other vulnerable groups and eventually universal health coverage will be a central part of this future.

Chapter 23

The future: younger and future leaders

Nigel Crisp with contributions from John Paul Bagala, Clarisse Bombi, Susana Edjang, Ndwapi Ndwapi, Kelechi Ohiri, and Nana Twum-Danso

For this chapter we asked six younger and future leaders to answer four questions:

- What do you see as the key features of health and health care in sub-Saharan Africa today?
- What are the encouraging signs of improvement and the trends that need to be supported?
- What are the worrying signs and concerns about the future?
- What is your vision and your hope for the future?

This group of leaders are very realistic and straightforward about the difficulties of the present situation in their responses to these questions. They offer their own analysis and, often, their own solutions in what is fundamentally an optimistic view of the future. They stress many of the same themes as the leaders writing in earlier chapters but, perhaps unsurprisingly, they place greater emphasis on innovation and technology, and on creating plural systems with more investment and action from non-governmental players. They don't all agree with each other but there is a shared perception of the importance of leadership and of the need for Africans to take control of their own destinies. There are three women and three men in this group; three are from West Africa and one each from the East, Centre, and South. Three are doctors; there is also a nurse, a physiotherapist, and the President of the African Federation of Medical Students' Associations. Four live and work or study in their own countries, whilst two have global roles.

What do you see as the key features of health and healthcare in sub-Saharan Africa today?

There is a great deal of agreement amongst the contributors about the situation today.

Nana Twum-Danso writes:

> In the past few decades many sub-Saharan African countries have witnessed substantial gains in life expectancy attributable to an increasing standard of living and with it, improved access to better nutrition, healthcare, education, safe water, sanitation, and other basic services. Indeed, there is much to celebrate.
>
> However, this overall assessment masks the large inequities within countries—the urban/rural divide and variation by wealth quintiles continue to grow. Further, some demographic groups such as pregnant women and newborn children are being left behind in the race to achieve Millennium Development Goals Four, Five, and Six. The early wins—vaccine-preventable diseases, diarrhoea, malaria—are being made but for conditions that require functioning health systems and overcoming deep-seated socio-cultural beliefs and practices (e.g. maternal and neonatal health) there is still much to be done.

Susana Edjang puts it bluntly:

> Although progress has been great, Africa, as a group, will not meet the health-related MDGs (MDG4 on child mortality, MDG 5 on maternal mortality, and MDG 6 on aids, tuberculosis, and malaria). There is pervasive and growing inequality of health outcomes and poor civil registration and vital statistics data. Often we don't really know who is dying and the cause of death. In Africa, only four countries have functioning vital registration systems: Egypt, Mauritius, Seychelles, and South Africa.

Ndwapi Ndwapi is even blunter:

> The resource burdens of HIV/AIDS have essentially mortgaged the future of health systems' development for generations to come . . . there are some smouldering epidemics: maternal mortality; under-five mortality; road traffic accidents; drugs and alcohol. These epidemics are fuelled by poverty (e.g. HIV/AIDS and TB), but also by increasing wealth and urbanization. There are complications of young womanhood (teenage pregnancy, single parent households, lack of birth control, lack of safe abortion services, intergenerational sex). Sexual reproductive healthcare issues need to be openly and rationally addressed.

Kelechi Ohiri continues the theme:

> News about health in Africa is always sobering. The common narrative of health and healthcare in sub-Saharan Africa is one of heavy disease burden and frequent epidemics and needless, preventable deaths. The HIV epidemic very quickly assumed an African face, with sub-Saharan Africa being most severely affected, with nearly 1 in every 20 adults (4.9%) living with HIV and accounting for 69% of the people living with HIV worldwide. Most African countries are not on track to meet the MDGs.

John Paul Bagala emphasizes the links between health and poverty, writing:

A vicious cycle exists between health and the financial status of the biggest majority of persons in Africa. One will have poor health because he/she is poor and cannot afford healthcare and he/she will be poor because of the poor health that doesn't allow him or her work and earn a living that could enable him/her to access better healthcare. There is a clear separation between the few individuals who can afford healthcare and the much larger group living on less than $2 a day who face challenges in accessing and footing their health care bills.

These younger and future leaders describe the way in which disease patterns are changing and the problems associated with the increase in non-communicable diseases.

Clarisse Bombi writes:

The epidemiological landscape is characterized by the transition from communicable to non-communicable diseases. Hypertension, diabetes, and cardiovascular disorders are increasing as a growing proportion of the population become overweight and/or obese. This imposes changes in the healthcare delivery system and mechanisms that must adapt to respond to these changes.

Nana Twum-Danso says:

Another important feature to note is the epidemiologic transition that many countries in sub-Saharan Africa are currently undergoing. Non-communicable diseases or 'diseases of the wealthy', such as hypertension, hypercholesterolemia, diabetes mellitus, and cancer, are becoming increasingly more prevalent as life expectancy increases and we become wealthier. Yet, our health systems are still designed primarily to manage acute episodic illnesses, such as malaria, diarrhoeal illnesses, and injuries, rather than chronic diseases that require continuity of care. Outside of maternity care and immunizations during the first year of life, our health systems generally do a poor job of keeping track of individual patients, their medical histories, prior treatments, and complications.

She adds:

A visit to the medical records' office in most clinics and hospitals in sub-Saharan Africa is all you need to understand how dire the situation is. Without a functioning medical record system and an orientation towards continuity of care, it is no wonder that both health providers and their patients manage chronic diseases so poorly. It is not uncommon for doctors to prescribe newly diagnosed hypertensive patients one month's worth of medicines without clear instructions on follow-up and yet be surprised when they end up in the emergency room with a stroke within a year.

She concludes:

Technological innovations such as electronic medical records and mobile health could certainly help solve this problem but the more fundamental challenge is the orientation of health providers towards chronic disease management, namely screening and primary prevention, to reduce the incidence of clinical disease coupled with treatment and rehabilitation to reduce morbidity, mortality, and disability.

Ndwapi Ndwapi writing about the same point says:

Although the HIV/AIDS pandemic continues to preoccupy healthcare systems, the infrastructure, training, and clinical approaches that have been developed to address HIV/AIDS can and should be used to address non-HIV conditions such as diabetes, hypertension, and heart disease. The clinical protocols and policies that have been put in place for HIV/AIDS care should serve as a model for similar protocols for treatment of common non-HIV disorders. As HIV-infected people recover and have the prospect of living longer, their non-HIV conditions will require appropriate care: it would be a tragedy if patients who have benefited from HIV therapies eventually succumb to non-HIV conditions prematurely.

Health workers

Clarisse Bombi, writing from her own experience as a nurse in Cameroon, draws attention to staffing and reforms in human resources:

These reforms have seen the nurse occupy different positions and play different roles. In one the nurse is the team leader and the other the nurse is a team member. In the wake of the implementation of primary healthcare, and through the years of the economic stagnation, some divisions (e.g. midwifery) were closed in the training schools and recruitment into the public service was frozen. The implications were far reaching: staff went on retirement, died, or left for greener pastures abroad without replacement.

She describes how nurses headed most of the frontline health services and:

It was not uncommon to find a single nurse offering consultation, antenatal clinics, immunization both at fixed and outreach posts, compiling statistics, drawing up annual activity plans for the vertical programmes, etc. They were the team leaders even if it was a one-man team; they were polyvalent nurses. The situation has not changed much though. As one moves up the health pyramid, there are doctors in the sub-divisional hospitals, the district hospitals, and regional hospitals to make the diagnostic and therapeutic decisions, thus making the nurse assume the role of a team member and no longer the ultimate decision maker.

She points out there is inequitable distribution of the few health personnel:

Most of them prefer to work in the big urban centres where they have more opportunities to do something extra to earn some extra money to make up for the low salaries. The rural health facilities are consequently grossly understaffed, creating an apparent shortage. There is the glaring near absence of mental health nurses and rehabilitation nurses as the consequence of the little attention that has been accorded to these areas.

She also draws attention to corruption:

One of the millennium development goals has to do with governance. Corruption in the health sector has been receiving a lot of attention recently. The Cameroon

Government ordered the putting in place of anticorruption committees in the health facilities. Nurses are members of these committees. Controlling the doctors remains a major challenge for them.

Wider economic, social, and political perspectives and the determinants of health

Kelechi Ohiri puts these problems into the wider social and economic perspective:

A double disease burden is emerging as the incidence of non-communicable diseases steadily increases, with lifestyle diseases like diabetes, heart disease, hypertension, and cancer becoming more common. In many countries, a triple burden of disease already prevails, due to the high prevalence of injuries and trauma-related deaths. These situations are further aggravated by the poor state of other socio-economic determinants of health, including low literacy rates and harmful cultural practices. These may undermine the uptake of many health messaging campaigns and interventions. Geographical and environmental factors such as tropical climates and remote localities hinder efforts to improve health outcomes.

He describes this in the historical context:

Colonial-era healthcare systems were designed for the treatment of well-known threats to health, such as malaria and other infectious diseases. Unlike the evolution of the education sector, historically health systems were disproportionately designed and operated to cater to the health needs of colonizers and the local elite, with few indigenous caregivers being trained with the skills necessary for proper healthcare delivery. Whereas many changes have been made since colonial times, present-day health systems have inherited and maintained many aspects of that era's approach to healthcare delivery, such as: the predominant focus largely on curative care, with very little focus on prevention and healthy living; access remains better for the well-off, whereas those in the lowest income quintiles lack access to basic care.

He continues by drawing attention to the financing of systems:

Many African health systems lack proper health coverage schemes, creating a lack of financial risk protection and causing the majority of health expenditures to still come from out-of-pocket payments. Many underserved populations are accustomed to poor access and availability of services. The elite and affluent segments of the population often utilize their option to obtain health services abroad, while the base of the pyramid must tolerate the sub-standard healthcare services where available and when affordable. Underlining many of the problems with healthcare is widespread poor quality of care and lack of government responsiveness to the healthcare needs of the population. Inadequate oversight, lack of capacity, and obscurity of responsibility amongst many regulatory bodies create gaps and overlaps in healthcare regulation.

He concludes, however, that:

There are some grounds for hope even though the current state of the health systems in many countries within sub-Saharan Africa has stymied the health of the population and hindered overall economic growth. To give due credit, many health systems are making significant improvements and championing efforts for further gains in health outcomes. Although most health indicators are not yet at target levels, several new approaches and trends in healthcare delivery have the potential to positively impact many African health systems.

John Paul Bagala also stresses the importance of the wider determinants of health:

The main contributors to poverty in Africa are the low levels of good quality education in many African communities, keeping the literacy levels low and thus many individuals fail to compete for well-paying jobs. The low levels of employment, even for the few who have managed to acquire education, remains a challenge to many in Africa. Lack of jobs is attributed to most of the scholars opting to becoming job seeking rather than being job creators.

He writes that:

Governments not fulfilling their responsibilities and playing their respective roles of improving the infrastructure, which would modify the working environment of their citizens, also remains a key contributing factor to the reduced levels of employment. This, accompanied with corruption and misappropriation of funds, leaves many people lacking the necessities they would have obtained regardless of the few resources.

He says that:

No single silver bullet will break this poverty–poor health cycle: diverse efforts from bottom to top, commitment, self-mobilization, and inputs contributed by the individuals who fall victims of circumstance are key in breaking the cycle; a multi-sector intervention with a skill mix approach in reaching out and delivering healthcare to the lower cadres addressing the cause of the poverty that is leading to poor health also needs not to be neglected.

He continues by citing the impact of population growth:

The population in Africa is increasing at a fast rate compared to the rate of growth of the economy that should support it. This nature of population growth has increased the demand with limited supply for healthcare services due to the limited number of health workers, the few health centres, which are less equipped, and drug shortages, thus leaving the unmet need of healthcare services.

He concludes:

The key contributors of the fast-growing population are the high fertility rate of the sub-Saharan African women, lack of knowledge, and the conflicting cultural beliefs in societies, which have significantly contributed to the low uptake and usage of the population control measures and services like family planning. Population growth still remains a key threat to health and healthcare in many sub-Saharan African communities that needs urgent attention.

Finally, in describing the current situation Susana Edjang draws attention to the changing political environment:

Health is at the centre of the national, regional, and the global agendas that bilateral, multilateral, and global partnerships pursue in the continent. This is in great part a direct result of the MDGs. This might, of course, change with the post-2015 agenda as the health goals and indicators might be broadened or collapsed.

She continues:

At the same time there are more Africans and Africans in the Diaspora in leading positions at global health institutions outside Africa. For example, in the UN UNAIDS with Michel Sidibé, UNFPA with Babatunde Osotimehin, and Phumzile Mlambo-Ngcuka with UN Women. In addition, there is increased visibility of African women in leadership positions in health in governments across Africa, such as Agnes Binagwhaho in Rwanda [author of Chapter 17] and Awa Marie Coll-Seck in Senegal, and global civil society, such as Joy Phumaphi, Chair of Global Leaders Council of Reproductive Health and Executive Secretary of the African Leaders Malaria Alliance.

She adds:

We have also seen the elevation of health issues, in particular women's issues, to the top of the political agenda. Across sectors, Kandeh Yumkella, Director-General of UNIDO championing the link between sustainable energy and women's health, and Kumi Naidoo, Executive Director of Green Peace, linking women's health and rights to climate change's adaptability and mitigation efforts. In the last 5 years, the voices of some Heads of State and Governments have been heard on issues such as adolescent health and rights and unsafe abortions. Having women Heads of State and Government (Liberia, Malawi) and Chairing the African Union are steps in the right direction.

What are the encouraging signs of improvement and the trends that need to be supported?

The younger and future leaders describe a very wide range of encouraging and positive trends. The following contributions describe trends that cover the whole region, as well as some that apply specifically to their own countries.

Nana Twum-Danso takes the wider African perspective and writes that:

Strong leaders establishing a compelling vision for the future, enabling an actionable plan, mobilizing resources, and holding people accountable for results are just a few of the encouraging signs I see in countries such as Ethiopia, Malawi, Rwanda, and Sierra Leone that are making substantial progress in improving the health of their populations [for further information see Chapters 14, 5, 18, and 23]. Sub-Saharan Africa needs more of these types of leaders, not just at the highest political levels, but also in the technocratic bureaucracies in capital cities and provincial towns, as well as in the health facilities.'

She writes:

We need strong leaders who empower managers to be effective, who in turn provide the enabling environment for health providers to do the jobs they have been trained to do in a reliable way so that each patient gets the right care at the right time and populations get the appropriate promotional and preventive care on a regular basis.

Susana Edjang also takes the Africa-wide perspective:

Many countries are increasing the percentage of their GDP and government budgets that they spend on health. The levels are nowhere near the Abuja target but many countries have increased steadily their per capita expenditure on health.

She also describes:

the increasing visibility and action of business leaders and philanthropists on health issues. Examples include Aliko Dangote [Africa's richest man] and Jim Ovia [CEO of Zenith Bank] during the Nigerian floods in 2012; Toyin Saraki through the Wellbeing Foundation, the Motsepe Foundation, and the Nigerian Private Sector Health Alliance led by the CEOs of the major Nigerian banks, including the CEO of Access Bank, Aigboje Aig Imoukheude, and Jim Ovia. There is also the increasing visibility and mobilization of civil society on health issues through the Africa Coalition on Maternal, Newborn, and Child Health or AMREF, and at the country level through groups like Nigeria Health Watch.

She continues:

There are innovations in products and approaches across the board such as the development and empowerment of community health workers and other middle cadre level health workers; the development of mPedigree software to identity counterfeit drugs; the use of the Coca-Cola supply chains to distribute health supplies and medicines—to name only a few examples. This has been accompanied by reductions, in some communities, in the mortality and morbidity of the most vulnerable, often women and children.

She adds:

Although the region is experiencing a critical shortage of health workers, Africa has the youngest population in the world and is the only region in the world where the youth population will expand. However, 60% of young people are unemployed. By 2050, this population is expected to double and be equivalent to one-quarter of the global health workforce. There is an excellent opportunity to engage youth into healthcare jobs and I hope our leaders do something about it.

The situation in Botswana

Ndwapi Ndwapi addresses his own country as part of the bigger picture:

The discovery of new exploitable mineral deposit across Africa has not escaped Botswana and Southern Africa. While it will be a number of years before many of these deposits are brought to production, the anticipation of these opportunities is driving the flow of Foreign Direct Investment and growing the economies. There is a full realization that health systems will need to be overhauled, not just to support an increasing number of foreigners who come with international investment, but also the local populations. Many of our countries have thriving and invigorated democracies in which the citizenry has never been more aware of its entitlement to good healthcare as a basic responsibility of the State.

He writes:

There is a need for greater transparency in decisions made affecting healthcare, and citizens must be encouraged to actively participate in their medical care, and to demand the best possible care within the economic constraints of their particular country. There should be established monitoring and evaluation, e.g. quality improvement, which should be carried out on a routine basis, with results being published for public review and comment.

He writes:

In Botswana, the majority of the population is under 40 years of age. Young people are not afraid to engage technology. The IT industry is one of the fastest growing in the economy. These same young people are ready to transform out-dated paradigms that no longer serve the society as a whole—technologically and culturally. They must be encouraged to do so.

He concludes:

Other trends that should be encouraged are improved governance in some countries, including greater responsiveness to the needs of communities. Since the turn of the century there has been a critical mass of political will to address major health issues (e.g. male circumcision, malaria, TB, as well as HIV/AIDS). This has been further encouraged by evidence-based policies, propping up the boldness to try out new strategies (e.g. Malawi with option B +) [see Chapter 5 for further information]. We have also seen home-grown innovations that need to be supported, such as the fielding of community health workers at the household level. The advent of major home-grown solutions is a coming of age of African health leaders that will usher in many decades of increasing self-determination.

Cameroon

Clarisse Bombi writes about Cameroon that:

There is more attention being paid to promotional health. There is a whole section that has been dedicated to health education and health promotion in the heath sector strategic plan. There is also an area on nutrition. People are being educated on healthy lifestyle and eating healthily. These efforts have to be encouraged and sustained because old habits die hard.

At the same time, she writes:

Public–private collaboration is improving. The state is providing equipment like refrigerators to the private health facilities to enable the storage of vaccines. The private health facilities are also accepting to provide preventive services like immunization without charging any fees. Efforts are also being made to organize the traditional healers and to seek ways and means by which they can collaborate with the mainstream/contemporary health facilities. They have been trained to recognize diseases with epidemic potential and report to the mainstream health facilities so that they can be investigated.

She describes a number of very practical improvements:

A move has been taken to re-start the training of midwives. The public service has also started recruiting nurses and doctors. Attention is being focused on mental health and rehabilitation. Moves are also being made to curb the flurry of training schools to ensure that staff is of good quality. Curricular of training schools are also being adjusted to include issues of contemporary interest and no longer stereotyped. Staff members are also being trained to be multifunctional with less specialization.

She writes that:

The recent move to construct and equip referral hospitals, imaging centres, and dialysis centres is to be commended. Nurses will need to receive special training to work in these specialized centres. However, the health centres and the district hospitals need to be constructed and equipped also. Only 20% of the patients are referred from the health centre to the district hospital and an even lower percentage is referred from the district hospital to the regional hospital.

She also warns about the need for better governance:

The financial motivation mechanisms put in place need to be made to function better. Also non-financial motivation methods like decoration of nurses, appointment of nurses to posts of responsibility, provision of housing for nurses should also be instituted and made to work. The anti-corruption committees are definitely an important step forward in the fight against corruption in the health sector. The composition of these committees should empower the nurse more. These committees should be made to function better.

Sub-Saharan Africa

John Paul Bagala returns to the wider perspective and sees many encouraging signs:

Many global and local partners support the delivery of healthcare in sub-Saharan Africa. These partners have tried to bridge the gap of the increasing demand with the limited supply of the healthcare services by the government. Both knowledge and financial support have been brought close to the people with effective and improved strategies of monitoring the usage of these resources and services. The sustainability of these efforts and services, brought on board by the different partners, should not solely be the role of the partners but it should be the role of the government being supported, the partner, and the local community who are the final beneficiaries of the services. There is great need to create an ideal and conducive environment that enables the operation of the partners and to greatly support the implementation of their activities.

He warns, however, that:

Many donors and partners in African countries have discontinued their work due to the misuse of funds that are meant to benefit the lay people in the communities, political and civil unrests causing insecure working environments and unfavourable government policies. All these barriers need to be addressed to streamline and improve the international partnerships.

He sees progress with the determinants of health:

We need to appreciate and recognize the efforts that have been made to increase access to universal education in the different communities in sub-Saharan Africa. Having a literate and educated population will significantly lower the disease rates and improved health standards of the different African communities.

He also sees progress with health services:

The provision of health services is increasing enormously. Many governments are recognizing the benefits of investing in health, as having a healthy population is a key contributor to economic development and the primary step in eradication of poverty. We need to give credit where it is due. This may not be achieved in a fortnight; however, moving a single step is much better that folding our hands with nothing done. Putting the health facilities and structures in place is a great achievement, support then is needed to staff and equip the health facilities. Additionally, there is the need to build the capacity of young researchers and support staff so that Africa can be in position to identify solutions to its own problems and challenges.

Kelechi Ohiri sees opportunities in the fact that healthcare in Africa is so under-developed:

A criticism of the African health sector has been that the poorly formed systems and the lack of structure act as immense obstacles toward improvement. Contrary to this frame of mind, the lack of defined structures and systems is potentially one of the greatest strengths. Many Western health systems are locked into a mode of operating based on the historical systems put in place, rendering them unable to easily change political or operational processes to reflect more modern and cost-efficient practice methods. Healthcare in many developing countries, on the other hand, is positioned to leap frog development phases by capitalizing on new technologies and embedding novel models of care delivery into its structures. Innovative solutions, such as mobile health technologies and creative business models—such as high-volume low-cost care systems and cross-subsidization cost financing—can be used in part to shape African healthcare delivery, policy, and regulation.

He writes that:

Several key areas are poised for impact and are driving the gradual rehabilitation of many African healthcare systems. The changes in healthcare financing, as many countries gradually move away from heavy out-of-pocket spending, is rendering care affordable for many for whom formal healthcare was previously out of reach. A number of countries are moving toward universal health coverage, as there is an increasing shift toward spending governments' own resources for health. Since governments' funding for healthcare is often limited, healthcare delivery in resource-constrained environments engenders innovation toward low-cost options. Moreover, ensuring cost-effective use of available resources has generated increasing interest in fiscal space analyses, creating opportunities to measure allocative efficiency and improved health spending policies.

He continues that:

Another key area receiving increasing attention from governments and development partners alike is the health private sector. Traditionally, healthcare in Africa has been largely focused on public facilities and governments' ability to exercise control over the activities of these facilities. However, the fact that about 60% of health services and 40% of healthcare facilities in Africa come from the private sector means that a fresh approach to healthcare delivery is needed to have a significant impact on health outcomes. Creative approaches have included the networking of providers to achieve economies of scale and improve quality of care, or high-volume low-cost models of care that utilize cross-subsidization of costs between high- and low-income populations.

He notes that:

All the improvements being made in the African health sector depend on health workers: from the low-skilled community workers to highly-trained specialized physicians. The health labour force and the development of sound healthcare practices are also showing some promising trends. There has been an increase in South–South health learning engagements, where governments, organizations, and individuals in developing countries exchange ideas and expertise to improve healthcare delivery. Formal and informal South–South collaboratives, such as the Joint Learning Network, provide opportunities where effective solutions to some of the most daunting health problems can be taken from one geography and appropriately adapted to another. The increase of international knowledge and learning exchange has also been precipitated by the number of returning African diaspora across all sectors. While, admittedly, the rate of returning health diaspora is currently a mere trickle, the returnees are creating opportunities to add technical know-how and expertise in their respective fields.'

What are the worrying signs and concerns about the future?

These younger and future leaders also see a wide range of worrying signs and concerns from immediate service issues to wider political and environmental matters. There is much agreement about the importance of leadership, the continuing and changing disease burden, and the lack of capacity and resources to address these issues.

Clarisse Bombi is concerned about ageing and family structures but also about the private sector and traditional healers:

As the healthcare is improving, the people are living longer so we are going to have an increasing population of older people coming to put more strain on the health system. Also the family sizes are becoming smaller and many families have one or all their children living and working abroad. The old people used to go and stay with their children, they may now have to open old people's homes and take them there as it happens in the West. The lack of interest by the private healthcare providers to provide preventive services, because most of these are free, is a major source for concern. The continuous threat posed by the increasing numbers of traditional healers who operate without strong collaborative measures is also a great cause for worry.

She is very concerned about the whole healthcare system:

The weak health systems, the near absence of a health systems' strengthening component in the plan of most vertical programmes suggests that the 'vertical' versus 'integration' debate will go on for a long time. The quality of training delivered by the approved training schools continues to be a major concern. Nothing is done to retain the home trained doctors and nurses to check the brain drain. The school curricular is not revised and updated to meet the needs of the changing epidemiological profile. Mental health nurses, public health nurses, and rehabilitation nurses are still in short supply. The urban/rural imbalance in the distribution of health personnel remains and will continue for a long time.

She adds:

New health facilities are being created without respecting the appropriate requirements and procedures. Many of those promised have not been constructed. Some constructed have not been equipped and not adequately staffed so they cannot function properly. Salaries remain low. Revenue set aside to be used for incentives is not paid. The actions of the anti-corruption committees are not assessed. The over-bearing attitude of the doctors and the hierarchical gradient that exists between the nurses and the doctors makes it difficult for the nurses to make pronouncements on the corrupt practices of the doctors.

John Paul Bagala writes that:

The uncontrolled population growth with its accompanying effects continues to be a big threat for the future. Breaking the cultural barriers, extensive community awareness, and sensitization on the values of having small manageable families and the methods that can be used to control population growth and unintended pregnancies are key breakthroughs that should be emphasized.

He is also concerned by the continued Brain Drain:

Africa has tried its very best to train its own sons and daughters to deliver healthcare to fellow African; however, it remains a worrying sign of unimproved healthcare delivery if the few who are being trained leave their respective communities and there is no account of the resources invested in them. The more the concerned individuals keep a deaf ear and pay no attention to this concern, it remains a big threat since the demand for the health workers is continually increasing with the increasing population in Africa and there is room for them to go in the developed nations and practice.

His final concern is about leadership:

Many African leaders are not portraying and representing the voices of the people they lead, instead they go after personal satisfaction and interests. This remains a big challenge in many African countries. This kind of leadership leads to unequal distribution of resources with some areas having adequate and others inadequate healthcare delivery. With this kind of leadership, many people are left not reached and this often represents the greater part of the population.

Politics, inequality, and accountability

Kelecho Ohiri writes:

The promising trends in sub-Saharan Africa health and healthcare are poised to take many countries' health systems to an improved future, but the existing problem areas must be addressed before substantial improvement can be seen. Agenda setting for healthcare in Africa still occurs largely in the 'global health space' in a top-down manner where governments and local agencies are only consulted after-the-fact. While governments are sometimes included in the agenda development process, it is still the global health community that drives the process in-country. Increased ownership and origination of health agendas by governments and competent in-country bodies would diminish many of the complications that arise when development partners and donor organizations attempt to implement policies on-the-ground.

He continues:

Another disturbing aspect of African healthcare is the political climate for healthcare planning and decision-making. Within countries, there are political and policy decisions that have significant impact on healthcare, e.g. decentralization, social safety nets, taxation, and external tariff policies. While developing national plans for areas such as these, the input of the health sector is typically not sought, creating a discrepancy between broad national plans and the role of the healthcare in economic and social development. Similarly, increased cohesion between development partners and governments is critical to successful execution of health improvement plans. The complex nature of most African health systems—with multiple levels of governance and opaque systems of reporting—makes attempts at navigating the system alone largely futile. National governments need to be aware of all health projects taking place under their jurisdiction. Just as different branches and ministries of government must better collaborate when determining cross-sectional national agendas, increased cohesion between development partners and government is critical to achieving improved program results.

He concludes:

Finally, among the numerous obstacles facing the African health sector, the capabilities within the sector are not prepared for the challenges of the future. There is a lack of investment into the health sector in terms of both financial and human capital. For lack of financial investment, part of the issue stems from the lack of, or unavailability of, data and information on health provider and facilities' services and operations. On the human capacity issue, few healthcare professionals are properly trained and equipped to deliver high-quality patient-centred care. Heightened investment into financial and knowledge/training resources are required to take African health systems from where they are now to the ideal state they aspire to reach in the coming years.

Susana Edjang is concerned by:

The pervasive inequity of access, quality, and results at all levels that threatens to undermine all the progress on health indicators achieved thus far. She also cites 'traditionalism' as a problem: the resistance of groups of African health professionals in powerful positions to be pragmatic by empowering lower cadre health professionals, or addressing issues concerning minority religious groups, women, or sexual minority groups. Prejudices impact on inter-country and regional collaboration. For example, in country X there were a lot of complaints about nursing tutors from Y country. When we went to investigate the reason for those complaints, we found the main issue to be that the tutors were Muslim and from a very unpopular country. Another example is the number of male nurses across African institutions versus the number of female nurses. Attitudes and action against gender-based violence are also a problem. The average age of an African is 19, and the average of a President is 61. If you extrapolate this to the health sector, you have an idea of the ideological disconnect that there might be between suppliers and seekers of healthcare.

She is also concerned by:

Keeping mental health marginalized from the wider health agenda, e.g. understanding of mental health issues and its implications, the number of psychiatrists or psychiatric nurses or clinical officers.

And finally by:

The impact that climate change might have in the spread of infectious diseases, urban health problems, poverty, and forced migration.

Ndwapi Ndwapi writes that:

We are still far from reaching the point of zero new HIV infections. This means that the prospect of a future HIV/AIDS epidemic that will devour resources at an even greater pace is real. The disease burden in general is also on the rise. We are also seeing an increasing gap between the rich and the poor, resulting in greater incidence of abject poverty and all the ills that come with it, such as malnutrition. This is happening at a time when the post-2008 world economy has caused shortages in donor funding after more than a decade at historic levels, leaving many developing countries, especially those deemed 'middle income', financially disorganized.

He notes that:

In many countries, there is unfortunately too much emphasis on 'bricks and mortar', at the expense of focusing on core, fundamental problems in the delivery of healthcare, e.g. making healthcare staff accountable for their performance, training healthcare staff, and establishing standards of quality care. A 'culture of responsibility' must be nurtured, and both government and the public should demand accountability, both from government and from providers of medical care. In middle- and low-income countries, a two-tier system of healthcare is becoming the norm, in which government employees and their families are provided a higher level of care than that available to the vast majority of poorer citizens. As a result of this stratification of care, healthcare workers (as government employees) do not have a stake in the quality of care that they provide poorer citizens.

He believes:

Accountability has been further eroded by the brain flight from African countries to the West and other rich nations, and from the public sector to the private sector. This has not been matched by greater innovation in training less traditional (and therefore less internationally appealing) cadres, as opposed to continuing to be a production ground for traditional cadres that are highly sought after in rich countries.

Finally, he writes:

Leaders must find new ways to develop more democratic representation of the youth. Low voter registration points to a lack of engagement and trust within the political process—especially among youth. There must be new avenues created for the young people to spark their active participation in civil concerns and democracy. Gender inequalities need to be openly addressed—particularly the growing trends of transactional sex.

Nan Twum–Danso adds to the list:

Fragmentation, especially in public health, is the order of the day. 'Vertical' programmes, especially infectious disease control programmes funded primarily by external donors, continue to dominate the public health landscape in sub-Saharan Africa. While attempts at 'diagonalization' or integration of vertical programmes into existing health systems have increased in the past decade, the reality at the implementation level (i.e. frontline health provider and district health administrator) is still a basket of distinct programmes, projects, funding, timetables, training workshops, guidelines, protocols, indicators, and reporting forms that compete for limited time and attention.

She adds that:

This problem appears to be getting more acute as 'global health' becomes increasingly attractive to more people in rich countries and they generate more funds to accelerate the achievement of the Millennium Development Goals and the post-2015 development goals, whatever they may be. Without local leaders playing a central role in defining their populations' needs and priorities, and coordinating/integrating all the 'global health' assistance (and in some cases even declining it), the risk of duplication of effort, waste of resources, and delivery of poor quality care is heightened.

What is your vision and your hope for the future?

Clarisse Bombi writes simply:

> I dream of a Cameroon where essential healthcare is available and accessible to everyone in every part of the country regardless of age, sex, financial status, religious orientation, or ethnicity.

John Paul Bagala writes:

> It is my vision for every man, woman, and child in Africa to access better improved healthcare and to live a healthy life with a fully developed potential, socially productive and potentially constructive.

Kelechi Ohiri describes his vision in more detail:

> The vision for future African healthcare is driven by innovation and productivity in the sector. In this future, health outcomes have improved across the continent in absolute terms and in an equitable manner. The discourse and agenda on health in Africa has moved away from the current development agency driven discourse to focusing on systems and conversations within and across countries. In this future, a strong emphasis is placed on data collection, analysis, and monitoring as evidence-based interventions become the foundation of project implementation. Health systems in the future are more responsive, with governments possessing the tools and will to build systems that cater to the needs of the population.

He continues:

> To consistently and successfully execute a patient stay such as childbirth or any more complex conditions, much work needs to be done. To ensure that adverse events such as maternal or infant deaths are reduced to a minimum, an aggressive change agenda needs to be devised and carried out. Collaborative planning and agenda-setting, transparency of data and information, and adequate resource investment into both public and private health sectors are pivotal parts toward achieving the future needs of the healthcare industry.

Ndwapi Ndwapi addresses specific goals in his vision for his country:

> Botswana currently has free medical care for all citizens, but also provides private health insurance for government employees, who constitute approximately half of the jobs in the country. The best way to encourage the best possible medical care for all citizens, regardless of insurance status or socio-economic status, is to mandate that all inpatient care shall be provided only at government facilities to all citizens. Consequently, everyone in government, from permanent secretaries down to the doctors and nurses, will become advocates of quality medical care at government hospitals, since they and their families may someday require care at such facilities.

He continues:

> In Botswana, where one-third of the population is HIV positive, requiring interaction with the health system indefinitely, technology must be innovatively engaged to improve efficiencies. With human resources and capacity at all levels unable to meet the

ever growing demand for services, improving technological systems and solutions must be at the forefront if we stand a chance to succeed.

Susana Edjang's vision is that:

Africa has the necessary critical mass of high quality African health institutions and critical mass of health professionals. There are improved opportunities for professional development within the profession such as the opportunity for clinical officers to become doctors if they wish. There is increased investment from African governments and regional institutions on African research, increased investment from African-based businesses and philanthropic groups on health commodities and medicines and where innovations and innovative approaches are scaled up.

She adds, very much in tune with one of the core messages of this book:

Greater visibility of African leaders and populations as transformative leaders.

Finally, Nan Twum-Danso writes:

My hope for the future is that African countries play a more central role in defining the 'global health' agenda and priority setting. With increasing national wealth, African countries need to contribute an increasing proportion of their funds to health so that they have more control over what is prioritised, funded and implemented.

She continues:

Countries must balance investments in health more equitably across acute and chronic diseases in response to the epidemiological transition. They need to invest more in human resources for health and the other building blocks of functioning health systems so that healthcare becomes an attractive profession for young, smart, hardworking people to join and health facilities become the first port of call for the population when sick. They must also strengthen the social sector beyond healthcare, specifically basic education, sanitation, safe water, safe housing, and safe energy.

Finally, she concludes:

Africa must develop more visionary leaders at all levels of the health system to steer us in the direction of health and wellbeing. We need to have a more vibrant civil society with informed and engaged patients/consumers who will demand more from their leaders, and by extension from their health systems, and hold them accountable.

Chapter 24

The future: vision and challenges

Francis Omaswa and Nigel Crisp

The final chapter draws together the major themes from throughout the book and identifies the lessons that can be learned for Africa and for the rest of the world. It concludes by offering a vision for the future, which can be achieved if Africans 'claim their own future', if there continues to be sufficient global solidarity to support health around the world, and if the countries of the continent develop a clear vision of 'health made at home'.

The major themes

The first section of the chapter explores some of the themes that have emerged strongly from leader after leader in earlier chapters. There are clear patterns that are distinctly African, such as the emphasis on community, the improvisation and innovation in service delivery and staffing, and the existence of a very wide mix of healthcare providers of all sorts. It is interesting to note that health leaders in Europe and America are just beginning to talk about the importance of using all the assets in the community as they face up to trying to control costs in their expensive systems. Africans have been doing this for years.

There is an enormous amount here to build on for the future. There are, however, also obvious problems that cannot be ignored, such as the status of women, inequalities more generally, male- and doctor-dominated hierarchies, and, all too often, corruption. There are other things that are both opportunities and threats: population growth is a major threat but the large numbers of young people could be an opportunity if handled appropriately; similarly, the lack of health infrastructure is devastating in the short term but also provides a clean sheet for development in the mid-term.

The second section of the chapter, written mainly by Francis Omaswa from an African perspective, addresses the future and concludes by addressing three big questions:

◆ What should Africans be doing for themselves to lead improvement in health in their own countries—and thereby creating change and claiming the future?

◆ What do they need from the rest of the world in the spirit of global solidarity?

◆ What is the vision for health and health services in Africa for the future and how will this contribute to improving health globally?

In answering these questions we recognize, as we did at the beginning of the book, that we are dealing mainly with sub-Saharan Africa and that this is made up of many different countries. We therefore attempt to be very careful in what we attribute to Africa and Africans as a whole and what is only relevant to certain societies and locations. We start the chapter with public health and, specifically, the promotion of health and prevention of disease and the role of the family and the community.

Health is made at home

> Health is made at home and only repaired in health facilities when it breaks down. Be clean, eat well, and do not share accommodation with animals. This is a message from the Director General of Health Services.

Francis Omaswa writes that in 2000, as Director General of Health Services in Uganda, he had this statement recorded and played several times a day on radio stations throughout the country until mid-2005. His starting point was that most human beings are born completely normal and healthy, devoid of birth defects, and can live in good health for long periods of time until old age without losing their health and without needing healthcare to restore it. Indeed, it is worth remembering what the human body is capable of doing to maintain its wellbeing and defend itself from health risks. Western medicine describes this as homeostasis; there are similar concepts in other medical and healing traditions.

The primary responsibility for maintaining uninterrupted health through the life course must rest on the shoulders of individuals, households, families, and communities. The mothers, fathers, clan, other cultural and religious leaders, and local administrators are the faces of the key actors.

Each individual, as Francis Omaswa argued as Ugandan Director General, should appreciate and celebrate the fact that they have health, not take it for granted, and should work hard to protect it. A key role of the health system should be to ensure that individuals continue to remain healthy and do not lose their health and will not need avoidable healthcare. This can be achieved by promoting and embedding awareness, also known as health literacy, and health-seeking behaviour into the routine life of the population, identifying and highlighting health risks and either removing them or facilitating behaviour that favours health. In the West, as we know, people are too often disempowered by the health system, having intentionally or otherwise 'outsourced' their health to the professionals and the institutions.[1]

The Participatory Poverty Assessment Studies carried out in Uganda showed that Africans don't need to be convinced about the importance of health. When poor people were asked what caused their poverty, 67% said poor health. When the question was reversed to 'what is the most likely effect of poverty to you?' the most frequently cited answers were 'poor health and death'.

However, effective and educated demand for better health services from African populations is generally weak. Families have to be encouraged to immunize children fully, attendance at ante natal clinics is poor, diseases are reported late, and, worse still, patients do not demand good quality healthcare. They will visit a clinic and on finding no health workers and no drugs just shrug their shoulders and go home and seek other remedies. They do not stand up to demand an explanation as to why the services are not provided.

Francis Omaswa's experience echoes Miriam Were's account in Chapter 8 of working with Kenyan villagers in the 1970s to eliminate the 'oral–faecal' link. Her dialogue with villagers, starting with 'Who is to solve these problems?' shows how villagers began to overcome their passivity and to recognize that they could take on health-promoting roles themselves. Her work shows that it is possible to change norms of behaviour by working with the community as a whole. She argues that in traditional settings, which have strong ties between families and community members, these norms are very much more robust than if an individual simply acquires a new behaviour pattern by his or her self.

Other writers such as Uche Amazigo in Chapter 9 and Hannah Faal in Chapter 13 describe how they used the strength of these communities to deliver services, whether through engaging older village women as health advocates and advisers or through accepting the community's choices over who should be the drug distributors as part of the community directed treatment programme. Chisale Mhango, too, describes in Chapter 5 how he enlisted the support of traditional leaders to change attitudes and behaviour about maternal health in Malawi. Agnes Binagwaho takes this further in Rwanda by ensuring that communities own their part of the *Mutuelle* health insurance system and determine many of the rules for its use.

Throughout Africa there are now increasing numbers of community health schemes in existence or being developed with, for example, a global campaign for a million community health workers for sub-Saharan Africa.[2] It is a campaign we support as part of a wider approach to creating a fully functioning health service that can support these workers to achieve their full potential.[3] Interestingly, there is a new scheme in New York whereby community health workers, modelled on the African experience, are being introduced to fill a gap. It is not just Africa that can learn from these pioneers.[4]

These accounts deal largely with traditional African communities, mainly in rural areas, and it may be asked what relevance these community based approaches have at a time when many such communities are breaking up under the twin pressures of urbanization and the development of Western-style economies, and when many people have been displaced due to social unrest or violence. People may be losing their traditional roots for these and other reasons: nevertheless, communities of different sorts are developing—whether as communities of Ugandans, let us say, in Johannesburg or as communities of interest linked together by email or Facebook. *Mothers to Mothers* or *M2M* is a wonderful example where mothers with HIV provide support and advice to pregnant women with HIV, helping them to avoid passing it on to their babies.[5]

Traditional ties persist, *Ubuntu* (I am who I am because of you) is deep in the psyche of many Africans; whilst at the same time, new and different sorts of communities develop. The lessons from these community approaches have continuing relevance in Africa and renewed relevance in other parts of the world, such as the UK, where traditional communities have largely disappeared but others, more diverse and less geographically restricted, are appearing.

These approaches are consistent with the principles of the Alma Ata Declaration of 1978, which was intended at the time to guide future developments in health but has largely been side-lined in favour of a more top-down professional-orientated and hospital-based approach.[6] The Declaration was re-affirmed by the WHO at the 30th anniversary in 2008 and the examples in this book show its continuing importance. These bottom-up community based approaches to population health create the bedrock on which more formal services can be established.

There are, of course, limits to a purely community based strategy, particularly in the growing urban populations where there is high mobility and, often, crime and violence. Different, more direct interventions are needed in these areas as governments and agencies try to deal with the multiplicity of inter-related problems. In making progress on tackling HIV/AIDS in South Africa, for example, the government has had to support interventions in urban slums as well as in more stable, if equally poor, rural areas.

It is also important to recognize that whilst these community bonds often provide the opportunity for improving health, they can also work against improvement. Lack of money and poor access to services mean that many people's first resort for help is to their family or to a traditional healer. This may also be culturally much easier. As Miriam Were says, traditional healers are perceived to care about people, unlike practitioners of Western medicine with its impersonal focus on body systems and diseases. People can easily walk away discouraged and empty handed from what can be perceived as an alien service. The right approach is surely to seek to integrate traditional healers into wider health systems, as has been attempted in many places. This will, as Catherine Odora-Hoppers implies in Chapter 15, allow for the sharing of insights and practices, and the development of services that are both culturally and scientifically appropriate.

Another principle of the Alma Ata Declaration that is well understood by the leaders writing in this book is that health is connected to everything else. The policy of most African Governments is to embed health in its wider development plans and to address health issues as being essentially cross-sectoral. Authors in this book frequently talk about the need to engage others from outside the health sector in order to improve health. They naturally adopt the 'health in all policies' approach advocated by the WHO and now being adopted in countries around the world.[7]

Governments also have a very important role in legislating to improve health. South Africa now has one of the most progressive policies on tobacco control globally. However, as Luis Sambo points out in Chapter 6, there is very much more to do to tackle the determinants of health and provide safe and healthy physical and social environments for African populations. Nutrition is a huge issue, as are health and safety at work and traffic accidents. Economic globalization may have much to offer Africa but the introduction of fast foods and a sedentary Western lifestyle are not amongst them.

Looking to the future in the last chapter, the younger and future leaders, as well as their elders, remind us that disease patterns are changing and that long-term conditions and chronic or non-communicable diseases will become a central focus of attention in the next few years, and that the neglected issues of disability and mental health need to be given priority. People with mental health problems are cared for well in some communities but the overriding picture is of neglect bordering on abuse, with too many instances of people chained up or caged as the only means of containing their illness. There is, as we write, a gathering momentum around the importance of tackling mental health globally and a growing body of literature about how to do so.[8]

Even as these other concerns come onto the agenda, HIV/AIDS will still be a dominant concern in some countries like Botswana, where Ndwapi Ndwapi writes of 'the resource burdens of HIV/AIDS having essentially mortgaged the future of health systems' development for generations to come'.

Perhaps the most significant issue that needs to be addressed is the position of women in many societies in Africa. Their lower status means that they are amongst the poorest and the most affected by ill health and disability, as well as domestic and war time violence.[9] They are also, however, the health promoters and protectors in the family and have the potential, when enabled to do so, to have enormous impact on the health status of their countries and continent. As Bience Gawanas argues in Chapter 10, following the work of the Commission on women's Health, 'women's health is the foundation for social and economic development in the African Region'.

Health systems

Health systems in most African countries are weak and, in some cases, almost non-existent. The examples of Rwanda, South Africa, and Ghana, described in earlier chapters, show how these countries are methodically working to strengthen all the components of their systems and provide universal health coverage for all their citizens. We will not repeat what has been said earlier but draw attention here only to three key areas: human resources; science and technology; and, underlying all the others, governance.

Human resources

Author after author has highlighted the importance of human resources and the critical shortages that impede improvement. Gottlieb Monekosso has described in Chapter 14 how education systems have developed over the last 50 years. Further strengthening is needed. Africa educates and trains too few health workers and loses many of the most highly educated to other countries and to NGOs. There are problems with the recruitment and retention of health professional, particularly in poor and rural locations where their services are most needed. There are also major issues with pay and conditions of service.

Nurses very often feel under stress and disempowered, as Clarisse Bombi argued in the last chapter. Nurses are the largest part of the workforce in sub-Saharan Africa and as Elisabeth Oywer says in Chapter 11 'Without nurses therefore, nobody can begin to talk about health systems in Africa'. We believe that nurses have been undervalued and under-developed in Africa and that in the future there needs to be much more emphasis on developing nurse leadership, as well as improving education and training.

Making the best use of the available health workers, however, is an area where in many ways sub-Saharan Africa leads the world. Skill mix change and team work need relatively little discussion as they have come up repeatedly throughout the book. As Chapter 11 shows there is now evidence about what needs to be done to achieve a successful skill mix change or task shifting—or, indeed, how to make it fail.[10] Skill mix changes or task shifting are very often seen as temporary measures put in place until, for example, more clinicians are available. It seems to us that this is undoubtedly the right approach in some cases but not in others. Why would one interfere with an arrangement that is working well simply because more highly trained health workers are available? Why would African countries automatically follow the path trodden by Western countries of ever-increasing specialization and costs? Decisions like this need to be based on evidence not on a priori assumptions about the roles of different professions.

By contrast, we believe that countries should be proud of things they are doing and in which they are leading the world. We believe that increasing demand for healthcare and escalating costs will mean that other countries will inevitably follow this African pathway—and, as we have noted, some are already doing so.

Science and technology

These approaches to health workers have already demonstrated real transformative power. Much less has been said in this book about the potential transformative power of technology. This is partly because most of the accounts in this book describe events at a time when technology had less of a role. However, it is also because the examples we have today are mostly still relatively isolated one-off applications. We can only begin to glimpse what integrated technology may enable us to do and the impact it might have. In even five years' time the position will look very different indeed. Human resources' innovations are, by contrast, much more integrated. We have a sense of the shape of the future workforce and of how truly integrated inter- and trans-professional education and training is shaping up by looking at countries like Ethiopia, described in Chapter 11, and others around the world.[11]

Today there are many individual examples where technology is making a difference. The African NGO AMREF, for example, has upgraded the training of thousands of nurses in Kenya through a distance-learning project. It is now using mobile phone technology to train the community health workers who are the successors to those trained by Miriam Were in the 1980s and 1990s. Phones throughout Africa are used for tasks such as making clinic appointments and follow-ups, transmitting test results, and checking for counterfeit drugs by reading barcodes. Email and videos support patient consultations and allow isolated clinicians to seek advice from colleagues in the great medical centres of the world.[12] Africa and other developing regions, without the legacy of earlier infrastructure, are adopting many applications earlier than more industrialized countries.

There are national eHealth associations developing in many countries to share learning and promote new practices. The eHealth Foundation, chaired by Archbishop Tutu, and other global organizations are promoting the use of eHealth and seeking to help develop standards for performance and inter-operability.*

Not all technology is related to eHealth and mHealth, and there is very important work underway in the development of low-tech equipment, processes, and devices produced by Africans and others working in Africa. These range from diagnostic tests to non-reusable needles and from refrigerator boxes for vaccines that can be used in remote sites to anti-microbial coated female condoms and insecticide-treated mosquito nets.

There are some surprising combinations of low and high tech. The community distributors of ivermectin, described by Uche Amazigo, each has a 7-foot stick, which has the bottom section painted one colour, the next section in another colour, the next section another colour, and the top section in a fourth colour. They stand it next to each villager in turn. Small children who are only as tall as the first colour are given one tablet; bigger children who reach the second colour get two and so on. It is a very simple and elegant method for determining dosage. By contrast, workers in a related Sightsavers' programme who are mapping the prevalence of trachoma in rural areas are given an android phone so that their results can be uploaded to the cloud every day. Both technologies are essential tools in eliminating these neglected tropical diseases.

The bio-sciences have played a vital part in many of the accounts in this book; most obviously in the development of ARVs, treatments for other diseases, and vaccines. They will undoubtedly have a very large role to play in the future with the development of further vaccines, as well as new treatments for the 'diseases of the poor' and tackling the growing threat from anti-microbial resistance worldwide. Most of these have been developed outside Africa or by Westerners leading research in Africa; with notable exceptions such as the work on Community Directed Treatments described in Chapter 9; but African-based science and research is beginning to be properly established.

Professor James Hakim, a distinguished researcher from Zimbabwe, told us that Africans were not involved in research as investigators during the colonial era, although they contributed as technicians. Some played significant roles,

---

* Strive Masiyiwa, President of Econet, and Nigel Crisp are both Ambassadors for the Foundation.

such as Dr Christian Barnard's assistant who, although not medically trained, was physically involved in carrying out heart transplants during the first experimental stage.

Africans began to be investigators in the 1960s and 1970s as they took up roles in medical schools and institutes. Initially most were co-investigators working alongside researchers from resource rich settings. Over time, however, some started to be principal investigators in their own right. They have been able to work in a number of important and well-established research centres: including CAPRISA in Durban, Africa Centre (north of Durban), MRC (Gambia), MRC (Entebbe), KEMRI (Kenya), Retro-C (Cote d'Ivoire), and NMRI (Tanzania).

James Hakim's hope for the future is that, as the pool of strong African mentors grows, it will be possible to see a more rapid increase in training researchers to be independent investigators. More African research institutions are now headed by Africans who have achieved their posts through competitive applications. African universities are pushing for candidates as lecturers to have PhDs. Strong transparent partnerships are developing with, for example, institutions in the US, Europe, and Australia, which will empower African researchers. His fears, however, are that international funding for research is stagnating and this is leading to a stop/start approach to development, which will damage the infrastructure needed for successful research.

Science and technology, changes in human resources policies, and the engagement of the community are all key elements in creating low-cost, high-value health systems in the future. Researchers and consultants are beginning to make these links as they search for solutions to meeting both the aspirations of growing populations in expanding economies around the world and the continuing demands of the ageing populations of the West.[13] Africa is well placed to put all the pieces together thanks to its history of innovation over many years.

Governance

Underlying everything else are the problems with governance alluded to by former Commissioner Bience Gawanas and other leaders. Improvements are needed in many countries both for *governance of* the health system itself but in *governance for health* amongst all the other organizations and institutions that affect health and its determinants. There is research evidence that shows that this is crucial to improving health and health systems.[14] It supports the large amount of anecdotal evidence of the way in which poor governance and corrupt practices and corrupted systems affect the care that people receive.

Most African countries recognize the rights of their citizens to health and to healthcare. Their constitutions commit their governments, as the stewards of the public interest, to make sure that arrangements are put in place for the provision of basic health services and for creating conditions that enable the population to be as healthy as is possible. Health leadership by African governments and ministers of health are critical to the ability of Africa to respond to population health expectations. The study on ministerial leadership pointed out the central role of governments and ministers of health. At the same time the study identified the potential of other health bodies and institutions, outside ministries of health, which have the potential to support governments to keep the national health agenda visible and could act as accountability agents.

There are very many non-government and not-for-profit organizations providing health services in Africa. Faith-based organizations, in particular, provide 40–50% of health services in many African countries. Their continuing role appears to be very important for the future in these countries. There are also many other non-state providers, such as traditional healers and pharmacies and other shops, mostly operating for profit at a small scale.

The for-profit private sector is expanding, with existing and new actors looking for the new and greater opportunities that economic growth is bringing. We have not dealt with this much in this book, which has been up to this point largely looking backwards. The main exceptions are, first, the Rwandan example in Chapter 17 where small private enterprises are being stimulated into existence by the government within the overall national framework. The other main exception is in South Africa, where there is a very large incumbent private sector that serves a small part of the population very expensively and sits firmly outside the national framework—and, for the most part, seems to be resisting engagement or incorporation into the framework.

These Rwandan and South African examples broadly mark out the extremes of the different policies that governments can adopt towards the growing for-profit sector. Does a government want to engage and embrace the for-profits within a national framework as in Rwandan (a more European model) or to allow them complete freedom of positioning as in the current South African (or United States) model? Whatever their policy towards engaging the for-profit sector in the formal health system, all countries will undoubtedly see a rapid growth driven by entrepreneurs in electronically enabled apps and services that offer greater choice and power to patients and citizens. At this stage of development there is little or no evaluation as to which of them will improve health and to what extent they will do so. These, of course, are questions that apply equally across the world and not just to sub-Saharan Africa.

As with technology, the various different manifestations of the private sector will undoubtedly play a much larger role in Africa and the position will look very different in the next few years. This is a feature that many of the younger and future leaders picked up on in the last chapter.

The future

We turn to the future in the remainder of this chapter and address the three big questions we raised at the beginning. In doing so we understand that there are enormous risks as well as opportunities facing Africa. As well as huge economic, demographic, and environmental challenges, there are traps to fall into in following the Western trajectory on health and health systems. There are also traps of Africa's own making.

Francis Omaswa writes:

> I listed five factors in Chapter 2 that could cripple African development: high levels of poverty, high population growth, a high level of dependency at community level, the loss of the 'can-do-attitude,' and the pervasive 'given up' attitude that tolerates the unacceptable. I also noted the current 'hopeful Africa' with high levels of economic growth, in a global setting where the push for equity and social justice is stronger than ever before and there is palpable global solidarity in addressing global and local challenges.

The MDGs and the current discussions on what will follow them post-2015 are testimonies to this hope. Global responses to pandemics such as SARS, swine and avian flu, and to natural disasters such as the typhoon that struck the Philippines islands are other illustrations of global solidarity in action. Africa is much better placed now to eradicate poverty, disease, and ignorance than when the new leaders made their *clarion call* for it at independence 50 years ago. There is evidence that the world is ready to help when we hear leaders of the World Bank, USA Global Health Initiative and USAID Forward, the Commission on Africa and others talk of promoting ownership and capacity building in Africa and raising the possibility of eradicating extreme poverty within a generation. There are now plans for what is called *convergence* with health outcomes and indices converging around the world over the next 35 years.[15] These are bold ambitions.

This second opportunity for Africa is here with us and is talked about widely among African leaders as the African Renaissance. The talk doing the rounds is that time came for the dragon (China), the elephant (India), and the tigers (South East Asia); now it is time for the lion (Africa). The changes are visible country by country.[16]

Yet the journey will not be smooth sailing. Africa is still gripped by poverty, the weak capacity of its institutions, governance shortcomings, corruption, inadequate energy and infrastructure, and low public demand for accountability from their leaders. It is pertinent at this point to recall the statement by President John Kufour of Ghana:

> We should bear in mind however that the renaissance is not an event or project whose success must be measured at a predetermined time. It must be seen as a whole movement, a whole crusade that will result in unearthing all that is beautiful, adorable and unique of Africa.[17]

'This is Africa, what do you expect?' Thirty years ago, Francis Omaswa writes, my wife and I made an adventurous decision to go to work in a remote mission hospital in the Ngora district of Uganda, moving from the University Teaching hospital in Nairobi where we had spent three years as high-flying specialists in anaesthesiology and cardiothoracic surgery. Uganda had gone through the worst of times. Frequently things did not work and the local people laughed it all off saying, 'This is Uganda, what do you expect?'.

After the initial shock, we persuaded the same people that together, we would convert that hospital into a place where things work so well that the same statement will be used to denote the consistency of the excellence of our performance. 'This is Uganda, what do you expect? Only the best.' Two years later, with the support of the local people and the Association of Surgeons of East Africa, that hospital became a highly performing institution.

In 2003, I was invited by the newly elected President of the African Union Commission Alpha Konare as a keynote speaker on health at a meeting to help him to set his priorities upon taking the leadership of the AUC. I spoke on the theme 'This is Africa, what do you expect? Only the best'. My statement was well received with an ovation signifying the conviction that Africa is willing and capable of pursuing and achieving excellence with consistency. I may be a few years early in saying this, but this should be the level of our ambition.

Creating change and claiming the future—what Africans should be doing for ourselves

Today, Africa is hopeful again and its countries are moving steadily and irreversibly towards transformation from Highly Impoverished Country status to becoming middle and upper middle income countries. In order for this to happen, Africans need to take charge of their destiny and reclaim their role as agents of change. The new *clarion call* has to become 'If not by us, by whom? If not now, when? If not here, where?'. African home-grown food, culture, and solutions are good. We do not always have to copy and, where we do copy, the importance of contextualization and adaptation should be born in mind.

First of all, Africans must acknowledge that both the problems and solutions are primarily our responsibility. We must own our destiny. 'Until and unless we Africans, individually and collectively, feel the pain and the shame of our condition, we will not have the commitment to take the actions needed to right the situation'. Armed with this spirit of ownership and a sense of duty, accompanied sometimes by shame or anger, Africans should identify and set standards and boundaries for what is acceptable and unacceptable, and conduct their affairs strictly and with zeal within these boundaries.

This is ultimately all about creating better functioning democratic societies and improved governance. It will require the development of tripartite partnerships between:

1 African populations represented by households, organized communities, and civil society groups, who should articulate their needs and be assertive in demanding solutions and services. The legitimacy of those who govern should be predicated on how they respond to population needs. Elections should be won and lost on these issues.

2 Knowledge generation, translation, dissemination, and public use will be critical. Therefore, entities such as universities, science academies, research centres, and think tanks, whose role is to study and identify appropriate and responsive solutions in close collaboration with communities, should play more proactive and aggressive roles than they do at present. There has been relative and unacceptable complacency amongst the 'techno-professionals', as I discussed in Chapter 2. Africa will not transform without the active participation of these people and their institutions. Their ability to team up with both communities and politicians will be critical to Africa's future.

3 The political class and governments who are responsible for creating the enabling environment of law and order, freedom of speech and association, resource allocation and oversight of timely implementation, as well as official engagement with the international community in representing Africa in multilateral and bilateral forums.

Many of the younger and future leaders made similarly powerful points about the way society has to change. Clarisse Bombi discussed the hierarchical attitudes that held back nurses from fulfilling their potential, whilst Susana Edjang cited 'traditionalism' as a problem: 'the resistance of groups of African health professionals in powerful positions to be pragmatic by empowering lower cadre health professionals, or addressing issues concerning minority religious groups, women, or sexual minority groups. Prejudices impact on inter-country and regional collaborations'. As Nana Twum Danso concludes: 'We need to have a more vibrant civil society with informed and engaged patients/consumers who will demand more from their leaders, and by extension from their health systems, and hold them accountable.'

Second, Africa needs to sustain the high levels of economic growth, which is critical to the future development of Africa. According to *The Africa Competitiveness Report 2013* 'the continent is seen both as an investment destination of choice and as a region marked by greater prosperity and development. Talk of an "African economic renaissance" continues to grow: the continent has experienced an average growth rate of more than 5 percent over the past decade, when much of the developed world still struggles to recover from crisis.' The Region has grown at an average 5% over the last decade.[18] The African Development Bank has stated that 34 sub-Saharan African countries have discovered viable deposits of oil, other minerals, and natural resources in the recent past.[19]

Evidence of this economic growth can be seen in the streets of almost all African capitals. I travelled to many cities in the past where there was visible apathy, dirty buildings—some unoccupied, empty streets and self-imposed curfews. Today in the same cities the streets are bustling, there are traffic jams, and people are moving with a purpose in their lives.

Whilst Africa is rising, this economic growth is still insufficient to bring about the changes that we want. The tax base in most sub-Saharan African countries cannot sustain the provision of basic essential social services, such as health and quality education. Africa in the medium term will continue to need external support as African economies grow and the tax base expands to levels that can sustain the provision of basic social services from internally generated resources. Whilst this is happening, African countries need to lay foundations that will encourage rapid and balanced economic growth. These include good governance, accountability, law and order, freedom of expression and association, human and institutional capacity, energy, roads, inclusive social policies, and fair tax laws.

Third, Africa must harvest the demographic dividend by investing in its youth. Most African countries have a huge youth bulge with 50% of populations below 15 years of age, and 60% below 20 years of age. It is, therefore, critically important and urgent for Africa to design and implement policies that can transform this large young population into a demographic dividend and avert a possible demographic disaster in the event that the positive potential of our youth is not realized. High-quality education is the answer and also the entry point; alongside measures to stem the rapid population growth. This means inclusive life-long education starting with early childhood development and nutrition that sets the foundation for the child's brain to develop cognitive skills; universal primary education that provides competence in the three 'Rs' namely reading, writing, and arithmetic, thus enabling all citizens to navigate their way round the community and surrounding world; universal secondary and vocational education for life skills and increased productivity; and transformative tertiary education to produce sufficient numbers of highly skilled technicians, professional leaders who are change agents and can represent Africa effectively at the international level.

Finally, Africa must grasp the opportunity presented by the new information and communication technologies to rapidly expand the reach of services and access to individuals, households, and communities. Healthcare professionals now have tools for their own development and for supporting each other in their quest to reach every person in every village in Africa with skilled care.

On a personal note, I launched The African Centre for Global Health, and Social Transformation (ACHEST) with colleagues in 2008 to respond to the need for Africans to take full advantage of the 'hopeful Africa' by inspiring African leaders and populations to take ownership and to be accountable, and to advocate for our international friends to provide the support that Africa needs to transform through enhanced ownership and accountability. ACHEST's vision is one of 'Africa as a people-driven continent enjoying the highest attainable standard of health and quality of life.' And the mission is 'To develop, test, and promote evidence-based and technically sound policies and strategies and to apply these to build professional and institutional capacity for programme implementation that are owned and driven by African populations themselves.'[20]

The message is simple: sustainable change is endogenous, for any change to take root, it is necessary for it to be owned and driven by motivated beneficiaries. As Miriam Were says in Chapter 8, 'if it does not happen in the community, it does not happen in the country and if it happens in the community, it happens in the nation'. Or as Thoraya Obeid has said, 'Only that change that comes from the communities themselves is sustainable'.

ACHEST is only one organization. We need more such institutions in Africa to work together to support the changes we need to see happen and grasp the opportunity to *claim the future*. The Strong Ministries for Strong Heath Systems study report concluded that 'Every country needs to cultivate and grow a critical mass of individuals, groups, and institutions that interact regularly among themselves and with their governments, parliaments, and civil society as agents of change, holding each other and their governments to account, as well as providing support. Networking among in-country players will be essential to promote cross learning and support.'[21] At the African regional level and at international level, there should be active networking between these national and transnational institutions.

Global solidarity—what Africa needs from the rest of the world

The ideal globalized world of the future will be one where there is interdependence, joint learning, and co-development between nations, institutions, and communities beyond nations. Partnerships, collaboration, and solidarity will be the name of the game. Nigel Crisp has written a book on '*Turning the World Upside Down*' that describes some of the things that richer countries can learn from low- and middle-income ones and advocates for joint learning and *co-development*. This will be resisted by some individualist and nationalistic tendencies and profiteers. However, I believe that they will be outnumbered by proponents of the common good.

What Africa needs from the rest of the world at this time corresponds with, and is a mirror image of, what Africans should do for themselves. The world needs to perceive Africa and Africans is a different way. First, the world needs to trust Africans and give them space. President Barack Obama on his first visit to Africa in Accra stated 'Africa's future is up to Africans'. Two of the five Objectives of the Africa Commission are: 'To offer a fresh and positive perspective for Africa and its diverse culture in the 21st century, which challenges unfair perceptions and helps deliver changes'; and 'To understand and help fulfil African aspirations for the future by listening to Africans'.[22]

A paradigm shift needs to take place where the rest of the world stops perceiving Africa as a continent for pity, unable to take care of its people and in need of external resources and ideas. I have personally experienced situations where I have been treated as a person in need of help simply because I am African. In other cases surprise has been expressed if I have done well '*beyond expectation*' because I am African. To illustrate, at one time, after I gave a talk at the Royal College of Physicians in London, one of the participants approached me and complemented me by saying 'that was very good; you are confident and seem to know what you are talking about. It is not common to see people like you from your continent'.

There are many Africans like me all over the African continent if you care to look for them. What is needed is to support these individuals and their institutions to build the capacity to play the role of change agents in their respective countries and communities. This is now beginning to happen. For example, the government of the USA through the Global Health Initiative (GHI) states, 'GHI strengthens U.S. government engagement with partner countries to support national ownership and priorities that are aligned with GHI objectives'[23] and the USAID Forward strategy among others is to undertake a 'critical shift in the way of administering assistance, placing emphasis on public–private partnerships and working with local government and CSO's to ensure sustained results.[24]

There are also developments in relationships with other countries. Brazil for example, which has itself been the recipient of aid in the past, has developed a new approach based on mutuality and partnership. It is also able to offer technical assistance based on its own experience of development and of dealing with similar problems. This sort of South to South partnership is likely to grow further in years to come. We have yet to see, however, the sort of *co-development* Nigel Crisp advocates—and based on mutual respect and mutual learning—shaping the partnerships with the more traditional donors of the West.

International partners need to see the new Africa as a people-driven continent where people know what they want and demand it. They need to learn how to work with African leaders who are confident and not see them simply as people to teach and patronize, as has frequently been the case in the past. The good news is that I have been privileged to work with lots of colleagues from all over the world who have treated me as an equal and valued partner. Those who patronize exist but are few and will get fewer. My own professional upbringing from the very beginning has been a story of faith, trust, and mutual respect from mentors and colleagues from inside and outside Africa, and many of these professional relationships have resulted in strong personal and long family bonds crossing generations.

I have noted with appreciation the fact that the appetite for institutional collaboration with African institutions by developed country partners is insatiable. This is good news for Africa; but Africans need to be well prepared for these partnerships and collaborations, enabling African institutions to build their own capacity. Support to Africa should have a focus on training individuals and teams, and developing African institutions and experts who are not half-baked but are equal in to their counterparts in the rest of the world. This was the approach taken by the UK in, for example, helping Makerere University achieve world class status in the 1960s.

This is what is needed for facilitating joint global learning co-development and improving understanding between the people of the world. It doesn't always work like this. I have seen developed countries provide grants to Northern institutions and individuals to carry out studies in Africa. I have described some of the challenges with these studies; namely, inappropriate design, analysis, conclusions, and recommendations. We need to get away from this and to use more and more local institutions and consultants with the ability to contextualize these studies. Studies on African issues should be led by those who understand Africa best. These should ideally be African-based individuals and institutions although, of course, partnerships with Northern-based institutions and individuals should not be excluded. Whilst developed country governments and institutions are increasingly supporting the capacity building of African institutions through grants and partnerships, there are northern institutions that see strong African institutions as a threat to their own survival.

Africa urgently needs good quality foreign direct investment in order to accelerate economic growth, enlarge the tax base, and raise the local resources needed to free Africa once and for all from dependence on charity from other countries. The return on investment in Africa is high, if sometimes risky, and many entrepreneurs and foreign-based multinationals are seeking to take advantage of this. Africans themselves need to invest in their own countries as there are risks inherent in a foreign-dominated economy. Partnerships, once again, are important in promoting the growth of business and industry.

At a number of G8 meetings such as at Gleneagles UK, pledges have been made by developed countries to increase Official Development Assistance (ODA) to Africa. However, many of these pledges remain unfulfilled. Only a handful of countries in the Nordic region, Ireland—and in the near future the UK—have fulfilled the commitment to providing 0.7% of their GDP to ODA. On top of this, there are issues with compliance with the Paris Declaration on Aid Effectiveness. Why, I wonder, is there not a *Marshall Plan* for Africa, as advocated by Minister Binagwaho in Chapter 18? This would be a plan for investment and growth not, as now, a handing out of charity with strings attached.

Some donor countries concerned by corruption and weak governance in African countries are backtracking on commitments to budget support to governments. In the process, implementation is slowed down and the country's implementation capacity is weakened as donors set up implementation units manned by their own staff or led by agencies from their own countries. It is far better to face up to country governments and address weakness to budget support in the short run, rather than bypassing the use of existing systems and institutions. As well as supporting governments to be more accountable and efficient, development partners need to help develop the capacity of non-government actors, which can work constructively with governments both as supporters and as accountability monitors along the lines described above in the Strong Ministries for Strong Health systems study report.

The vision for health and health services in Africa—and its contribution to improving health globally

We believe that the vision for health and health services in Africa needs to contain three elements:

- Social, economic, and health policies that support health improvement and promotion at all stages of life—resting on the foundation that *health is made at home.*

- Health services available to every member of the population, *leaving no one behind*—now generally promoted under the heading of *Universal Health Coverage.*

- A systematic and practical commitment to quality—in the spirit of: *This is Africa, What do you expect? Only the best.*

Taking these in turn, little more needs to be said about the first point. There are good foundations in much of Africa to establish and develop further appropriate public policies across government and society. This places a great responsibility on governments because even when individuals know what to do or what to eat, and which byelaws to follow, they still need access to the healthy food, clean water, adequate housing, education, and the other key determinants of health.

The current shortages of health service infrastructure mean that most countries do not have to dismantle an out of date legacy of hospital and professional dominance, and can start from a clean slate. It is critical and essential, that African countries do not seek to copy the policies and systems of high-income countries but plan to develop their own based largely on their own internal needs and strengths.

Turning to the second point, Universal Health Coverage, sub-Saharan Africa should take encouragement from the resolution of the UN General Assembly in December 2012 that: 'Urges Governments, civil society organizations and international organizations to promote the inclusion of universal health coverage as an important element in the international development agenda and in the implementation of the internationally agreed development goals, including the Millennium Development Goals, as a means of promoting sustained, inclusive and equitable growth, social cohesion and well-being of the population and achieving other milestones for social development, such as education, work income and household financial security.'[25]

There are now existing models of what can be achieved in Rwanda, Ghana, South Africa, and elsewhere. Many African countries have defined a minimum, basic, or essential package of services that are prioritized from the national burden of disease surveys and are expected to be available at designated levels of the healthcare system, as near to the households as possible and with a referral system to higher levels of care. Africa stands the best chance of improving health indices with available country and donor resources if priority is placed at the household and community level. Primary and community services, delivered by a wide range of actors, should be emphasized, rather than hospitals—although they too will be needed. The governance of communities should be the entry point for enforcing compliance with health bye laws that address priority elements of the defined health package. Examples include attendance at antenatal clinics, immunization of children and pregnant women, household hygiene including latrine coverage and use, access to safe water, food security, all children attending school, marriage laws including avoiding early marriages, registration of births and deaths, and others as locally determined. When Francis Omaswa grew up in colonial Uganda, the local chief took care of all this and was supported by clan heads. Today the same could be achieved by strengthened local government arrangements that have basic health as a key component of the roles of the administrators at all levels.

Funding, of course, is crucial to establishing universal health coverage. Not surprisingly, many people have been sceptical about whether most African countries can afford it. We understand these arguments very well but would counter them with three main points. First, universal health coverage is not an all or nothing concept. It can be built towards by setting out a basic package of services available to particular segments of the population in the first instance. Over time, this starting package can be extended, both in scope and to other parts of the population. The Commission on the Macro-economics of Health set out just such a basic package for the cost of $35 per person in 2001.[26] Countries may not be able to afford $35 per person but they can make a start and with the support both of donors and expanding economies can grow the package over time.

The second point is that Rwanda, Ghana, and South Africa, as described in this book, are well down this route, as are others countries. They recognize that this takes time, but they have demonstrated the progress that can be made. They have also all understood our third point—there are costs in not doing this. Investing in the health of the population is a sensible economic decision. The Commission on the Macro-economics of health made the argument that investment in health, handled in the right way, is an investment in future wealth and prosperity. More recently, the Commission on Investing in Health has updated the economic case for investment in health.[27] It needs to be taken seriously.

The continued early mortality and disease in the poorest countries of the world is a human tragedy but it is also an economic disaster. We have in our generation the opportunity to do something lasting about this.

Francis Omaswa writes:

> Advocacy for UHC is urgently needed. If health is accepted as a human right and backed by all the declarations at the UN and included in the constitutions of most countries, why is there not outrage at the many Africans and other people who go without basic healthcare all over the world? The successful advocacy to get increased access to treatment for HIV and AIDS remains a lesson for us: where there is sufficient demand it is possible to get governments and the international community to respond positively. I would like to see Africans and partners in the international community mobilize and demand for UHC. This is urgently needed, it is practical and it is affordable. We only lack the will. It is not just political will that is lacking; we all need to move away from tolerating the unacceptable.

Finally, we turn to quality. Access to health services—quantity without quality—is unacceptable and does not work. There is a danger as we write these words in early 2014 that global policies to promote universal health coverage may ignore this vital point. Advocacy for universal health coverage has to include embedded quality. The danger, as was described in South Africa in Chapter 18 and seen in other countries, is that there will be a commitment to universal access but that the services are so poor that all but the most desperate avoid them. This is a mistake, which Minister Motsoaledi is determined to ensure is not repeated under his plans for National Health Insurance in South Africa.

Francis Omaswa has talked about wanting 'only the best' in Africa. It is important to remember and emphasize that good quality is not always more expensive than poor quality. Agnes Binagwaho of Rwanda understands this well in arguing that beautiful things don't necessarily cost more than poorer looking things. The Japanese thinker Kano distinguishes between three levels of quality. One is about eliminating defects: getting rid of all the errors, the duplication, and the waste of equipment and of peoples' time that is all too evident in many African (and other) health systems. The second level is about achieving the same goals but with fewer or cheaper inputs. Many African health systems are adept at doing this, in particular through flexible skill mix approaches or task shifting and stronger reliance on clinical judgment. The third level of quality is adding a new feature or service to the existing package. The first two levels save money, whilst the third may add cost.

Africa undoubtedly needs investment to pay for the third level of quality but it, equally undoubtedly, needs to pay attention to the first two levels. Waste and inefficiency have devastating effects in poorer countries, whilst they can more easily be tolerated in richer ones (although they should not be).

Quality and processes of quality improvement need to underpin action on health and health services in Africa as elsewhere. Quality is not only a desirable end in itself but the pursuit of it through quality improvement process is a means of implementing policies and closing the gap between the actual level of achievement and the desired goals. There are already impressive examples of using well-tested quality improvements in this way.[28] In Ghana the Catholic Health Service and the Ministry of Health, with technical support from the Institute of Health Improvement, have delivered very impressive reductions in child mortality through their *5s alive!* Programme, which is now being rolled out nationwide.[29] Similar approaches in other countries have led to impressive improvements.[30]

The importance of quality cannot be over-emphasized in the African context. It is about being able to achieve the most with currently available and often limited resources. It is about empowering staff to eliminate waste, in a way that enables them to do everything the right way at all times. The poorer the country, the more quality is needed as waste is less affordable. There are many other African countries that are currently implementing quality improvement approaches with the support of the government of Japan and the USAID. In East Africa there is a Regional Centre for Quality of Healthcare based at Makerere University. Cultivating and institutionalizing the culture of quality in the health system is the bedrock of an efficient and responsive health system as it provides flexible and versatile problem-solving approaches that are scalable and with capacity to build the 'can-do' attitude among the health workforce.

Final words from the editors

As editors it has been a privilege to work on this book with so many outstanding fellow authors. This is, as we said at the beginning, a celebration of people who have achieved so much in such difficult circumstances. They all acknowledge the solidarity and help they have received from outside Africa, but ultimately it is these leaders who have taken personal responsibility to make change happen. They have been there every day in their own countries, putting together all the pieces of external help and making use of the assets they have to hand to make change and inspire hope for the future.

As well as joining in this celebration, we hope that readers will take away three clear messages:

- African health leaders are claiming the future—in Africa, but also by sharing their insights and knowledge globally and contributing fully to improving health throughout the world.

- Africa is a continent rich in people and resources that still requires global support and solidarity to develop—not primarily in aid, but through investment, collaboration, partnerships, and co-development. Why is there not a modern *Marshall Plan* for Africa as Agnes Binagwaho has proposed?
- The future improvement of health and healthcare in Africa needs to rest on three foundations—an understanding that 'health is made at home'; the determination to offer access to health services for everyone; and an insistence on the pursuit of quality; a framework that applies equally to other continents.

References

1 **Crisp N.** Patient power needs to be built on strong intellectual foundations. *BMJ* Sept 2012; **34j5**:e6177.

2 One Million Community Health Workers. The Earth Institute, Columbia University, 2013. <http://1millionhealthworkers.org/>.

3 WHO and Global Health Workforce Alliance. *Scaling Up, Saving Lives.* 2008.

4 **Crisp N.** Turning the World Upside Down. <http://www.ttwud.org/>.

5 Mothers 2Mothers. Empowered Mothers Nurture Healthy Families. <www.m2m.org>.

6 Report of the International Conference on Primary Health Care—Alma Ata, USSR, 6–12 September 1978. World Health Organization, Geneva.

7 **Cook S, et al.** *Health in all policies: securing quality, implementing policies.* Ministry of Social Affairs and Health, Finland, May 2013.

8 **Patel V, Saxena S, De Silva M, Samele C.** *Transforming Lives, Enhancing Communities, Innovations in Mental Health.* World Innovation Summit for Health, Dec 2013. <http://www.wish-qatar.org/home.

9 WHO/AFRO. *Addressing the Challenge of Women's Health in Africa: Report of the Commission on Women's Health in the African Region.* 2012.

10 All Party Parliamentary Group on Global Health. *All the Talents—how new roles and better teamwork can release potential and improve health services.* London, 2012.

11 **Frenk J, et al.** Education of Health Professionals for a new century: transforming education to strengthen health systems in an interdependent world. *The Lancet* Dec **4**, 2010; **376**: 1923–58.

12 **Wooton R, et al.** (eds). *Telehealth in the Developing World.* RSM, 2009.

13 KPMG. *Necessity is the mother of innovation.* January 2014.

14 **Balabronova D, McKee M, Mills A.** *'Good Health at Low Cost' 25 Years On.* London School of Hygiene and Tropical Medicine, 2011.

15 **Jamison DT, et al.** Global Health 2035: a world converging within a generation. *The Lancet,* Dec **3**, 2013, 10.106/SO140–6736(13)62105–4.

16 **Dowden R.** *Africa: Altered States, Ordinary Miracles.* Portobello Books, 2008.

17 New Partnership for Africa's Development. Speech to New Economic Platform for African Development meeting. 14 Oct 2010. <www.nepad.org>.

18 World Bank and World Economic Forum. *The Africa Competitiveness Report, 2013.* <http://www3.weforum.org/docs/WEF_Africa_Competitiveness_Report_2013.pdf>.

19 World Economic Forum. *The Africa Competitiveness Report*, 2013. <http://www.weforum.org/reports/africa-competitiveness-report-2013>.

20 The African Centre for Global Health and Social Transformation (ACHEST). <www.ACHEST.org>.

21 **Omaswa F and Bouford J.** *Strong Ministries for Strong Health Systems*. ACHEST, Jan 2010.

22 Report of the Commission for Africa. *Our Common Interest*. March 2005.

23 US Global Health Initiative, 2013. <www.ghi.gov>.

24 United States Agency for International Development. USAID Forward Progress Report 2013, Washington, DC, USA. <http://www.usaid.gov/sites/default/files/documents/1868/2013-usaid-forward-report.pdf>.

25 UN Documentation: General Assembly. Resolutions. 67th UN General Assembly, 12 Dec 2012.

26 WHO. Report of the Commission on Macroeconomics and Health, 2001.

27 **Jamison DT, et al.** Global Health 2035: a world converging within a generation. *The Lancet*, Dec 3, 2013, 10.106/SO140–6736(13)62105–4.

28 **Ciampa PJ, et al.** Addressing poor retention of infants exposed to HIV: a quality improvement study in rural Mozambique. *J Acquir Immune Defic Syndr* 2012; **60**(2):e46–52.

29 The Institute for Healthcare Improvement (IHI). <http://www.ihi.org/offerings/initiatives/ghana/Pages/default.aspx>.

30 **Franco LM, et al.** *Results of Collaborative Improvement: Effects on Health Outcomes and Compliance with Evidence-based Standards in 27 Applications in 12 Countries*. USAID, Dec 2009.

Appendix 1

Africans on the world stage

Other great African health leaders

We chose the African health leaders in this book to be broadly representative of countries and activities, avoiding over-concentration on particular countries or areas of expertise wherever we could. There are many others who would have merited inclusion and we can't name all the many national and local leaders who have played significant roles in their own countries; some, of course, who have played leading roles are relatively unknown outside their sphere of influence and unknown to us.

We also can't identify all those people from outside health who have had a major impact on health across their own countries or globally. One obvious example is Kofi Annan of Ghana who as Secretary General of the United Nations played a leading role in mobilizing the international community in the battle against HIV/AIDS: calling it his personal priority and issuing a *Call to Action* in April 2001. Another is President Olusegan Obasanjo of Nigeria who convened African Heads of State and Governments to a series of summits in Abuja on Malaria, HIV, TB, and other infectious diseases and was the UN Special Envoy for Africa in 2008 and has been a catalyst in driving Africa's economic transition. Others who might well be included in the future are the new group of African philanthropists who are beginning to turn their attention to health.

We list in this Appendix those Africans who have held major global or regional responsibilities for health as regional directors of the WHO or in leading major global programmes. We have omitted the contributors to this book who have held these global or regional posts—Advocate Bience Gawanas, Honourable Professor Gottlieb Monekosso, Dr Luis Sambo, and Dr Francis Omaswa—because their biographies appear in the list of contributors.

Dr Anarfi Asamoa-Baah—Deputy Director-General, WHO (2007 to date)

Dr Anarfi Asamoa-Baah, from Ghana, was appointed as WHO Deputy Director-General in January 2007. He is a medical doctor who specializes in public health, with post-graduate degrees in health economics, and in health policy and planning, from the UK and USA, respectively.

Dr Asamoa-Baah was instrumental in developing health sector reforms in Ghana and in establishing the Ghana Health Service. He was also a pioneer of the sector-wide approach process to health development. Between 1988 and 1998, Dr Asamoa-Baah served as a WHO Consultant on Primary Health Care and health systems' strengthening. He also served as a member of the Scientific and Technical Advisory Committee (STAC) of the WHO Special Programme for Research and Training in Tropical Diseases (TDR), and on the Expert Committee of the Expanded Programme on Immunization.

Dr Asamoa-Baah's career within WHO began in 2000 when he was appointed as Executive Director for External Relations and Governing Bodies; he subsequently served as Executive Director for Health Technology and Pharmaceuticals; Assistant Director General of Communicable Diseases; and as Assistant Director-General, for the HIV/AIDS, Tuberculosis, and Malaria programme; before becoming Deputy Director General in 2007. As Deputy Director-General, Dr Asamoa-Baah leads the formulation of specific strategies and advises programmes on WHO policies and operations. He is also Co-Chair of the WHO Global Task Force on Primary Health Care.

Professor Adetokunbo Lucas, Founding Director of the Division for Tropical Disease Research Programme (TDR), WHO

Professor Lucas did his medical training in Nigeria and the UK, and is an international leader in the field of tropical parasitic and infectious diseases. He founded and directed the WHO Tropical Disease Research Programme and later became involved in programmes for the prevention of maternal morbidity and mortality.

In his 10 pioneering years at TDR from 1976 to 1986, Professor Lucas developed a model approach for global networking amongst scientists, research laboratories, and pharmaceutical firms. This network was very successful in developing new drugs for malaria, leprosy, African sleeping sickness, onchocerciasis, and lymphatic filariasis.

Professor Lucas subsequently served as chair of Carnegie Corporation's grant programme concerned with strengthening human resources in developing countries for four years and also chaired the Global Forum for Health Research. He became a professor at the Harvard School of Public Health and served as Coordinator of the Harvard Executive Leadership programme for Ministers of Health. He has remained very active into his 80s and his many subsequent roles and activities include representing West and Central Africa on the Governing Board of the Global Fund for Fighting AIDS, Tuberculosis, and Malaria during its startup phase.

Mrs Daisy Mafubelu, Former Assistant Director-General WHO (2007–10)

Mrs Mafubelu was the coordinator of the African group on health matters based at the Geneva mission of the Republic of South Africa. In this capacity she represented and negotiated on behalf of the African Region, which enabled the African region to articulate common positions on matters of regional interest. During her period in office she managed to increase the cohesion of the African region and represented Africa on the bureau of the conference of the parties of the framework convention on tobacco control.

Her background is in management within the South African Health Service, where she played a significant role in the transformation of the public health services. She was Director of Human Resources and later a Deputy Director-General of Health. She was involved in the reform of nursing in South Africa and had a particular interest in reproductive health, research, child health, immunization, gender, and in women and health.

Dr Margaret Mungerera, President World Medical Association (2013–14)

Dr Margaret Mungerera is a Ugandan Senior Consultant Psychiatrist who assumed leadership of the World Medical Association for the year 2013/14. She is the first African and also the first woman to occupy this office. She has served several terms as President of the Uganda Medical Association and is a strong advocate for improving conditions of service for all health professionals.

Dr Faoumata Nafo-Traoré, Executive Director of Roll Back Malaria (RBM) (2010 to date)

Dr Nafo-Traoré, a former Mali Minister of Health and Minister Social Affairs, Solidarity and the Elderly, brings to the RBM Partnership a wealth of expertise in maternal and child health, malaria control and health systems strengthening, as well as significant leadership experience in facilitating global, regional, and country-level partnerships.

Dr Nafo-Traoré has helped strengthen the health sector across Africa in serving the health community in different capacities: as President of the Assembly of ECOWAS Ministers of Health, as a member of the Board of GAVI (Global

Alliance for Vaccines and Immunization) and as a member of the UNAIDS/ WHO technical working group.

In her recent positions, she facilitated efforts to implement the Paris Declaration on AID effectiveness and the UN reform Delivery as One initiative (2006–12). She also nurtured a policy dialogue among ministries and diverse sectors of the society to anchor health in key national agendas and increase domestic funding for health. She worked with bilateral, multilateral, and national actors to develop a health sector plan, which proposed, inter alia, strategies to manage a human resources crisis and improve health information systems.

Dr Babatunde Osotimehin, Executive Director, United Nations' Population Fund (2011 to date)

Dr Babatunde Osotimehin became the fourth Executive Director of UNFPA, the United Nations' Population Fund, in January 2011. He had previously been Nigeria's Minister of Health and, earlier, Director-General of Nigeria's National Agency for the Control of AIDS.

Dr Osotimehin is a physician and public health specialist, educated in Nigeria and the UK, who was a professor at the University of Ibadan before being elected Provost of the College of Medicine in 1990. He was Chair of the National Action Committee on AIDS, from 2002 to 2007.

As Executive Director he has participated in the Cairo Population Conference, Beijing Women's Conference and United Nations special sessions on AIDS. Dr Osotimehin received the Nigerian national honour of Officer of the Order of the Niger (OON) in December 2005.

Joy Phumaphi, Vice President of the World Bank (2007–09) and Assistant Director-General of WHO (2003–07)

Joy Phumaphi, a former Botswana Minister of Health, has held many very important leadership roles outside her country. She has been an Assistant Director-General at WHO and, subsequently, held the position of Vice President and Head of the Human Development Network at the World Bank.

She is currently the Executive Secretary of the African Leaders Malaria Alliance (ALMA). During her tenure, ALMA has grown to include 39 heads of state, pioneered innovative financing for malaria drugs and commodities, and led the development and implementation of an accountability mechanism that regularly updates the heads of state on progress towards the malaria goals.

Mrs Phumaphi is a member of the Global Leaders' Council for Reproductive Health, the Africa American Institute, and a trustee of the Children's Investment Fund Foundation. She is a distinguished African American Institute Fellow and has been Commissioner in the UN Secretary-General's Commission on HIV/AIDS and Governance in Africa. She chairs ACHAP (African Comprehensive HIV/AIDs Partnership), a partnership between the Botswana Government, Merck, and the Gates Foundation.

Dr Comlan Alfred A. Quenum, Regional Director WHO (1965–84)

The late Dr Quenum was born in 1926 at Ouidah in Dahomey, now known as the Republic of Benin, and was the first African to serve as Regional Director of the African region of WHO.

He did his medical training in Senegal and France before being appointed professor of histology and embryology of the medical faculty of Medicine of Dakar. He represented his country at the World Health Assembly in 1963 and 1964 and was appointed as regional director from the following year.

Dr Ebrahim Malick Samba, Regional Director WHO (1995–2005)

Dr Ebrahim Malick Samba is a Gambian public health specialist who was the WHO Regional Director for 10 years from 1995.

Dr Samba trained in Ghana, Ireland, and Scotland before returning to Africa. As a clinician and a public health practitioner, he gained international recognition for the innovations he initiated in public health programmes and interventions. In 1980, Dr Samba became the Director of the Onchocerciasis Control Programme (OCP) in West Africa, a position he held until 1994. Under his guidance, the OCP became the showpiece of the World Health Organization (WHO), its donors, and other beneficiary countries.

In 1995, Dr Samba was elected Regional Director of the WHO African Regional Office (AFRO), and made responsible for developing a policy framework to combat disease throughout the continent. He was re-elected in September 1999.

Michel Sidibé, UNAIDS Deputy Executive Director (2009 to date)

Mr Sidibé is from Mali, holds advanced academic degrees in economics, international development, and social planning, and became Executive Director of UNAIDS in January 2009.

He began his career with the UN in 1987 when he was recruited by UNICEF to work in the Democratic Republic of Congo and subsequently at its headquarters in

New York. He managed large and complex programmes for immunization, malaria, community development, and support for marginalized and vulnerable populations, as well as model HIV programmes for the prevention of mother-to-child transmission, civil society empowerment, and the protection of human rights.

Mr Sidibé joined UNAIDS in 2001 as Director of Country and Regional Support department, immediately following the first Independent Evaluation of UNAIDS and has since played a major role in the organization, engaging personally with key global and national leaders to implement sustainable and strategic action in response to AIDS.

Mr Sidibé has advocated for unifying the long-term objectives of health systems' strengthening and reversing the AIDS epidemic. His other significant career achievements include pioneering the first movement for girls' education in Africa, managing an immunization programme for 30 million people in the Democratic Republic of Congo, securing a humanitarian corridor for the provision of life-saving medication during the aid embargo in Burundi, negotiating the successful release and rehabilitation of child soldiers from Eastern Congo, and convening one of the first agreements on price reductions for anti-retroviral drugs in Africa.

Dr Francisco Songane, Director of the Partnership for Maternal, Newborn, and Child Health (2004–09)

Francisco F. Songane is a former Minister of Health from Mozambique (2000–04) and was, until 2009, the Director of the Partnership for Maternal, Newborn, and Child Health.

Trained in Mozambique, the United States, and England, as an obstetrician and gynaecologist, he was a district medical director and teacher, as well as the director of the country's second-largest hospital. As Minister of Health of Mozambique, he is credited for using a partnership approach for averting the outbreak of disease during the floods of 2000 and 2001, as well as for the conclusion and operational launch of the country's health-sector strategy. He worked to introduce innovative interventions into the Mozambican health system, including a Hepatitis B vaccine, trials on a candidate malaria vaccine, and use of a more effective cholera vaccine, as well as introducing anti-retroviral therapy into the public system—an example that has been shared globally.

Dr Songane's extensive involvement with the international community has included serving as Board Member of GAVI. He was also a member of Task Force 4 of the UN Millennium Project analysing the practicalities of achieving the goals related to maternal and child health. He is a Member of the Board of Trustees of the International Vaccine Institute, and serves on several Advisory Committees.

Index